The Art of Cooking for the Diabetic

MARY ABBOTT HESS, R.D., M.S.
AND
KATHARINE MIDDLETON

FOREWORD BY NORBERT FREINKEL, M.D.
Past President, American Diabetes Association

A SIGNET BOOK

SIGNET
Published by the Penguin Group
Penguin Books USA Inc., 375 Hudson Street,
New York, New York 10014, U.S.A.
Penguin Books Ltd, 27 Wrights Lane,
London W8 5TZ, England
Penguin Books Australia Ltd, Ringwood,
Victoria, Australia
Penguin Books Canada Ltd, 10 Alcorn Avenue,
Toronto, Ontario, Canada M4V 3B2
Penguin Books (N.Z.) Ltd, 182–190 Wairau Road,
Auckland 10, New Zealand

Penguin Books Ltd, Registered Offices:
Harmondsworth, Middlesex, England

Published by Signet, an imprint of Dutton Signet,
a division of Penguin Books USA Inc. This is an authorized reprint
of an edition published by Contemporary Books, Inc.

First Signet Printing, January, 1993
10 9 8

 REGISTERED TRADEMARK—MARCA REGISTRADA

Printed in the United States of America

Dedication

This book is dedicated to the memory of Katharine Middleton, the co-author of the original edition of this book. Completing the revised edition was her dream, and there was nothing I could have done to honor her that would have meant as much as to see that dream realized. In her 80th year Kay was honored with a Certificate of Merit from the American Diabetes Association and was elected to the national Home Economists in Business Hall of Fame.

Contents

III Recipes

Foreword

The second edition of *The Art of Cooking for the Diabetic* continues in the proud tradition of its predecessor. In the first edition, the late Katharine Middleton and her collaborator Mary Abbott Hess sought to develop a volume "with loving care and much attention" and in "response to the many questions" that they were asked by the patients with diabetes whom they had been counseling. Their goal was to demonstrate that the joys of the gourmet table need not be denied to the patient with diabetes, provided that creative dining could be combined with responsible "know-how" about nutrition and meal-planning. The success with which they met this goal can best be gauged by the "instant success" which the first edition achieved and its enormous acceptance by patients and their families. Now, fully a decade later, the second edition scores again. It has been completed by Mary Abbott Hess and provides a fitting monument to Katharine Middleton—a remarkable pioneer in diabetes education with whom many of us on the Chicago scene were privileged to interact.

The second edition is beautifully updated. All of the chapters have been rewritten to incorporate the latest in contemporary nutritional thought. A new glossary contains some lucid definitions that truly provide the reader with "Word Power." New chapters on fiber, fats, and non-caloric sweeteners attest to the recent explosive developments in these areas. The changing lifestyles of the 1980s are acknowledged by helpful tips concerning such eclectic pursuits as "eating out," "brown bag food," "traveling safely" and even "supermarket skills." Finally, the informational data base achieves practical fruition with 350 splendidly creative recipes. Seventy-five of these are wholly new and consonant with the prevailing advocacies for more seafood, fiber, and fowl in our diets. The recipes are mouth-watering, imaginative, and calculated to tempt the palates of those without diabetes, as well as the patients with diabetes whom the authors have served so long and so well. Indeed, the recipes elevate *The Art of Cooking for the Diabetic* into a "state of the art" compendium on how to dine well, contentedly, and always knowledgeably.

Norbert Freinkel, M.D.
C.F. Kettering Professor of Medicine
Director, Center for Endocrinology,
    Metabolism and Nutrition
    Northwestern University Medical School
Director, Endocrine-Metabolic Clinics
    Northwestern University Medical Faculty Foundation
    Chicago, Illinois
Past-President, American Diabetes Association

Acknowledgments

Many of the individuals whose lives were enriched by knowing Kay Middleton generously contributed their time, interest, and expertise to make this book a part of her legacy.

Many thanks to:

Margaret A. Powers, R.D., M.S., C.D.E., Director of Nutrition, Diabetes Center, Northwestern Memorial Hospital, Chicago, for suggestions from her experience as a diabetes educator and for reviewing the manuscript.

Jeanette Hoyt, R.D., M.S., of the Food & Nutrition Services Department, Rush-Presbyterian St. Luke's Medical Center, Chicago, for recipe calculations and technical review of the manuscript.

Barbara Grunes, superstar recipe developer and friend.

Anne Hunt and the staff of Hess and Hunt, Inc., Nutrition Communications/Counseling, for all kinds of assistance and support.

Jane Grant Tougas for editorial aid.

Kristine A. Stewart, James A. Washington III, Susan Black, David Siegal, and Rachel Elizabeth Hess for typing the manuscript.

My family—Peter, Rachel, and Leslie—for encouragement and love shown to both authors.

Carolyn Williams, D.T.R., for assisting in calculation of the recipes.

Marion J. Franz, R.D., M.S., C.D.E., and the International Diabetes Center for sharing their materials.

The American Dietetic Association for permission to use the exchange lists.

The Quaker Oats Company and the National Turkey Federation for recipes.

Jane Jordan Browne, our fine literary agent.

Jean-Marie Brownson, a former student of whom I am very proud, who did the food styling for the cover photo, and Bill Hogan, a wonderful photographer.

Mary Abbott Hess, R.D., M.S.

The Art of Cooking
for the Diabetic

Introduction

Only a decade ago, the diet prescribed for individuals with diabetes was quite different than the diet most people ate. Following a "diabetic diet" meant avoiding sugar in all forms and relying on "special diet foods," most of which did not taste good. Times have changed. The United States Department of Agriculture, American Dietetic Association, and other organizations are telling the general public to eat just like those with diabetes! The Dietary Guidelines for Americans, promoted by the federal government advises everyone to:

- Eat a variety of foods
- Maintain desirable weight
- Avoid too much fat, saturated fat and cholesterol
- Eat foods with adequate starch and fiber
- Avoid too much sugar
- Avoid too much sodium
- If you drink alcoholic beverages, do so in moderation.

The diet that promotes health and prevents disease is good for all of us—whether or not we have diabetes. For diabetics, the consequences of not following the guidelines are more serious than for generally healthy individuals. Eating suitable meals at regular mealtimes helps avoid emergencies and complications. And this isn't so hard to do. While moderation and portion control are important, the philosophy of diabetic management is far more liberal than it was a few years ago. Even sugar can be used, though in small quantities.

Diabetes mellitus requires ongoing medical and nutritional monitoring. Your needs will certainly change over time. The more you understand about diabetes, the more productive your appointments will be with your physician and diet counselor and the better you will feel because you are in control of your own health.

In these pages we explain the role of the diet in diabetes management. The section titled "Word Power" in the Appendix of the book gives simple explanations of the terminology of diabetes mellitus that will help you understand the information. The chapters on sugars, sugar substitutes, fats, and fiber will answer many of your questions and help you make choices at the supermarket and in your kitchen. We will explain how these substances in foods affect your blood sugar and blood fat levels.

The chapters in Part II, "Living with Diabetes," give practical advice on how to deal with common situations. Should I eat differently when I exercise? What can I eat in restaurants? When I drink alcohol, should my diet be changed? What are some things I can bring for lunch at work? When I see a new food at the market, how can I tell if it is okay for me to eat? These and many other questions are answered in Chapters 6 through 13.

Every recipe has been calculated and converted to exchanges so that you can fit them into your meal plan. This information is listed in a chart following each recipe. Cholesterol (Chol) and fiber values are given as well as calorie (CAL), and carbohydrate (CHO), protein (PRO), fat, and sodium levels.

If you have been told to limit your sodium intake, instructions are on the bottom of each recipe to help you do that. In all recipes we have used minimal amounts of salt, sugar, and fat. The recipes and dietary advice in this book are good for everyone.

The food industry has responded to consumer demands for more healthful foods. Many prepared foods and meals now have reduced levels of sugar, fat, and salt. Foods with increased levels of fiber—breads, muffins, cereals, and grains—are being introduced by many food companies. You will have lots of company when you eat sugar-free soft drinks, puddings, low calorie salad dressings, and high fiber cereals.

The final section of the book is the Appendix. In addition to "Word Power," you will find lists of books and other resources that we recommend for those wanting additional information.

The first edition (1978) of *The Art of Cooking for the Diabetic* was enormously successful and garnered rave reviews in both the popular press and professional journals. As authors, we were gratified by the comments of individuals who told us that our book had helped them understand how to control their diabetes or lose weight, and that the recipes were delicious. This book is written with the same loving care and shares the art of cooking, especially for the diabetic. With it, you can eat wisely, and very, very well.

Part I
Diet in Diabetes Management

Diet is the foundation of good control and management of diabetes mellitus. The restriction of certain foods and the moderation of total caloric intake are musts for all diabetics. Some cases of diabetes, especially in overweight people, can be controlled by diet alone, without oral medication or insulin. Generally, meals are well balanced, moderate in portion size, limited in simple sugars, and spaced throughout the day to lessen the need for insulin production by the pancreas. Many diets for diabetics are modified by the doctor or dietitian to meet other individual, medical needs such as sodium restriction.

The goal of a diabetic diet is to provide all of the nutrients needed by the body. Vitamin supplements should not be taken unless specifically prescribed by your physician. In fact, vitamin C (ascorbic acid) in pill form may interfere with accuracy in testing of the urine for sugar.

When people eat, their food is digested and much of it is changed into glucose, a kind of sugar the body uses for fuel. The bloodstream carries the glucose to cells where it is used for energy. Glucose is absorbed by the cells with the help of the hormone insulin. Normally, the body produces all the insulin it needs both for immediate energy and to store extra glucose and fat for later use.

When you have diabetes, your body does not make enough insulin or the insulin it does make is not used properly. Without insulin, digested food, in the form of glucose, builds up in your blood. Cells can't get the energy they need, because insulin isn't available to move the glucose into the cells where the sugar is used as fuel.

There are two major types of diabetes mellitus:

• Insulin-dependent (IDDM, Type I, juvenile-onset)
• Non-insulin-dependent (NIDDM, Type II, adult-onset)

Individuals with insulin-dependent diabetes do not make insulin. When the body has no insulin and cannot use glucose for energy, it begins to burn fat. When fat is burned for energy, acid wastes called *ketones* are formed. The ketones build up in the blood and cause a serious condition called ketoacidosis. Those with insulin-dependent diabetes must take insulin to avoid this life-threatening condition. This insulin must be injected. If taken as a pill, it would be digested and made inactive.

Those with non-insulin-dependent diabetes make some insulin, but either there is not enough insulin or it does not work properly. This type of diabetes can sometimes be controlled by limiting the type or amount of food they eat and by increasing their exercise. Oral hypoglycemic agents (diabetes pills) help some people to make more insulin or to use their own insulin better. The pills do not replace insulin; they work only when a person's body needs a "boost" to make its own insulin. Non-insulin-dependent diabetics sometimes need insulin injections to regulate their blood glucose levels on a temporary basis.

The management of diabetes has three parts:

• food
• activity
• medication (if needed)

Food raises blood glucose and blood fat levels, and both of these cause problems for those with diabetes. Activity and medications (insulin injections or oral hypoglycemic agents) lower both blood glucose and blood fat levels. A balance of food, activity, and medication is the way to good management of diabetes.

This book discusses your food needs and provides information and recipes that will help you make wise food choices. Chapter 8, "Exercise and Sports," discusses the effect of activity on diabetes. Your physician will be the primary source of information about medications and other medical concerns.

The American Diabetes Association, Inc., and the American Dietetic Association, in their joint publication *Exchange Lists for Meal Planning*, have identified three nutritional goals of diabetes management:

Goal 1: Appropriate blood glucose and blood fat levels. Learn to balance the food you eat with your activity level and with the insulin in your body so that your blood glucose and blood fats (cholesterol and triglycerides) stay as close to normal as possible. By stabilizing blood glucose levels you can prevent ketoacidosis (diabetic coma) or, if using insulin, too low a blood glucose level (insulin reaction). It is important to match the amount of food you eat with the amount of insulin in your body, whether your body still produces insulin on its own or with the help of diabetes pills, or your insulin comes from injections. You will feel better, and you may reduce or prevent the complications of diabetes.

Blood glucose monitoring can show you the effects of foods or activities on your blood glucose levels. You can measure your own blood glucose using a finger-stick device and test strip. A monitoring record will help you match your meal plan to other aspects of your diabetes management.

People with diabetes run a greater risk of developing heart disease than other people because diabetics often have high levels of blood fat. Chapter 4, "A New Look at Fats," discusses blood fats and their control.

Goal 2: Reasonable weight. Eating the right number of calories will help you reach and stay at a reasonable body weight. Calorie needs also depend on your size, age, and activity level. Your diet counselor may change your meal plan to raise or lower calories to help you attain or maintain an appropriate weight. Eating the right number of calories is important for many reasons. For example, eating too many calories causes weight gain, which will worsen Type II diabetes and increase the risk of high blood pressure and heart disease. Your body makes and/or uses insulin best when you are at your desirable weight. Eating too few calories causes a different problem. Children and teens with diabetes must eat enough calories to grow properly. Pregnant and nursing women must eat enough calories to provide for proper development of their babies.

Exercise is very important, too. It is helpful while trying to lose weight, and it is also good for your heart and blood vessels. You can increase your activity level by walking, biking, or just taking the stairs instead of an elevator. If you wish to begin an intensive exercise program, check with your health care team first.

Goal 3: Good nutrition. It is important to eat a variety of foods that contain vitamins, minerals, carbohydrates, protein, and fat. Most foods contain a mixture of these nutrients. Carbohydrates, protein, and fat all contain calories, which are used for energy. Carbohydrate, which has four calories per gram, is the major source of energy. Protein also has four calories per gram, but protein is needed for growth and replacement of body cells. Fat is the storage form of energy and is higher in calories—nine calories per gram of weight. Insulin is needed to burn the calories from carbohydrate, protein, and fat. When you eat foods containing energy nutrients, you will also get the vitamins and minerals needed to maintain health.

The principles of good nutrition are important to everybody who wants to maintain health and prevent disease. For people with diabetes, however, the risks associated with poor dietary choices are much greater.

Reaching the three goals above is not easy. For most, some dietary changes are necessary. If you choose from the recipes in this book, you will have a head start, because the recipes have reduced amounts of fats, sugars, and salt and have increased fiber where possible. You can also follow these five principles of good nutrition:

1. **Eat less fat.** The average American adult eats too much fat. Too much fat can cause heart and blood vessel disease. To reduce dietary fat, limit the frequency of consumption and the portion size of foods that contain fat,

such as cold cuts, nuts, gravy, salad dressing, margarine, butter, and cheese. Drink skim or low-fat milk and substitute lean meat, fish, and poultry for high-fat meat. Refer to Chapter 4, "A New Look at Fats," for more information.

2. **Eat more carbohydrates (starches and breads), especially those high in fiber.** Carbohydrate foods are a good source of energy, vitamins, and minerals. Fiber in foods may help to lower blood glucose and blood fat levels. Dried beans, peas and lentils, whole-grain breads, cereals and crackers, and fruits and vegetables are good sources of carbohydrates and fiber. Foods that are high in fiber are noted in the Exchange Lists with a special symbol ![symbol] . The benefits of fiber are discussed in Chapter 5, "Fantastic Fiber."

3. **Eat less sugar.** Most people, including those with diabetes, should eat less sugar. Refined sugar has lots of calories, no vitamins or minerals, and it can cause tooth decay. Foods high in sugar include desserts such as frosted cakes and pies, sugary breakfast foods, table sugar, honey and syrup. One 12-ounce can of regular soft drink has nine teaspoons of sugar! Chapter 3, "The Great Sugar Masquerade," tells you what you need to know about sugar. If you want to replace some sugar in your diet, read the section titled "Sugar Substitutes."

4. **Use less salt.** Most of us eat too much salt. The sodium in salt can cause the body to retain water, and in some people it may raise blood pressure. Foods that are high in sodium, such as processed and convenience foods, are noted in the exchange lists with a special symbol ![symbol] . The sodium level of every recipe in this book has been calculated for you. If you are on a low-sodium diet, follow the instructions at the end of each recipe.

5. **Use alcohol in moderation.** It is best to avoid alcohol, but if you like to have an alcoholic drink now and then, ask your dietitian how to work it into your meal plan. If you take insulin, it is important to eat food with your drink. For guidance on the safest drinks for you, read Chapter 10, "Alcohol for Diabetics?"

It seems like a lot to know and do. Your doctor and/or dietitian will help determine your needs and will work out a nutrition prescription that fits your caloric needs and food habits, as far as is possible. Learning more about your diet, by reading this book and other information about diabetes care, will make you more knowledgeable and confident.

1
The Diabetic Meal Plan

Your meal plan is one of your most important tools for controlling diabetes. The plan should be tailor-made for you by your diet counselor, usually a registered dietitian, to reflect your food preferences and habits, and the type of insulin you take.

The most common type of meal plan uses the food exchange lists, but your diet counselor may decide that another approach, such as Basic Nutrition Guidelines, Simplified Exchanges, a High-Fiber Plan, Caloric Counting, No Concentrated Sweets, or a Point System, is more suited to your needs.

The meal plan is a guide that shows the number of food choices (exchanges) or types of food you can eat at each meal and snack. The plan is designed so that you will eat more than half of your total daily calories as carbohydrate, and you will eat less fat and protein.

Your meal plan must be tailored to the type of diabetes that you have and its nutritional treatment.

For those with insulin-dependent diabetes, consistency is the most important nutrition principle. Eating times, amounts of foods, and types of food eaten at each meal should be about the same from day to day because the food you eat is planned to balance your insulin injections and your activity. The exchange lists can help provide consistency so that the food and insulin work together to regulate blood glucose levels. If the meal plan and insulin are out of balance, wide swings in blood glucose can occur, causing you to suffer from insulin reactions or from the symptoms of high blood glucose.

Most people with non-insulin-dependent diabetes are overweight. Thus, the most important nutrition principle for people with this type of diabetes is weight control. It is still important to eat a balanced diet, even while losing weight. Your dietitian will help determine the number of calories needed, set weight goals, and give you tips to help you reach those goals. An exercise program is usually advised.

Many people ask if they can eat the same food as the rest of their family. The diabetic's meal plan is essentially a basic nutritional pattern that would be ideal for most people; however, many people do not eat in such a healthy way. It is very hard to change habits, especially about food. Just remember to make changes gradually, set short-term goals, and reward yourself with non-food rewards when you are successful.

To make your meal plan work, you will need to eat what is prescribed. Serving sizes are very important. If you eat too much or too little food, your blood glucose regulation and your weight will be affected. You will need to measure or weigh your food for the first week or so, until you learn to judge serving sizes. Suggestions on measuring serving sizes are included in Chapter 13, "Kitchen Tips for Controlled Diets."

Your meal plan may need to be changed as time goes on; changes in lifestyle such as work, school, vacation, or travel will require adjustments. Your weight may change; your eating habits may change; your activity may change—any of these changes may require a new meal plan. As children grow, they need more calories, and when they reach adulthood they need fewer. Review your meal plan regularly with your dietitian. Ask questions and learn about new nutrition information. Regular nutrition counseling can help you make positive changes in your eating habits and provide the education and support you may need to be confident and in control of your diabetes management.

Three situations require special instructions for insulin-dependent diabetics. Knowing what to do in advance will reduce stress; being prepared will prevent emergencies.

1. **Plan for sick days**. Before you become ill with the flu or a cold, ask your doctor, dietitian, and nurse for a special sick-day plan. It is important to:

- take your usual insulin dose;
- test your blood glucose regularly and check your urine for ketones;
- try drinking small sips of regular soft drinks, sweetened tea, sweetened gelatin, popsicles, fruit juice, or sherbet if you can't keep solid food down;
- drink lots of liquids;
- call your doctor immediately if you can't keep any food down.

2. **Prepare for insulin reactions**. If you have symptoms of low blood glucose, test your blood to determine your blood glucose level. Be sure to carry something with you at all times to treat low blood glucose. Most diabetics carry glucose tablets or hard candy to raise blood glucose if it becomes too low.

3. **Plan for exercise**. You may need to make some changes in your meal plan or insulin dose when you begin an exercise program. Check with your dietitian or doctor about this. Be sure to carry with you some form of carbohydrate (such as dried fruit or glucose tablets) to treat low blood glucose.

Additional information on these topics is available from your dietitian or doctor and in Chapter 8, "Exercise and Sports."

Follow the advice of your dietitian and physician. Regardless of the type of meal plan, this book will answer many of your questions and provide wonderful recipes that fit into any of the meal-planning approaches. If your meal plan doesn't follow the Exchange System, ask your diet counselor to mark this book and modify it to fit your needs. If you have multiple dietary restrictions, a combination diet, or specific food intolerances, this step will be especially important.

2
The Exchange System

The most popular way to teach diet management to people with diabetes uses the Food Exchange System because it stresses moderate, regular food habits and allows the individual to choose from a wide variety of foods.

The Food Exchange System was developed in 1950 by a committee set up by the American Diabetes Association, Inc., the American Dietetic Association, and the Chronic Disease Program of the U.S. Public Health Service. The food exchanges underwent major revisions in 1976 and again in 1986 on the basis of new knowledge of nutrition and food composition. The current exchange lists are concerned with total caloric intake and modification of fat intake as well as carbohydrate and protein values.

If you have been on a diabetic diet based on prior versions of exchanges, you will see some differences. We hope that this book will help you understand the new exchanges and make an easier changeover to these new lists. Check to make sure that your dietitian or doctor approves of your using the new exchanges. If your doctor or dietitian prefers that you stay on the old exchanges, and you have good control over your diabetes condition, then skip our lists and go on to other chapters of the book and the recipes. The nutritive values given for each recipe will still be useful to you.

What Is an Exchange?

Before we tell you about the food exchange lists, let's explain what is meant by the word *exchange*. You know that you can trade or exchange 5 pennies for one nickel or 10 dimes for a dollar bill. Right? Okay. In food exchanges, you may exchange one measurement or amount of food for another food in the same group. For example, look at List 4: Fruit Exchanges. Your diet for breakfast may tell you to have one fruit exchange. So you have been having ½ cup of orange juice day after day. Want a change? Look over the list. Select any fruit you want in the serving amount given for one fruit exchange for that fruit and exchange it for the ½ cup of orange juice.

The Food Exchange System is based on six exchange lists: starch/bread, meats, vegetables, fruits, milk, and fats. There are also some special lists. Foods are grouped within each list on the basis of similar amounts of carbohydrate, protein, and fat. For example, one fruit exchange is CHO 15 g, PRO 0 g, FAT 0 g, Calories 60. This is equivalent to ½ cup of grapefruit juice but only ⅓ cup of prune juice because prune juice has more sugar than grapefruit juice. By varying portion sizes, we come close to our goal of 15 grams of carbohydrate for each food on the fruit list.

Keep in mind that there will be some surprises. Corn, for example, is a vegetable, but it appears on the starch/bread list. That is because corn is starchy and its carbohydrate value is much closer to bread than to most vegetables. Foods from the starch/bread list are sometimes called *starch exchanges* and sometimes called *bread exchanges*—but they mean the same thing.

Each list contains many foods. When your meal plan is determined, the number of exchanges for each meal will be planned. If, in the morning, for example, you are allowed two bread exchanges, you might choose ½ cup cooked oatmeal plus one piece of toast, or 1 cup of oatmeal or two halves of a toasted English muffin. In other words, you may choose two different items from the bread list or double the serving of one item to use up your two starch/bread exchanges. This applies to all other exchange lists, too.

Your diet counselor will give you a meal plan, listing the food exchanges you are to eat at each meal. It is important to eat all of the food planned at each meal and to eat those meals at approximately the same time each day. No holdovers allowed! In other words, don't save up your exchanges from one meal to eat at another time. Why? Because your body cannot properly use a big load of food at one time, and your medication is prescribed to help process food taken at a specific time that matches the time the insulin is most active.

We have added some foods to the basic lists. We checked the nutritive values of each added item with several sources, including the newest tables of food composition and nutrient labeling on packages. Then we calculated the proper portion size for one exchange for each food. After the six food group lists, you will find lists of "free" foods, ones you may use without counting exchanges because they have few calories. Also included are lists of popular combination foods that provide exchanges from several lists, as well as a section on foods that have more sugar or fat than desirable for regular use but are acceptable for occasional use in measured portions if your diabetes is in good control. We have also included exchanges for a list of additional foods, mostly ethnic food choices, that do not usually appear on diabetic exchange lists. And in Part II you'll find a list of exchanges for popular fast foods. Rather than approaching your diabetes as a limiting factor, the lists will show you that there is an endless variety of foods from which you can choose.

With each list you will find a discussion of how to use it. The material in this chapter is a summary of many questions we have been asked in our years of counseling individuals with diabetes mellitus. The discussion also includes a brief consideration of the nutrients contributed by each group. This addition was irresistible to us as nutrition educators.

The following Exchange Lists (© 1986 American Diabetes Association, Inc., American Dietetic Association) have been reprinted with the permission of the American Diabetes Association and the American Dietetic Association. The Exchange Lists are the basis of a meal planning system designed by a committee of the American Diabetes Association and the American Dietetic Association. While designed primarily for people with diabetes and others who must follow special diets, the Exchange Lists are based on principles of good nutrition that apply to everyone.

List 1: Starch/Bread Exchanges

Each item in this list contains approximately 15 grams of carbohydrate, 3 grams of protein, a trace of fat, and 80 calories. Whole-grain products average about 2 grams of fiber per serving. Some foods are higher in fiber. Those foods that contain 3 or more grams of fiber per serving are identified with the fiber symbol 🌾

You can choose your Starch Exchanges from any one of the items on this list. If you want to eat a Starch food that is not on this list, the general rule is that:

* ½ cup of cereal, grain, or pasta is one serving
* 1 ounce of a bread product is one serving

Your dietitian can help you be more exact.

Remember that the use of brand names is not a product endorsement by the publisher or the authors. Brand names are used only so that you will know what product we are identifying; you may then substitute a similar type of product using the same measure.

Cereals/Grains/Pasta

Barley	⅓ cup
Bran cereals, concentrated (such as Bran Buds, All Bran) 🌾	⅓ cup
Bran cereals, flaked 🌾	½ cup
Bulgur (cooked)	½ cup
Cooked cereals	½ cup

Cereals/Grains/Pasta

Cornmeal (dry)	2½ tablespoons
Flour	2½ tablespoons
Grapenuts	3 tablespoons
Grits (cooked)	½ cup
Other ready-to-eat unsweetened cereals	¾ cup
Pasta, cooked (spaghetti, noodles, macaroni)	½ cup
Puffed cereal	1½ cups
Rice, white or brown (cooked)	⅓ cup
Shredded wheat	½ cup
Wheat germ	3 tablespoons

Dried Beans/Peas/Lentils

Beans and peas (cooked) (such as kidney, white, split, black-eyed)	⅓ cup
Lentils (cooked)	⅓ cup
Baked beans	¼ cup
Chick peas, garbanzos (cooked)	¼ cup

Starchy Vegetables

Corn	½ cup
Corn on cob, 6 inches long	1 cob
Lima beans (cooked)	½ cup
Peas, green (canned or frozen)	½ cup
Plantain	½ cup
Potato, baked	1 small (3 ounces)
Potato, mashed	½ cup
Squash, winter (acorn, butternut)	¾ cup
Yam, sweet potato, plain	⅓ cup

Bread

Bagel	½ (1 ounce)
Bialy	1 (1 ounce)
Bread sticks, crisp, 4 inches long × ½ inch	2 (⅔ ounce)
Croutons, low-fat	1 cup
Dried bread crumbs	3 tablespoons
English muffin	½
Frankfurter or hamburger bun	½ (1 ounce)
Party rye	4 small rounds
Pita, 6 inches across	½
Plain roll, small	1 (1 ounce)
Raisin, unfrosted	1 slice (1 ounce)
Rye, pumpernickel	1 slice (1 ounce)
Tortilla, 6 inches across (not fried)	1
White (including French, Italian)	1 slice (1 ounce)
Whole wheat	1 slice (1 ounce)

Crackers/Snacks

Animal crackers	8
Graham crackers, 2½ inches square	3
Matzo	¾ ounce
Melba toast	5 slices or 10 rounds
Oyster crackers	24
Popcorn (popped, no fat added)	3 cups
Pretzels	¾ ounce
Rye crisp, 2 inches × 3½ inches	4
Saltine-type crackers	6
Whole-wheat crackers, no fat added (crisp breads, such as Fin, Kavli, Wasa)	2–4 slices (¾ ounce)
Zwieback	3 slices (¾ ounce)

Starch Foods Prepared with Fat

(Count as 1 Starch/Bread serving, plus 1 Fat serving.)

Biscuit, 2½ inches across	1
Chow mein noodles	½ cup
Corn bread, 2 inch cube	1 (2 ounces)
Crackers, round butter type (such as Ritz)	6
French fried potatoes, 2–3½ inches long	10 (1½ ounces)
Muffin, plain, small	1
Pancake, 4 inches across	2
Stuffing, bread (prepared)	¼ cup
Taco shell, 6 inches across	2
Thin crackers (such as Wheat Thins)	12 (1 ounce)
Waffle, 4½ inches square	1
Whole-wheat crackers, fat added (such as Triscuits)	4–6 (1 ounce)

List 2: Meat Exchanges

Each serving of meat and substitutes on this list contains about seven grams of protein. The amount of fat and number of calories vary, depending on what kind of meat or substitute you choose. The list is divided into three parts based on the amount of fat and calories: Lean Meat, Medium-Fat Meat, and High-Fat Meat. One ounce (one Meat Exchange) of each of these includes:

	Carbohydrate (grams)	Protein (grams)	Fat (grams)	Calories —
Lean	0	7	3	55
Medium-Fat	0	7	5	75
High-Fat	0	7	8	100

You are encouraged to use more lean and medium-fat meat, poultry, and fish in your meal plan. This will help decrease your fat intake, which may help decrease your risk for heart disease. The items from the High-Fat group are high in saturated fat, cholesterol, and calories. You should limit your choices from the High-Fat group to three (3) times per week. Meat and substitutes do not contribute any fiber to your meal plan. Meats and meat substitutes that have 400 milligrams or more of sodium per exchange are indicated with this symbol .

Tips

1. Bake, roast, broil, grill, or boil these foods rather than frying them with added fat.
2. Use a nonstick pan spray or a nonstick pan to brown or fry these foods.
3. Trim off visible fat before and after cooking.
4. Do not add flour, bread crumbs, coating mixes, or fat to these foods when preparing them.
5. Weigh meat after removing bones and fat and after cooking. Three ounces of cooked meat is about equal to four ounces of raw meat. Some examples of meat portions are:
   2 ounces meat (2 Meat Exchanges) =
      1 small chicken leg or thigh
      ½ cup cottage cheese or tuna
   3 ounces meat (3 Meat Exchanges) =
      1 medium pork chop
      1 small hamburger
      ½ of a whole chicken breast
      1 unbreaded fish fillet
      cooked meat, about the size of a deck of cards
6. Restaurants usually serve prime cuts of meat, which are high in fat and calories.

For each food, the 1-ounce portion nutritive values are based on the cooked food with all separable fats removed. In other words, take your cooked meat, remove separable fat and bones, and weigh the edible, remaining meat. If you are allowed three Meat Exchanges at dinner, for example, you may weigh out a 3-ounce portion.

Diet counselors are not in complete agreement as to how the three meat lists are to be calculated for individualized meal plans. Some dietitians calculate strictly on the basis of lean meats, with extra fats available to be used for food from the Fat Exchange list or from medium-fat or high-fat meats. Others tell their patients to choose primarily lean meats, plus a few medium-fat or high-fat meats throughout the week, and then the meal plan is calculated on the basis of a somewhat higher fat value than the three grams of a lean meat. Your dietitian will explain how many lean, medium-fat, and high-fat meats you should choose. Our recipes give both nutritive values and the translation of that information into the correct exchanges.

The meat group provides many important nutrients. All foods from the meat lists supply protein, which helps to form and maintain all cells of the body.

Lean red meats are also the most important source of iron. Iron carries oxygen to the cells and is necessary for blood formation. Many women do not get enough of this mineral, and they develop iron-deficiency anemia. Iron is found in liver, red meats, egg yolk, dried peas and beans. Cooking in an old-fashioned black cast-iron pot or skillet, one not coated with enamel, can also increase the iron content of the diet.

Also necessary for proper blood formation and the prevention of another type of anemia is vitamin B_{12}, which is found only in foods of animal origin. Most foods in the meat group help meet dietary needs for B_{12}, but vegetarians and others who select vegetable sources of protein (dried beans, peas, peanut butter, etc.) may need dietary supplements.

Zinc is a mineral needed in tiny amounts. Scientists have found that it combines with insulin for proper storage of the hormone. Zinc influences our ability to taste foods and is necessary for metabolism. This nutrient is provided by meats, poultry, liver, seafood, eggs, and dried peas.

Meats, dried peas and beans, and peanut butter supply potassium, as do many fruits and vegetables. Potassium helps

Lean Meat and Substitutes

(One Exchange is equal to any one of the following items.)

Beef:	USDA Good* or choice grades of lean beef, such as round, sirloin, and flank steak; tenderloin; and chipped beef 🥩 ; tripe	1 ounce
Pork:	Lean pork, such as fresh ham; canned, cured, or boiled ham 🥩 ; Canadian bacon 🥩 ; tenderloin	1 ounce
Veal:	All cuts are lean except for veal cutlets (ground or cubed). Examples of lean veal are chops and roasts	1 ounce
Poultry:	Chicken, turkey, Cornish hen (without skin), capon, turkey	1 ounce
Fish:	All fresh and frozen fish	1 ounce
	Crab, lobster, scallops, shrimp, clams (fresh, frozen, or canned in water 🥩)	2 ounces
	Oysters	6 medium
	Tuna 🥩 (canned in water)	¼ cup
	Herring (uncreamed or smoked)	1 ounce
	Sardines (canned and drained)	2 medium
Wild Game:	Venison, rabbit, squirrel	1 ounce
	Pheasant, duck, goose (without skin)	1 ounce
Cheese:	Any cottage cheese	¼ cup
	Grated Parmesan	2 tablespoons
	Diet cheeses 🥩 (with fewer than 55 calories per ounce)	1 ounce

*USDA Good meat is now called USDA Select.

Lean Meat and Substitutes
(One Exchange is equal to any one of the following items.)

Other:	95% fat-free luncheon meat	1 ounce
	Egg whites	3 whites
	Egg substitutes with fewer than 55 calories per ¼ cup	¼ cup

Medium-Fat Meat and Substitutes
(One Exchange is equal to any one of the following items.)

Beef:	Most beef products fall into this category. Examples: all ground beef, roast (rib, chuck, rump), steak (cubed, porterhouse, T-bone), and meat loaf	1 ounce
Pork:	Most pork products fall into this category. Examples: chops, loin roast, Boston butt, cutlets	1 ounce
Lamb:	Most lamb products fall into this category. Examples: chops, leg, and roast	1 ounce
Veal:	Cutlet (ground or cubed, unbreaded)	1 ounce
Poultry:	Chicken (with skin), domestic duck or goose (well drained of fat), ground turkey	1 ounce
Fish:	Tuna (canned in oil and drained)	¼ cup
	Salmon (canned)	¼ cup
	Caviar, fish roe	1 ounce
Cheese:	Skim or part-skim-milk cheeses:	
	ricotta	¼ cup
	mozzarella	1 ounce
	diet cheeses (with 56–80 calories per ounce)	1 ounce
Other:	86% fat-free luncheon meat	1 ounce
	Egg (high in cholesterol, limit to 3 yolks per week)	1

Egg substitutes with 56–80 calories per ¼ cup	¼ cup
Tofu (2½ inches × 2¾ inches × 1 inch)	**4 ounces**
Liver, heart, kidney, sweetbreads (high in cholesterol)	1 ounce

High-Fat Meat and Substitutes

Remember, these items are high in saturated fat, cholesterol, and calories and should be used only three times per week.

(One Exchange is equal to any one of the following items.)

Beef:	Most USDA Prime cuts of beef; beef brisket, short ribs, corned beef	1 ounce
Pork:	Spareribs, ground pork, pork sausage (patty or link)	1 ounce
Lamb:	Patties (ground lamb)	1 ounce
Fish:	Any fried fish product	1 ounce
Cheese:	All regular cheeses , such as American, blue, cheddar, Monterey Jack, Swiss, feta, Gouda, brick, Camembert	1 ounce
Other:	Luncheon meat , such as bologna, salami, pimiento loaf	1 ounce
	Sausage , such as Polish, Italian, liverwurst	1 ounce
	Knockwurst, smoked	1 ounce
	Bratwurst	1 ounce
	Frankfurter (turkey or chicken)	1 frank (10/pound)
	Peanut butter (contains unsaturated fat)	1 tablespoon

Count as one High-Fat Meat plus one Fat Exchange:

	Frankfurter (beef, pork, or combination)	1 frank (10/pound)

maintain the acid-base balance of the body and is necessary for nerve and muscle activity, glycogen formation, and protein usage.

Specific foods in the meat group are excellent sources of other nutrients. Lean pork supplies considerable amounts of thiamine, seafoods supply iodine, which is also available to us through the use of iodized salt; the soft edible bones of canned tuna, salmon, and sardines provide calcium, although we get most of the calcium in our diet from the milk group. And then there is liver—rich in vitamin A and at least 12 other nutrients! But this nutrient package is also rich in cholesterol and is a poor choice if you have been advised to limit your intake of dietary cholesterol.

List 3: Vegetable Exchanges

Each vegetable serving in this list contains about 5 grams of carbohydrate, 2 grams of protein, and 25 calories. Vegetables contain 2–3 grams of dietary fiber. Vegetables that contain 400 milligrams of sodium per serving are identified with the 🖙 symbol.

Vegetables are a good source of vitamins and minerals. Fresh and frozen vegetables have more vitamins and less added salt than canned vegetables. Rinsing canned vegetables will remove much of the salt.

Unless otherwise noted, the serving size for vegetables (one Vegetable Exchange) is:

- ½ cup of cooked vegetables or vegetable juice
- 1 cup of raw vegetables

A small amount of a vegetable used as a seasoning or garnish need not be counted as a vegetable. For example, a slice of tomato or onion on a sandwich can be included without using up a Vegetable Exchange.

The National Cancer Institute now recommends that we eat more fiber, cruciferous vegetables, and foods rich in vitamins

Artichoke (½ medium)
Asparagus
Beans (green, wax, Italian)
Bean sprouts
Beets
Broccoli
Brussels sprouts
Cabbage, cooked
Carrots
Cauliflower
Eggplant
Greens (collard, mustard, turnip)
Kohlrabi
Leeks
Mushrooms, cooked

Okra
Onions
Pea pods
Peppers (green or red)
Rutabaga
Sauerkraut
Spinach, cooked
Summer squash (crookneck)
Tomato (one large)
Tomatoes, cherry (6-8)
Tomato sauce
Tomato paste (2 tablespoons)
Tomato/vegetable juice
Turnips
Water chestnuts
Zucchini, cooked

Starchy vegetables such as corn, peas, and potatoes are found on the Starch/Bread list.
For "free" vegetables see List 7.

A and C to reduce our risk of developing various kinds of cancer. Members of the botanical family of *Cruciferae* include brussels sprouts, cabbage, broccoli, cauliflower, rutabagas, and turnips. Greens, like mustard and turnip greens, are also in the family and are rich in vitamins and fiber as well. Broccoli, a favorite of many people, also rates highly in all of the suggested cancer-preventing substances. Check out the recipes found later in this book for delicious ways of serving the *Cruciferae* family to your family.

Brussels sprouts, peppers, broccoli, cabbage, and tomatoes are excellent sources of vitamin C needed for healthy tissues.

Dark green and deep yellow vegetables are particularly rich sources of carotene, which changes in our bodies to vitamin A. Vitamin A promotes growth, is needed for good vision, promotes resistance to infection, and maintains skin tone. The deeper the color of the vegetable, the better the source. For example, spinach is a better source of carotene than is iceberg lettuce.

Vegetables are also good sources of several vitamins of the B complex and a few minerals, as well as of dietary fiber. They add color, texture, and variety to meals. Plain or simply seasoned vegetables can fill you up without excessive calories.

List 4: Fruit Exchanges

Each item on this list contains about 15 grams of carbohydrate and 60 calories. Fresh, frozen, and dried fruits have about 2 grams of fiber per serving. Fruits that have 3 or more grams of fiber per serving have the symbol 🌾 . Fruit juices contain very little dietary fiber.

The carbohydrate and calorie contents for a fruit serving are based on the usual serving of the most commonly eaten fruits. Use fresh fruits or frozen or canned without sugar added. Whole fruit is more filling than fruit juice and may be a better choice for those who are trying to lose weight. Unless otherwise noted, the serving size for one fruit serving is:

- ½ cup of fresh fruit or fruit juice
- ¼ cup of dried fruit

Fresh fruits in season are generally the best choice for both flavor and texture. Whether you choose frozen, dried, or canned fruits, no sugar should be added. Read Chapter 3, "The Great Sugar Masquerade," for an explanation of the names of various sugars that may be added in the processing of fruit.

Canned fruits are quite popular, especially in the wintertime, when fewer fresh fruits are available. Canned fruits have widely varying carbohydrate content, depending on the liquid used in the canning process. Diabetics should not use fruit canned in regular syrup—light, medium, or heavy. Before the introduction of water- and juice-packed fruits, diabetics were told to use these fruits but to wash off the syrup. Well, it doesn't work! A fruit that sits for months in a heavy sugar syrup absorbs much of that sugar. If you were to use syrup-packed canned fruit that was washed, you would have to cut your serving size at least in half to have the correct carbohydrate value.

An acceptable alternative is flavorful juice-packed fruit, which has recently become widely available. Pineapple has been canned in unsweetened pineapple juice for years, but lately pears, peaches, and other fruits, packed in unsweetened white grape juice or unsweetened nectar, are available in supermarkets. The carbohydrate value of the juice must be figured in addition to that of the fruit. Drain and measure the juice, then count it as an additional fruit exchange or reduce the portion size of the fruit. By reducing the portion size you will still be using one fruit exchange. A serving of pineapple, for example, is two rings without any juice from juice-packed pineapple or one ring plus 2 tablespoons of the juice. Read our suggestions on "How to Read a Label" in Chapter 12 to learn how to estimate the nutritive values of the canned fruits.

Fruits are valuable sources of vitamins, minerals, and fiber. Vitamin C is necessary for the formation of healthy connective tissue and bones. Early symptoms of insufficient vitamin C in the diet include bleeding gums and the tendency to bruise easily. Most of us get almost all of the vitamin C (ascorbic acid) that we need every day from this food group. Citrus fruits, such as oranges, grapefruits, tangerines, and lemons, are the best food sources. Most Americans get vitamin C at breakfast, but other meals may also include rich vitamin C sources such as strawberries, mangoes, cantaloupe, or honeydew melon.

The functions of vitamin A are described in List 3: Vegetable Exchanges. Excellent fruit sources include fruits that are orange in color—apricots, mangoes, cantaloupe, nectarines, yellow peaches, and persimmons. Potassium is necessary for maintaining good cellular metabolic reactions, the nervous system, and energy metabolism. Certain medications can deplete the body of potassium, and eating high-potassium foods may be advised.

Fresh, Frozen, and Unsweetened Canned Fruit

Apple (raw, 2 inches across)	1 apple
Applesauce (unsweetened)	½ cup
Apricots (medium, raw)	4 apricots
Apricots (canned)	½ cup, or 4 halves
Banana (9 inches long)	½ banana
Blackberries (raw)	¾ cup
Blueberries (raw)	¾ cup
Cantaloupe (5 inches across)	⅓ melon
(cubes)	1 cup
Casaba melon (medium)	⅛ melon
Cherries (large, raw)	12 cherries
Cherries (canned)	½ cup
Crenshaw melon (medium)	⅛ melon
Figs (raw, 2 inches across)	2 figs
Fruit cocktail (canned)	½ cup
Grapefruit (medium)	½ grapefruit
Grapefruit (segments)	¾ cup
Grapes (small)	15 grapes
Guava	1 medium
Honeydew melon (medium)	⅛ melon
(cubes)	1 cup
Kiwi (large)	1 kiwi
Kumquats (medium)	6 kumquats
Mandarin oranges (canned)	¾ cup
Mango (small)	½ mango
Nectarine (1½ inches across)	1 nectarine
Orange (2½ inches across)	1 orange
Papaya	1 cup
Peach (2¾ inches across)	1 peach or ¾ cup
Peaches (canned)	½ cup or 2 halves
Pear	½ large or 1 small
Pears (canned)	½ cup or 2 halves

Persimmon (medium, native)	2 persimmons
Pineapple (raw)	¾ cup
Pineapple (canned)	⅓ cup or 2 slices
Plum (raw, 2 inches across)	2 plums
Pomegranate	½ pomegranate
Pumpkin (cooked)	¾ cup
Raspberries (raw)	1 cup
Strawberries (raw, whole)	1¼ cup
Tangelo (2½ inches across)	1 tangelo
Tangerine (2½ inches across)	2 tangerines
Watermelon (cubes)	1¼ cups

Dried Fruit

Apples	4 rings
Apricots	7 halves
Dates	2½ medium
Figs	1½
Lychees	8–10
Peaches	2 halves
Prunes	3 medium
Raisins	2 tablespoons or ½-ounce package

Fruit Juice

Apple juice/cider	½ cup
Cranberry juice cocktail	⅓ cup
Grapefruit juice	½ cup
Grape juice (purple, white, or red)	⅓ cup
Orange juice	½ cup
Pineapple juice	½ cup
Prune juice	⅓ cup
Tangerine juice	½ cup

List 5: Milk Exchanges

Each serving of milk or milk products on this list contains about 12 grams of carbohydrate and 8 grams of protein. The amount of fat in milk is measured in percentage of butterfat. The calories vary, depending on what kind of milk you choose. The list is divided into three parts based on the amount of fat and calories: skim/very low-fat milk, low-fat milk, and whole milk. One serving (one Milk Exchange) of each of these includes:

	Carbohydrate (grams)	Protein (grams)	Fat (grams)	Calories —
Skim/Very Low-fat	12	8	trace	90
Low-fat	12	8	5	120
Whole	12	8	8	150

Milk is the body's main source of calcium, the mineral needed for growth and repair of bones. Yogurt is also a good source of calcium. Yogurt and many dry or powdered milk products have different amounts of fat. If you have questions about a particular item, read the label to find out the fat and calorie content.

Milk is good to drink, but it can also be added to cereal and other foods. Many tasty dishes such as sugar-free pudding are made with milk (see List 8: Combination Foods).

The exchange list emphasis is on fortified milk, which is available in your market. Most milk sold in the United States is fortified with vitamin A (for growth, eye functions, resistance to infection) and vitamin D (for absorption and use of calcium). Milk has often been called a perfect food, but it isn't. In fact, no one food provides all the nutrients we need. Milk, for example, is low in iron and vitamin C (ascorbic acid), but its contributions are great in many other nutrients.

It is possible, but very difficult, to meet dietary needs for calcium and several of the vitamins and minerals if milk is not included in your daily meal plan. This is why most dietitians include milk unless the diabetic patient shows a specific intolerance, an allergy, or a great dislike of milk. Some people who are physically intolerant of milk can eat fermented milk products such as yogurt or cheese.

True allergy to food is very rare but intolerance to lactose, the sugar in milk, is quite common in adults, particularly in non-Caucasians. Lactose intolerance is caused by a diminished level or complete absence of lactase, the enzyme made by

Skim and Very Low-Fat Milk

Skim milk	1 cup
½% milk	1 cup
1% milk	1 cup
Low-fat buttermilk	1 cup
Evaporated skim milk	½ cup
Nonfat dry milk	⅓ cup
Plain nonfat yogurt	8 ounces

Low-Fat Milk

2% milk	1 cup
Plain low-fat yogurt (with added nonfat milk solids)	8 ounces

Whole Milk

The whole milk group has much more fat per serving than the skim and low-fat groups. Whole milk has more than 3¼ percent butterfat. Try to limit your choices from the whole milk group as much as possible.

Whole milk	1 cup
Evaporated whole milk	½ cup
Plain whole yogurt	8 ounces

the body that splits lactose into monosaccharides that can be absorbed from the digestive tract.

Most lactose intolerant adults can handle small amounts of milk (a few ounces) without much difficulty and can eat foods prepared with some milk as an ingredient. But larger amounts of milk cannot be digested. They pass through the digestive tract and, once in the colon, they absorb water and ferment. This can cause bloating, abdominal pain, diarrhea and gas. As distressing as those symptoms are, don't give up on milk immediately.

Since milk is a very nutritious food and an important source of calcium, what can people with lactose intolerance do? The problem is absence of lactase, so choosing low lactose dairy products or taking lactase in the form of tablets, liquid, or powder along with milk-based foods is the solution.

Increased use of hard, fermented cheeses helps protect the body's calcium status. These count as meat, not milk exchanges. Yogurt, kefir and similar fermented dairy products contain enzymes which break down the lactose so these foods are usually well tolerated. Products made from yogurt, such as frozen yogurts also can be tried. Low lactose milk, cottage cheese, and ice creams are available in many stores. Large portions of fermented milk products, like buttermilk, acidophilous milk, and sour cream are generally poorly tolerated. Again, except in severe cases, moderate amounts of dairy products are encouraged and should be built into meal plans, maybe splitting a milk exchange between 2 meals. These small portions help to protect bones and other body functions dependent on calcium.

Ask your dietitian to adjust your diet if you are unable to drink the milk in your plan. Most adult diets are planned with 2 cups of milk; children and teenagers usually drink 3–4 cups.

Diabetics are advised not to use commercial flavored yogurts because so much carbohydrate has been added for sweetening. Use only plain, unflavored yogurt. Turn to our recipes if you want to make delicious fruit-flavored yogurts (*see* Index).

List 6: Fat Exchanges

Each serving in the fat list contains about 5 grams of fat and 45 calories. The foods in the fat list contain mostly fat, although some items may also contain a small amount of protein. All fats are high in calories and should be carefully measured. Everyone should modify fat intake by eating unsaturated fats instead of saturated fats. The sodium content of these foods varies widely. Check the label for sodium information.

The amount and type of salad dressing to use is often very confusing. Generally, regular bottled salad dressings provide 1 Fat Exchange (45 calories) per tablespoonful. Reduced calorie dressings provide about 25 calories per tablespoonful, so you can have 2 tablespoons on your salad to count as 1 Fat Exchange. If you want to use more dressing, look for very low calorie (diet) dressings—some contain less than 10 calories worth, this can even be a free food. On the opposite side of the coin are the calorie dense dressings. Only 1 teaspoon of olive oil or corn oil provides 1 Fat Exchange. Ditto two teaspoons of mayonnaise or 1 tablespoon of lite mayonnaise.

Unless you have lots of calories and Fat Exchanges to use, try preparing some of our tasty, low calorie dressings and keep them in your refrigerator and save your fat exchanges for other uses in cooking, sauces, or spreads. Go on a treasure hunt in the salad dressing aisle of the supermarket after you read the chapters on fat and label reading. You will find a wide range of salad dressing options with different calorie, fat, and sodium levels. Take some low calorie salad dressings home and try them to find your favorites. When eating out, always ask for low calorie dressings and salad dressings "on the side" so that you can control portions.

In the recipe section of this book we have used polyunsaturated vegetable oil and margarine instead of butter in all but a few recipes. This decision was based on the increasing emphasis on cutting back on saturated fats to reduce risk of cardiovascular disease. Oil and margarine are also more economical

Unsaturated Fats

Avocado	⅛ medium or 2 tablespoons mashed
Margarine	1 teaspoon
Margarine, diet*	1 tablespoon
Mayonnaise	1 teaspoon
Mayonnaise, reduced calorie*	1 tablespoon
Nuts and Seeds:	
Almonds, dry-roasted	6 whole
Cashews, dry-roasted	1 tablespoon
Pecans	2 whole
Peanuts	20 small or 10 large
Walnuts	2 whole or 1 tablespoon pieces
Other nuts	1 tablespoon
Pistachios	15 medium
Pumpkin seeds, sesame seeds, pine nuts, sunflower seeds (without shells)	1 tablespoon
Oil (Canola, corn, cottonseed, safflower, soybean, sunflower, olive, peanut)	1 teaspoon
Olives*	10 small or 5 large
Salad dressing, mayonnaise-type	2 teaspoons
Salad dressing, mayonnaise-type reduced-calorie	1 tablespoon
Salad dressing (all varieties)	1 tablespoon
Salad dressing, reduced calorie (Two tablespoons of low-calorie salad dressing is a free food.) 🧂	2 tablespoons

Saturated Fats

Butter	1 teaspoon
Bacon*	1 slice

Chitterlings	½ ounce
Coconut, shredded	2 tablespoons
Coffee whitener, liquid	2 tablespoons
Coffee whitener, powder	4 teaspoons
Cream (light, coffee, table)	2 tablespoons
Cream, sour	2 tablespoons
Cream (heavy, whipping)	1 tablespoon
Cream cheese	1 tablespoon
Gravy	2 tablespoons
Salt pork*	¼ ounce

*If more than one or two servings are eaten, these foods have 400 milligrams or more of sodium.

than butter. Butter and bacon are used in our recipes only when they are necessary for flavor. You may substitute butter in other recipes if you wish.

All fats—animal or vegetable, hard or liquid—have nine calories per gram of pure fat. That means that they are more than twice as fattening as carbohydrates. So be careful to measure your fat exchanges or you will have trouble controlling your calorie intake. Be sure to read Chapter 4, "A New Look at Fats," for a complete explanation of the types of fats and their specific effects on your body.

While we emphasize the negative aspects of too much fat, foods high in fat play a role in providing essential nutrients. Margarine, butter, and cream contain vitamin A in a form that is easily utilized by the body. Vegetable oil is an excellent source of vitamin E, needed to prevent destruction of other vitamins and fatty acids. Nuts and seeds provide lots of dietary fiber as well as folacin, biotin, zinc, and magnesium—all important nutrients needed in very small amounts.

Nondairy Creamers

Powdered or liquid, nondairy creamers are also called *coffee whiteners* or *lighteners*. Many brands are available, and they differ greatly in food value. Read labels carefully. If the first ingredient is corn syrup solids, the product contains more sugar than any other ingredient. Because most of the fat in these products is highly saturated palm and coconut oils, they are not recommended for fat-modified diets.

A far better and less expensive way of "creaming" your coffee is to use 1 teaspoon of instant nonfat dry milk. In addition to saving money, the instant nonfat dry milk powder needs no refrigeration, provides calcium, and has only 10 calories per teaspoon. You may use 1 teaspoon per meal in your beverage without counting it as an exchange. When using dry milk powder in hot beverages, allow the tea or coffee to cool for a few moments before adding the powder or "sift" it in by sprinkling it from a shaker so that it will dissolve without a curdled appearance.

List 7: Free Foods

A free food is any food or drink that contains fewer than 20 calories per serving. You can eat as much as you want of those items that have no serving size specified. You may eat two or three servings per day of those items that have a specific serving size. Be sure to spread them out through the day.

Drinks

Bouillon or broth without fat	Cocoa powder, unsweetened (1 tablespoon)
Bouillon, low-sodium	Coffee/tea
Carbonated drinks, sugar free	Drink mixes, sugar-free
Carbonated water	Tonic water, sugar-free
Club soda	Postum

Miscellaneous

Nonstick pan spray	Wheat bran (1 tablespoon)

Fruit

Cranberries, unsweetened (½ cup)	Rhubarb, unsweetened (½ cup)

Vegetables
(raw, 1 cup)

Cabbage	Hot peppers
Celery	Mushrooms
Chinese cabbage	Radishes
Cucumber	Zucchini
Green onion	

Salad Greens

Cilantro	Romaine
Endive	Spinach
Escarole	Watercress
Lettuce	

Sweet Substitutes

Candy, hard, sugar free	Sugar substitutes (saccharin, aspartame)
Gelatin, sugar-free	
Gum, sugar-free	Whipped topping (2 tablespoons)
Jam/jelly, sugar-free (2 teaspoons)	
Pancake syrup, sugar-free (1–2 tablespoons)	

Condiments

Catsup (1 tablespoon)	Salad dressing, low-calorie (2 tablespoons)
Chili sauce (1 tablespoon)	
Horseradish	Salsa (2 tablespoons)
Mustard	Steak sauce (1 tablespoon)
Pickles, dill, unsweetened	Taco sauce (1 tablespoon)
	Vinegar

Seasonings

Seasonings can be very helpful in making food taste better. Be careful of how much sodium you use. Read the label and choose those seasonings that do not contain sodium or salt.

Basil (fresh)

Celery seeds

Cinnamon

Chili powder

Chives

Curry

Dill

Flavoring extracts (vanilla, almond, walnut, peppermint, butter, lemon, etc.)

Garlic

Garlic powder

Herbs

Hot pepper sauce

Lemon

Lemon juice

Lemon pepper

Lime

Lime juice

Mint

Onion powder

Oregano

Paprika

Pepper

Pimiento

Spices

Soy sauce

Soy sauce, low-sodium ("lite")

Wine, used in cooking (¼ cup)

Worcestershire sauce

List 8: Combination Foods

Much of the food we eat is mixed together in various combinations. These combination foods do not fall into only one exchange list. It can be quite hard to tell what is in a certain casserole dish or baked food item. This is a list of average values for some typical combination foods. This list will help you fit these foods into your meal plan. Ask your dietitian for information about any other foods you'd like to eat.

Here are the combination foods included in the booklet *Exchange Lists for Meal Planning* developed by the American Diabetes Association and the American Dietetic Association.

Combination Foods

Food	Amount	Exchanges
Casseroles, homemade	1 cup (8 ounces)	2 Starch, 2 Medium-Fat Meat, 1 Fat
Cheese pizza 🌾 , thin-crust	¼ of 15 ounces or ¼ of 10-inch	2 Starch, 1 Medium-Fat Meat, 1 Fat
Chili with beans 🌾 , 🌾 (commercial)	1 cup (8 ounces)	2 Starch, 2 Medium-Fat Meat, 2 Fat
Chow mein 🌾 , 🌾 (without noodles or rice)	2 cups (16 ounces)	1 Starch, 2 Vegetables, 2 Lean Meat
Macaroni and cheese 🌾	1 cup (8 ounces)	2 Starch, 1 Medium-Fat Meat, 2 Fat
Soup		
Bean 🌾 , 🌾	1 cup (8 ounces)	1 Starch, 1 Vegetable, 1 Lean Meat
Chunky, all varieties 🌾	10¾ ounce can	1 Starch, 1 Vegetable, 1 Medium-Fat Meat
Cream 🌾 (made with water)	1 cup (8 ounces)	1 Starch, 1 Fat
Vegetable 🌾 or broth-type 🌾	1 cup (8 ounces)	2 Starch
Spaghetti and meatballs (canned) 🌾	1 cup (8 ounces)	2 Starch, 1 Medium-Fat Meat, 1 Fat
Sugar-free pudding (made with skim milk)	½ cup	1 Starch

If beans are used as a meat substitute:

Dried beans 🌾 , peas 🌾 , lentils 🌾	1 cup (cooked)	2 Starch, 1 Lean Meat

List 9: Foods for Occasional Use

Moderate amounts of some foods can be used in your meal plan in spite of their sugar or fat content, as long as you can maintain blood glucose control. The following list includes average exchange values for some of these foods. Because they are concentrated sources of carbohydrate, you will notice that the portion sizes are very small. Check with your dietitian for advice on how often and when you can eat them. Generally, the best time to eat these foods is before exercise or with a meal, when the other foods in the meal will slow the absorption of the simple sugars.

Occasional Foods

Food	Amount	Exchanges
Angel food cake	1/12 cake	2 Starch
Cake, no icing	1/12 cake or a 3-inch square	2 Starch, 2 Fat
Cookies	2 small (1¾ inch across)	1 Starch, 1 Fat
Doughnut, plain, cake type	1 small	1 Starch, 1 Fat
Fig bars	1 large or 2 small	1 Starch
Frozen fruit yogurt	⅓ cup (1 stick)	1 Starch
Gingersnaps	3	1 Starch
Granola	¼ cup	1 Starch, 1 Fat
Granola bars, plain	1 small	1 Starch, 1 Fat
Ice cream, any flavor	½ cup	1 Starch, 2 Fat
Ice milk, any flavor	½ cup	1 Starch, 1 Fat
Ladyfingers	1 large or 2 small	1 Starch
Sherbet, any flavor	¼ cup	1 Starch

| Snack chips and puffs, all varieties | 1 ounce | 1 Starch, 2 Fat |
| Vanilla wafers | 6 small | 1 Starch, 1 Fat |

¹If more than one serving is eaten, these foods have 400 milligrams or more of sodium.

List 10: Additional Exchanges

We want diabetics to enjoy the same things as friends and family members do, as much as is possible. Commercial products, appropriately used, offer convenience and many easy options when there is little time to prepare food from "scratch." A great source of information on commercial products, with hundreds of foods, including ethnic foods, converted into exchanges is *Exchanges for All Occasions: Meeting the Challenge of Diabetes* by Marion J. Franz, R.D. The author is the director of nutrition for the International Diabetes Center in Minneapolis. Information on ordering this publication is listed in the appendix at the end of this book. Some of the useful exchange values in that book are listed here.

Ethnic and Other Popular Foods

Food	Amount	Exchanges
Beef or cheese enchilada	1	1 or 2 Medium-Fat Meat, 1½ Starch, 1 Fat
Beef ravioli	1 cup	2 Starch, 4 Medium-Fat Meat, 1 Vegetable, 1 Fat
Beef stew	½ cup	1 Starch, 1 Medium-Fat Meat
Chopped liver	1 ounce	1 High-Fat Meat
Eggplant parmigiana	1 cup	2 Medium-Fat Meat, 2 Vegetable, 1 Starch, ½ Fat
Fish sticks	4	1½ Starch, 1 Medium-Fat Meat
Fried rice	½ cup	1 Starch, 2 fat
Fruit bread, banana	1½ ounce slice	1½ Starch, 1 Fat

Ethnic and Other Popular Foods

Food	Amount	Exchanges
Gefilte fish	1 ounce	1 Lean Meat
Ground beef, drained	½ cup cooked	3 Medium-Fat Meat
Italian sauce, meatless	½ cup	1 Vegetable, 1 Fat
Matzo ball	1 medium	1 Starch
Onion rings, frozen	2 ounces	1 Starch, 1 Fat
Refried beans	⅓ cup	1 Starch, 1 Fat
Taco, folded and filled with meat, lettuce, tomatoes, cheese	1	1 or 2 Medium-Fat Meat, 1 Starch, 1 Vegetable

Years ago, individuals with diabetes were taught to avoid foods having sugar of any type. Today, restrictions tend to be less severe, making it easier to eat well and have a wider variety of foods from which to choose as long as blood sugar and weight remain in control.

A dietitian can translate the nutritional value of your favorite desserts into exchanges for you. Whether or not these foods can be fit into your meal plan is the next decision.

Recently, we converted some Kitchens of Sara Lee frozen desserts into exchanges. Even though they are made with sugar and most with butter, several can fit into the diets of some people with well-controlled diabetes. For example, a slice of pound cake, a chocolate fudge cake snack, or an individual cheese or raspberry danish contains 130–135 calories, and each is equivalent to one Starch plus one Fat Exchange. Other Kitchens of Sara Lee desserts may be appropriate in carefully measured portions for very special treats or occasional use. They do have sugar and saturated fats, but they are lower in calories than most home recipes that also contain sugar and fats. When we saw these values for fancy cakes, we began to hum "Happy Birthday. . . ." Be careful about other foods at the same meal and ask your doctor or dietitian if these treats are permitted.

Sara Lee Products

Food*	Amount	Exchanges
Chocolate Mousse Light Classic	1 slice (2 ounces)	1 Starch, 2½ Fat (200 calories)
Coconut Layer Cake	1 slice (⅛ cake)	1½ Starch, 2 Fat (220 calories)
Double Chocolate Layer Cake	1 slice (⅛ cake)	1½ Starch, 2 Fat (210 calories)
French Cheesecake Light Classic	1 slice (2½ ounces)	1 Starch, 2½ Fat (200 calories)
Strawberry French Cheesecake Light Classic	1 slice (2½ ounces)	1½ Starch, 2 Fat (200 calories)

Remember to check labels because recipes of commercial products change from time to time.

Be cautious with home recipes. Don't assume that Aunt Tillie's home recipe for a cookie has the same exchange value as either a recipe in this book or a commercial cookie. Aunt Tillie's recipe or even a cookie from a specialty store probably has a lot more butter and sugar and may be twice the size of one of our cookies or a commercial cookie. In other words, six small vanilla wafers equals one Starch plus one Fat Exchange, but only one homemade cookie may carry the same exchange value. If you must share Aunt Tillie's bounty, take the recipe to your dietitian, who can calculate the nutritive value and exchange values and determine whether or not the recipe is suitable. Sorry, Aunt Tillie!

Frozen Treats

Your supermarket offers many choices of sweets. Try the sugar-free gelatins and puddings, but read the labels carefully. Many treats can be found in the freezer case. We have identified products by brand name here so that you will know what to look for. We are not endorsing brands but rather trying to help you find the same products we have converted into ex-

Frozen Treats

Food	Amount	Exchanges
Chocolate Treat (Weight Watchers)	1 bar (2¾ ounces)	1 Starch, 1 Fruit (130 calories)
Crystal Light Bars (General Foods)	1 bar (1.8 ounces)	Free (14 calories)
Frozen Fruit Bars (Shamitoff)	1 bar (2½ ounces)	1 Fruit (60 calories)
Fruit and Juice Bars (Chiquita)	1 bar (2 ounces)	1 Fruit (50 calories)
Frozen Fruit'n Juice Bars (Dole)	1 bar (2½ ounces)	1 Fruit (70 calories)
Frozen Mousse (Zellers)	1 cup (4 ounces)	1 Fruit, 1 Skim Milk (130 calories)
Frozen yogurt (Columbo, Sealtest)	4 ounces	1 Fruit, ½ Medium-Fat Meat (100–102 calories)
Frozfruit Bar (strawberry and pineapple)	1 bar (4 ounces)	1 Fruit (68 calories)
Fruit Juice Bar (Weight Watchers)	1 bar (2½ ounces)	1 Fruit (50 calories)
Sandwich Bar (Weight Watchers)	1 bar (2¾ ounces)	1 Starch, 1 Fruit (130 calories)
Soft Frozen Yogurt, banana (Yoplait)	3 ounces	1 Starch (90 calories)
Sugar-Free Ice Pops with Juice (Popsicle)	1 bar (1¾ ounces)	Free or ½ Fruit (18 calories)
Sugar-Free Fudge Pops (Popsicle)	1 bar (1¾ ounces)	½ Starch (35 calories)
Tofutti (Lite Line)	3 ounces	1 Starch (90 calories)

changes. Your dietitian can help you evaluate which products are appropriate for you.

Avoid sweetened ice pops, frozen gelatin bars, pudding pops, and similar items. While they often contain fewer than 100 calories, they are almost all sugar and not suitable for diabetics.

Frozen fruit bars account for almost 20 percent of frozen "novelties," as they are called in the industry. Frozen fruit bars are low in fiber when compared to fresh fruits, and some have added sugar. The best choices are those without sugar that derive their sweetness from the fruit itself. Fruit and cream bars and bars made with coconut generally have more calories and fat than the pure fruit types.

3
The Great Sugar Masquerade

To most people, the word *sugar* means white table sugar or brown sugar. But there are really more than 100 sweet substances that can be described as sugars. All of these sweet substances are carbohydrates—an enormous family of nutrients that provide most of the energy in our diet. Carbohydrates come in four forms:

1. **Sugars:** The smallest and sweetest members of the carbohydrate family. Sugars are found in all sweets and in fruits.
2. **Starches:** Chemically, long chains of sugars that are usually not sweet. Starches are found in grains, cereal, potatoes, pasta products, and baked goods. After digestion, they are broken down into glucose for use in the human body.
3. **Indigestible Carbohydrates:** Cellulose and other fibers that give structure to food. Our body does not have the enzyme to break down these carbohydrates, so no sugar is released when we eat cellulose. See Chapter 5, "Fantastic Fiber," for information about the benefits of fiber.
4. **Sugar Alcohols:** Synthetic products made from sugars or cellulose. Although the digestive system metabolizes these sugar alcohols more slowly than it does sugar, these products end up in the body as glucose. The most popular ones are sorbitol, mannitol, and xylitol.

Although diabetics are cautioned about the use of particular carbohydrates, we know that everyone, even those with the most serious and difficult-to-control diabetes, must eat carbohydrates every day. This food family is an important source of quick energy, and our brain and nervous system require carbohydrates as their fuel.

The phrase *nutritive sweetener* on a label means the product contains a sweetener having calories. Conversely, *nonnutritive sweetener* means few or no calories are present; for example, saccharin or aspartame.

100 Sugars?

What about all those 100 sweet substances? Well, we don't need to know all their names, but there are several that every diabetic should know about, to be able to recognize hidden sugars on label ingredients lists. One trick is to look for *-ose* words like these:

Sucrose: Sometimes called *saccharose.* White sugar (cane or beet sugar), granulated, cubed, or powdered sugar gives us nothing but calories. Brown sugar, much less refined, is derived from molasses (sorghum cane), and gives us very small amounts of a few minerals. Raw sugar, very similar to brown sugar, is sometimes crystalline.

Fructose: Sometimes called *levulose.* Fructose is found in nature in fruits and honey. It is highly soluble and sweeter than any other sugar in equal amounts. You may see "high fructose syrup" on a label, which is a concentrated form of fructose. Fructose syrups are manufactured with 42, 55, and 90 percent fructose for different purposes.

Lactose: Sometimes called *milk sugar* because milk is its chief food source. Lactose is a combination of glucose and galactose.

Galactose: A simple sugar found in lactose (milk sugar).

Dextrose: Commercially obtained from starch. Dextrose is sometimes called *corn sugar* or *grape sugar.*

Glucose: Found chiefly in fruits, some vegetables, honey, and corn syrup. Starches break down to glucose, and all other sugars convert to glucose during digestion or metabolism. This is the form of carbohydrate that the body uses. The phrase *blood sugar* refers to the level of glucose in the blood.

Maltose: Comes from the breakdown of starch in the malting of barley. When starches are digested, they pass through a stage of being maltose before they end up as glucose.

Mannose: Comes from manna and the ivory nut. Mannose is used mostly by sugar chemists. Mannitol is derived from mannose.

Although these *-ose* sugars have different names, all are used to sweeten foods. And we must never forget that, whether we use them alone or with other ingredients, each of these *-ose* sugars is a carbohydrate; every gram gives us four calories. Concentrated sources of sugar must be limited by the diabetic because they require insulin for proper utilization by the body.

Other Familiar Sugars

In addition to the *-ose* group, there are other substances you need to recognize as sugars:

Brown sugar: Sugar crystals with some molasses for flavor and color. Brown sugar is over 90 percent sucrose.

Corn syrup: A liquid form of corn sugar, used in baking and infant feeding formulas. When crystallized, corn syrup may be called *corn syrup solids* or *corn sweetener.* It is relatively inexpensive and is used to sweeten canned fruits and in soft drinks. Corn syrup contains 42, 55, or 90 percent fructose; the rest is dextrose.

Dextrin: Results from the partial breakdown of starch.

Honey: Comes from floral sources from which bees collect nectar. Honey may be liquid, creamed, or in combs and is a more concentrated form of carbohydrate than table sugar. Some health food stores, farm stands, and magazines have told diabetics that they may eat honey instead of sugar because it does not require insulin to be metabolized. *This is not true.* Honey is converted to glucose like all other sugars, and insulin *is* required for metabolism. Don't be fooled! Honey is a carbohydrate.

Invert sugar: A sugar formed when the sugar molecule is split by acids or enzymes. Invert sugar is used in liquid form and is sweeter than sucrose; it helps baked goods stay fresher longer.

Maple syrup/maple sugar: Made from the sap of maple trees.

Molasses: A strong-flavored sweetener made from sorghum canes.

Raw sugar: A course, granulated, brown-colored solid made from sugar cane juice.

Turbinado sugar: Partially refined sugar that is crystals of sugar washed in steam.

Fructose as an Alternative Sweetener

Fructose, as mentioned earlier, is a natural sugar found in fruits and honey. When table sugar (a two-sugar fragment) breaks down in our body, it yields one unit of glucose and one of fructose. Fructose also is found in fruits and can be extracted from foods. It can be used for baking, canning, and freezing and is sold in both boxes and individual packets. Current label information tells us that:

1 teaspoon natural fructose sugar (SweetLite)
= 4 g CHO, 15 calories = ⅓ fruit exchange
1 packet fructose (Estee)
= 3 g CHO, 12 calories = ¼ fruit exchange

In Europe, especially in West Germany and Switzerland, pure fructose is accepted as a sweetener for use by diabetics. There, it is called *nonglucose carbohydrate.* Because many foods containing fructose are now being introduced in the United States, you should understand what fructose does and its advantages and limitations for use by diabetics.

Fructose is absorbed more slowly than glucose into the bloodstream. It does raise the level of sugar in the blood, but not as quickly to the same level as equal amounts of glucose. Unlike glucose, most fructose is metabolized in the liver, meaning it does not require an initial insulin response to move from the blood directly into the cells for metabolism. During metabolism, part of the fructose molecule may be changed into glucose. The rate of conversion of fructose to glucose varies among individuals. At this point, some insulin is required. But the entire process of fructose absorption and metabolism requires far less insulin than an equal amount of glucose requires.

Fructose is a carbohydrate and always must be used carefully, because it has the same caloric value as other sugars. Also, fructose is often included in foods that contain other carbohydrates that provide calories and raise blood sugar levels. Fructose in syrups contains variable degrees of glucose—it is never 100% pure fructose. The use of limited amounts of foods containing fructose seems to be safe; however, excessive use, or the use of fructose cake frostings and similar sweets, is unwise unless you are one of the rare diabetics with an exceptionally high caloric need.

Some medical research suggests that fructose consumption may increase uric acid production. This is a potential problem for people with gout. Present research data is limited regarding the long-term effect of high levels of fructose in the diets of diabetics. Because the use of fructose is still controversial, consult your doctor or diet counselor before adding it to your diet.

Foods with added fructose are never "free" foods, they must be substituted for fruits in your meal plan. You will be giving up fruit exchanges that will reduce your vitamin, mineral, and fiber intake. Read the label on a box or individual packet to find out the carbohydrate and calorie level in the amount you may wish to use. Because fructose is somewhat sweeter than other sugars, you may be satisfied using less.

Sugar Alcohols

Sugar alcohols: Have been adopted into the sugar family because, although they are chemically alcohols, they are made from sugar. Sugar alcohols are digested and absorbed much more slowly than other sugars, but they do end up in the body as carbohydrates and therefore must be counted in the diabetic diet.

You will see these names among commercial product ingredients:

Sorbitol: Commercially made from glucose. Sorbitol is used widely in the commercial manufacture of dietetic foods and sugar-free gum. Read labels and check the caloric level of products containing sorbitol.

Mannitol and dulcitol: Manufactured from mannose and galactose. Both are less sweet than sucrose.

Xylitol: Manufactured from xylose (wood sugar) found in corn cobs, straw, bran, wood gum, and the bran of seeds. Xylose has been identified in fruits such as cherries, pears, peaches, and plums. As with the other sugar alcohols, xylitol is absorbed slowly, but the amount absorbed by the body contributes calories. Some chewing gums contain xylitol because it is not supposed to cause tooth decay—a claim that is still under study.

We suggest caution in eating foods sweetened with sorbitol, mannitol, and xylitol. Many people, upon eating generous amounts of sugar alcohols, develop gastrointestinal problems such as diarrhea. For a diabetic, this can be especially serious.

Sweeteners in Recipes for Diabetics

Often, when our recipes needed a sweet taste we added a larger-than-usual measure of vanilla. Sometimes we added a sugar substitute to give a product a sweet flavor. Neither of these tricks, however, will work in baked products that need a real sugar. Regular sugars used in making cakes and cookies are required for sweetness and also for their chemical actions with the other ingredients that give baked products tenderness and lightness. As sugar cooks, it caramelizes, giving baked goods their nicely browned appearance.

Readers of the first edition of this book asked us why we used sugar or honey in our breads and rolls. Quite simply, yeast needs sugar in order to multiply and cause yeast breads to rise. Sugar substitutes don't work, and the amount of sugar or honey per serving is quite low. Don't worry about this.

Sugar substitutes don't combine with other ingredients to make the product light and tender; they just contribute a sweetish taste. They are valuable and useful in many recipes and certainly help to make the diabetic's menus much more interesting and varied without adding carbohydrates and calories. Unfortunately, they don't work well in baked foods because they undergo chemical changes in cooking and either lose their sweetness or tend to become bitter rather than sweet. One of the challenges to food technologists is to develop a good-tasting sugar substitute that withstands heat. Most of our recipes add the sugar substitute at the end of the directions to maximize the sweetening effect of the products.

Our extensive test-kitchen work proved to us that we can reduce the sugar in most baked sweets (cookies, cakes, etc.) with good results. In some recipes, part of the sugar can be replaced with sugar substitutes (Equal, Sweet'n Low, or Sugar-Twin). At present, the only heat-stable sugar substitute is saccharin. Our recipes were tested with Equal (aspartame) unless the specific food required baking or other long cooking that reduced the sweetening effect. In those recipes, we used Sweet'n Low (saccharin).

The current position of the American Diabetes Association, Inc., states, "In some individuals, modest amounts of sucrose may be acceptable, contingent upon metabolic control and body weight." Ask your dietitian or doctor if you may eat foods prepared with small amounts of sugar. If the sweetener is calculated into the recipe and is included in the exchange value—and if you eat only the portion size calculated—the food may be suitable for you.

Sugar Substitutes

Two types of noncaloric, nonnutritive, manmade sweeteners are being sold in the United States as this book goes to press: saccharin and aspartame. Cyclamate was withdrawn from the market a decade ago but may be back. Several nonnutritive sweeteners are in testing stages but have not yet received approval.

The American Diabetes Association, Inc., position statement says, "Particular nutritive and nonnutritive sweeteners are not encouraged but are acceptable. Use of various nonnutritive sweeteners is encouraged to offset the possible disadvantages that may result from the excessive consumption of a single agent."

Some nonnutritive sweeteners are mixed into small amounts of nutritive sweeteners (dextrose) because they are so concentrated that they can't be "sprinkled" if alone. Don't be concerned about a small amount of nutritive sweetener used as a filler in packets of nonnutritive sweetener.

Saccharin

The granddaddy of nonnutritive sweeteners, saccharin has been used for more than 100 years. Saccharin is a white, crystalline powder 375 times sweeter than table sugar. Very little saccharin is broken down by the body; it is excreted as saccharin in the urine.

Many saccharin products are made with sodium saccharin and are a less desirable choice for regular use for people on low-sodium diets.

Saccharin is available in three forms:

Tablets:　¼ grain saccharin = 1 tablet = 1 teaspoon of sugar in sweetness = 0 calories

Granular:　In packets, 1 packet = 2 teaspoons of sugar in sweetness = 4 calories

Sweet'n Low, a popular brand, is a sodium-free soluble saccharin. It is a blend of nutritive and nonnutritive sweeteners and contains a bit of dextrose.

Packets of SugarTwin and Weight Watchers Sweet'ner are made with sodium saccharin and contain some dextrose. 1 packet = 2 teaspoons of sugar in sweetness = 3 calories. One packet of Sweet'ner contains 16 mg of sodium—only a bit, but it does add up.

Boxes of Brown SugarTwin are made with sodium saccharin, caramel color, and artificial flavor. 1 teaspoon = 1½ calories.

Liquid: Sweet-10 and Superose are both sodium saccharin in water and have no calories.
10 drops = 1 teaspoon of sugar in sweetness
Sweet 10—1 tablespoon = ½ cup sugar sweetness
Superose—2 teaspoons = ½ cup sugar sweetness

The safety of saccharin has been much debated. In 1972, it was removed from the Generally Recognized as Safe (GRAS) list because of its potential link to bladder cancer (in male rats). When a ban was proposed, consumers, the American Diabetes Association, Inc., and the Juvenile Diabetes Foundation opposed the ban, and saccharin remained available. All products with saccharin carry a warning label that states: "Use of this product may be hazardous to your health. This product contains saccharin, which has been determined to cause cancer in laboratory animals."

Saccharin is banned in Canada, where cyclamate (another nonnutritive sweetener) is still sold.

Aspartame

Aspartame, a combination of two protein fragments or amino acids, is 180 to 200 times sweeter than table sugar. It was approved for use in 1974. The NutraSweet Company sells aspartame to food manufacturers under the brand name of NutraSweet. NutraSweet is the ingredient listed in sugar-free soft drinks, puddings, gelatin, cocoas, frozen desserts, drink mixes, etc. Aspartame for table use is called Equal.

Most people prefer the flavor of aspartame to the flavor of

saccharin. Many nondiabetics use aspartame-containing foods to reduce their calorie intake. Aspartame is now available to consumers in three forms:

Bulk: As an ingredient of processed foods as Nutra-Sweet. Read the label for nutritional information as products vary widely. NutraSweet is not sold directly to consumers in bulk but may be in the future.

Packets: 1 packet Equal = 4 calories = 2 teaspoons sugar in sweetness (6 packets Equal = $\frac{1}{4}$ cup sugar; 12 packets Equal = $\frac{1}{2}$ cup sugar). Equal in packets contains a small amount of dextrose in the form of dried corn syrup. When first introduced, Equal used lactose as a filler, but this has been changed because some people are lactose intolerant.

Tablets: 1 tablet Equal = 1 teaspoon sugar in sweetness and contains lactose as a binder.

Products containing aspartame have several labeling requirements. The label must state that aspartame should not be used in cooking or baking and that the product contains phenylalanine ("Phenylketonurics: contains phenylalanine"). Phenylketonuia (PKU) is a rather rare genetic disease characterized by a sensitivity to one of the amino acids in aspartame.

Aspartame is stable in dry foods but loses its sweetness when heated or held a long time in liquid form. Heating or keeping a soft drink sweetened with aspartame for several months will not result in an unsafe product, but it may lose its flavor.

Like saccharin, aspartame's long-term safety has been questioned, but the courts and governmental agencies have ruled that it is generally safe in amounts normally eaten. Certainly, you should avoid this, or any other food, if you have a sensitivity or negative reaction to it.

When the Searle (The NutraSweet Company) patent on aspartame runs out, other manufacturers are expected to produce aspartame and give it brand names other than Nutra-Sweet.

Other Noncaloric Sweeteners

Several other noncaloric sweeteners are being tested. Glycosides such as Stevioside are approved for food use in Japan; Acesulfame Potassium is used in the United Kingdom, West Germany, and Switzerland; Alltame is a protein-based sweetener 2,000 times as sweet as sugar that has been developed by Pfizer, Inc. None of these sweeteners has been approved by the Food and Drug Administration at this time, but watch for them. As new sugar substitutes come on the market, read the labels carefully to know how much to use.

The bottom line on nonnutritive sweeteners, sugar substitutes, is to use them in moderate amounts as necessary to sweeten and enhance your foods. You will want to use several types to take advantage of their flavors and cooking properties.

4
A New Look at Fats

It is important for diabetics to understand both fats in food and fats in the bloodstream. The amounts and types of fat in your diet are likely to influence the fats in your bloodstream, and that is where troubles can begin.

The average American gets about 37 percent of food calories from fats. Reducing fat to 30 percent of calories would be healthful for all of us. When fat is controlled, both the quantity and type usually need to be changed. It's easy to eat too much fat if we are not careful to choose lowfat foods and prepare them with a minimum of fat. While the fat in butter or margarine and around the perimeter of meat is quite visible, it's easy to underestimate the fat level in fried foods, cookies, ice cream, cheese, baked goods, sauces, and nuts.

Fats are vital to life. Nutritionally, they provide calories and energy; add palatability and flavor to food; provide fatty acids essential to growth; transport fat-soluble vitamins A, D, E, and K; and give a feeling of fullness and satisfaction after eating.

While some fat is essential to life, most of us eat too much. Too much fat in the diet, especially saturated fats and cholesterol (a fatlike substance), can promote heart disease, atherosclerosis, and cancer of the colon and breast. Certainly, too much of all types of fat can cause weight gain and obesity, which increase risks of gallbladder disease and a host of other medical problems. Some diabetics (Type II) who are overweight and can reduce their calories and weight can then produce enough insulin to control their diabetes without medication.

Your diet counselor will stress the importance of selecting primarily lean meats, low-fat milk and cheese, and carefully portioned foods listed on the fat exchange list. Why is there so much emphasis on fat?

The American Diabetes Association, Inc., and the American Heart Association have similar dietary recommendations— limit total fat to a maximum of 30 percent of calories and limit cholesterol to 300 milligrams per day. Reducing saturated fats and replacing some of them with polyunsaturated or monoun-saturated fats may slow the development of atherosclerosis. That is why the exchange lists separate the unsaturated from the saturated fats and why the recipes in this book specify margarine instead of butter.

Cholesterol is a fatlike substance found in foods of animal origin. It is made in our bodies, primarily by the liver, and is made in the bodies of other animals as well. Consequently, meats, poultry, and dairy products contain cholesterol in var-ied amounts, while grains, fruits, and vegetables never provide cholesterol unless it is added in processing or preparing those foods.

Every adult, whether diabetic or not, should know his or her blood cholesterol and triglyceride levels. Those with high-cho-lesterol levels should reduce the cholesterol supplied by food to see if they can reduce serum cholesterol by changing their diet—if not, medications may have to be taken. Each of our recipes tells you the milligrams of fat and cholesterol per por-tion. This information, plus careful reading of food labels, will help you reduce your fat and cholesterol intake.

Here is a listing of the cholesterol levels of typical portions of some popular foods:

While shellfish, shrimp, and crabmeat appear high in choles-terol, it seems that these foods contain a form of cholesterol that does not raise our level of blood cholesterol when we eat them. Egg yolk contains a large amount of cholesterol; if you

Food	Cholesterol (mg)
Fruits, grains, vegetables, nuts, seeds, vegetable oil, and margarines containing vegetable oil	0
Oysters (cooked)	45
Scallops	53
Clams	65
Fish, lean	65
Chicken/turkey, light meat (no skin)	80
Lobster	85
Beef, lean	90
Chicken/turkey, dark meat (no skin)	95
Crab	100
Shrimp	150
Egg yolk (one)	270
Beef liver	440
Beef kidney	700

eat lots of eggs, switch to egg whites only or egg substitutes and limit yolks to three per week for cooking and eating.

Fats in foods are mixtures of saturated and unsaturated fats. When we say a food is a saturated fat, we really mean that there are proportionately more saturated fatty acids than unsaturated ones. Saturated fats tend to raise blood cholesterol levels in some people, while unsaturated fats, both polyunsaturated and monounsaturated ones, tend to reduce blood cholesterol and triglyceride levels.

As you can see, palm and coconut oil are the two highest sources of saturated fat. Both of these fats are common ingredients in processed foods. Look for them on the ingredient panel of food labels. Granola type cereals, "creamers," baked products, and supermarket cookies often contain coconut oil. They should be avoided.

Oils and Fats

Type of Oil or Fat	Percentage of Polyunsaturated Fat	Percentage of Saturated Fat
Safflower oil	74	9
Sunflower oil	64	10
Corn oil	58	13
Average vegetable oil (soybean plus cottonseed)	40	13
Canola oil* (Puritan oil)	32	6
Peanut oil	30	19
Chicken fat (schmaltz)	26	29
Vegetable shortening	20	32
Lard	12	40
Olive oil*	9	14
Beef fat	4	48
Butter	4	61
Palm oil	2	81
Coconut oil	2	86

*Two oils are predominately monounsaturated fatty acids. Olive oil is 77% monounsaturated; Canola oil (Puritan oil) is 62% monounsaturated. To determine percentage of monounsaturated fats, add polyunsaturated and saturated fats and subtract that number from 100%; the remaining percentage is almost all monounsaturated.

What About Fish?

Fish is a terrific food for diabetics for many reasons:

- It is lower in fat than many meat choices (provided it is not fried).

- It is low in saturated fats and helps prevent atherosclerosis.
- Canned fish, especially those with soft edible bones (like canned salmon and sardines), are very rich in calcium. So are soft-shell crabs and smelts.
- It is rich in a certain type of polyunsaturated oil called omega-3 fatty acids that have been shown to decrease blood levels of triglycerides and cholesterol.
- It tastes so good.

Long-term studies show that people who eat at least seven ounces of fish each week (about two servings) are less likely to die of heart attacks. Eating fish, particularly the high-fat fish, at least twice a week is good advice. The types of fish richest in omega-3 fatty acids are salmon, tuna, canned sardines, mackerel, herring, trout, and shellfish.

Some people want to take a shortcut and take fish oil supplements instead of eating fish. As we write this book, many types of fish oils in capsule form are being promoted. If your doctor advises you to take fish oil capsules as a medication, you should certainly follow that advice. Much research is in progress and, at present, most experts recommend getting omega-3 fatty acids from fish rather than supplements. Fish oil supplements have a number of drawbacks. Very large amounts can cause blood clotting problems and may promote strokes. Large doses may provide toxic amounts of fat-soluble vitamins A and D. Like any fat, they provide calories and they are expensive. For some people, fish oil capsules cause indigestion and "fish breath."

A delicious serving of Grilled Salmon with Cilantro Spinach Sauce (pictured on the cover, *see* Index) has all the advantages of a wonderful fish meal and none of the potential health risks of supplements. Because of the new research and trends toward eating more fish, we have included many new fish recipes in this revised edition, particularly ones using salmon, mackerel, shrimp, and other shellfish.

To Lower Blood Fats

In addition to altering the amount and type of fats in your diet, we know that regular sustained exercise lowers levels of both triglycerides and cholesterol in the blood. Another way of lowering blood fats is to include more soluble fibers in your diet—oats, legumes, fruits, and vegetables.

If your body doesn't respond to dietary and exercise changes, medications may be prescribed by your physician. Since currently available medications for reduction of cholesterol levels have side effects, reducing blood fats through changes in the diet is preferable and safer.

5
Fantastic Fiber

Fiber is a Cinderella story in nutrition. Twenty years ago fiber was "roughage"—a nonessential part of the diet, an indigestible residue of carbohydrate. It was known that fiber aided elimination and relieved constipation. Scientists and people who worried about their bowels cared about fiber, but most people paid little attention to it.

Times have changed. Now fiber has been elevated in stature to one of the most important nutrients in the promotion of health and the prevention and treatment of disease. Most health authorities suggest that we increase the fiber in our diets, although a recent study of fiber research concluded that more evidence is needed before public recommendations should be made. Our day-to-day food choices can improve while scientists continue their debate. To understand the fiber story, it's important to know what fiber is, what it does, and how to get enough of it.

What Is Fiber?

Dietary fiber is the part of plant cells that are resistant to human digestive enzymes. Of the many types of fiber (celluloses, hemicelluloses, oligosaccharides, pectins, gums, waxes, and lignin), some occur in grains, others in fruits and vegetables, and others in dried peas and beans.

Unlike some animals that can make digestive enzymes to break the chemical bonds of fiber and release energy, we humans cannot completely digest fiber. We are learning that the body uses each type of fiber differently, so it is important to choose fibers from varied sources to garner maximum health benefits. Insoluble fibers such as cellulose pass through our digestive system relatively intact. Other fibers, the soluble ones, are partially digestible, and that is why they can do more for our body than aid elimination.

In 1984, a new method for analyzing dietary fiber content was accepted by the Association of Official Analytical Chemists (AOAC). Most dietary fiber is contained in the cell walls of plants, and dietary fiber is the total of some fibers that are soluble in water and others that are insoluble.

Prior to this time, only insoluble crude fiber was measured; these crude fiber values extracted the water-soluble fibers found in many fruits and vegetables, oatmeal, and dried beans and peas. We now know that the soluble fibers (gums, pectin) are among the most important for those with diabetes because they have positive effects in moderating blood sugar levels and reducing blood cholesterol and triglycerides. Unfortunately, the water-soluble fibers are quite difficult to measure. They were often extracted and discarded in the analysis process. New fiber values, those listed on the recipes, count dietary fiber—the total of all types.

Five Benefits of Fiber

1. In the digestive tract, insoluble fiber contributes bulk and absorbs water, making us feel full. This bulking action also has a laxative effect and aids in elimination. Fiber sources like salads and whole grains require chewing, and this allows time for the brain to get the signal that we have eaten and are no longer hungry.

Cellulose and the other insoluble fibers protect against constipation, irritable bowel syndrome, and diverticulosis, a condition affecting about half of people over the age of 60. Years ago, when a person had irritable bowel syndrome or diverticulosis, a low-fiber diet was prescribed. Now a high-fiber diet, including high-fiber cereals and bran products, is more likely to be advised.

2. Fiber also helps control weight because many low-calorie fruits and vegetables are rich in fiber and make us feel fuller than calorie-dense foods. Since most fiber stays in the digestive tract, it doesn't provide calories.

3. Increasing dietary fiber is particularly useful to diabetics because soluble fiber in the diet has been shown to reduce insulin requirements, thus improving control of blood sugar. Simultaneously, it decreases serum cholesterol and blood pressure.

The American Diabetes Association, Inc., in its 1986 position statement suggests that "Foods should be selected with moderate to high amounts of dietary fibers from a wide variety of foods. These foods include legumes, lentils, roots, tubers, green leafy vegetables, all types of whole grain cereals (e.g. wheat, barley, oats, corn and rye), and fruits. Fruits and vegetables should be eaten raw to maximize the fiber effect, and not pureed, which causes loss or reduction of the fiber effect." The exchange lists are marked to highlight food with three or more grams of fiber.

Another part of the statement points out that radical changes in fiber intake can alter insulin needs and that hypoglycemia can result if insulin dosage is not adjusted. Changes in fiber level should be gradual and monitored to see if blood sugar levels or insulin needs change.

4. Even people without diabetes are also advised to eat more fiber because soluble fibers (pectin, guar, locust bean gums, oat bran, and beans) have been found to lower blood cholesterol levels. When you order a bowl of oatmeal, you may have the company of lots of health-conscious people who are not diabetics. Everyone should try to prevent cardiovascular disease.

5. A fifth benefit is promoted by the National Cancer Institute. Diets high in fiber have been statistically correlated with reduced frequency of bowel cancers. Since diets high in fiber tend also to have less fat, it is hard to separate the independent effects of increased fiber. For example, when you substitute lentil soup for a steak, you reduce the fat and raise the fiber simultaneously. The effect is likely to be positive, but the relative importance of each change is hard to determine.

Nothing is all good, however. The other side of the coin is that fiber, in excess, can trap and bind minerals such as calcium, copper, selenium, and zinc so that they are not well absorbed. That is why vegetable sources of calcium—broccoli, for example—do not provide all of the calcium that food composition tables say they provide.

Much research shows that legumes—lentils, chick-peas, navy beans, split peas, pinto beans, and kidney beans—are capable of reducing cholesterol and sometimes triglyceride in the bloodstream as well. The soluble fibers in legumes are more beneficial than insoluble fibers in normalizing blood glucose responses after meals. The effect of oat bran fiber is similar to that of legumes in promoting these positive effects.

Here are 10 tips to boost your fiber intake:

- Increase your consumption of vegetables of all types, including plenty of raw vegetable salads and cut vegetables.
- Eat whole fruits and dried fruits with skins (apples, pears, etc.) instead of juice or canned fruits that have been peeled and have less fiber.
- Select breads with visible grain particles—whole wheat, pumpernickel, corn tortillas—instead of white bread.
- Choose high-fiber starches—corn, winter squash, lima beans, peas—often.
- Eat high-fiber cereals as starch exchanges—bran, shredded wheat, oat bran, wheat germ—and use high-fiber cereals in recipes.
- Have legumes several times a week in soups, casseroles, or salads.
- Eat the edible skins and seeds of vegetables—the skin of a baked potato, the seeds of a cucumber.
- Think nuts and seeds if you can afford the calories and fat exchanges.
- Eat brown rice instead of white rice.
- Look for fiber-rich crackers—Ry-Krisp, Wasa, Finn, and those with seeds to add fiber.

Since dried beans and peas are economical and have so many health benefits, their components are now being extracted to fortify less nutritious foods. Recently pea fiber has been added to increase the fiber content of some frozen muffins.

When you see on a food label that a food is fiber-rich, check the ingredient list to learn the source of the fiber. If you want only the gastrointestinal benefits, wheat bran is fine. But if you want the cardiovascular and blood sugar benefits, look for soluble fibers from legumes, fruits, and oat bran. On some ingredient lists, you will see "guar gums," a soluble fiber used as a thickener and stabilizer. While every bit helps, the amount of guar gum is usually very small.

Getting Enough Fiber

How much fiber do we eat? Probably about 10 to 20 grams each day. The National Cancer Institute suggests that the optimum intake of fiber is about 25 to 35 grams per day. In this edition of our book we have added many fiber-rich foods, particularly soups made with peas and beans. Every recipe has been calculated to include the amount of dietary fiber. Try to eat at least 8 grams of fiber at each meal. In the exchange lists, foods with 3 grams or more of fiber are marked. Eat them often.

Individual tolerances for fiber vary, so increase your intake gradually. Nature makes ample fiber available on a year-round basis. Fiber tablets or supplements are not necessary unless prescribed by your physician.

Part II
Living with Diabetes

6
The Adult with Diabetes

Many factors affect adults with diabetes—the nature and severity of the diabetes, family background, education, type of work, and finances. When your diabetes is first diagnosed, don't panic. Accept the fact, learn about diabetes, talk about it, ask your doctor and dietitian all kinds of questions, and read when and what you can. Many people, places, and resources are willing and able to help you, but the extent to which you take control will have a great deal to do with the quality of life that lies ahead for you. Your doctor and your dietitian will tell you that you are basically responsible for yourself. They can give you all the information you need, but you make all the decisions in your day-to-day care.

Because the foods you eat and your meal plans are truly the foundation of successful diabetes management, we urge you to learn about foods for the diabetic. You will be the one who makes food choices at every meal. You will be the one who eats, or doesn't eat, at the appropriate time. You will be the one who decides to stop at the cookie store or pass it by. And the decisions you make will have effects on your body. Choosing to be in control will reduce reactions, emergencies, and complications. We are not suggesting that this is easy—it's not. It's hard, and it doesn't go away. But it is controllable, and that's a whole lot better than some other diseases that you are blessed not to have.

Parents and other family members and friends can be very helpful. Their understanding and patience can encourage you.

But don't let anyone coax you into breaking the rules. Don't hide the fact that you are now diabetic. Stand up to it, talk about it, and you'll be surprised at the warm understanding that will surround you. As you become increasingly aware of your diabetes, enjoy a wide selection of foods (such as our recipes), and perhaps be a greater achiever than you have ever been before!

7
The Child with Diabetes

On "Sesame Street" Kermit the Frog sings the song "It's Not Easy Being Green." That song tells how difficult it is to be different. The child who has diabetes is different from other children, and that's not easy—for either the child or the parents. Almost every child at some point feels different, unacceptable to others and to himself or herself. Sometimes it's because he or she is too fat, too skinny, has acne, or wears glasses. Diabetes is a medical problem that is not easily understood by the children it affects or their peers. The treatment—by insulin and diet—restricts schedules, activities, and independence.

Dr. Deborah Edidin, a pediatric endocrinologist at Northwestern University works with children with diabetes and their parents each day. She advises parents to give their children "a good, nutritious diet, without junk food, and to be sure that they eat at the same times each day."

As children reach school age, they make many food decisions at school and when with friends, and need to know what they can and should eat. They have the independence to choose foods on their own. By this time, they have learned that their blood glucose monitoring reflects what they have eaten at previous meals. The cause and effect relationship becomes clear and reinforces good food choices. If they follow their diet, their blood sugar level is more predictable. If they eat too much or the wrong kinds of food, their blood sugar level gets too high.

Dr. Edidin points out that "Adolescence is a difficult time for many kids, particularly those with diabetes or other medical problems. It's important to acknowledge that it is very hard to have dietary restrictions that friends don't have and to have to take insulin each day. Since the developmental tasks of adolescence are autonomy and separation, empathy and flexibility are important. Teaching how fast foods fit into the diet and how to alter food intake and insulin levels for different situations based on blood glucose monitoring helps teenagers to be more successful in controlling their diet and their lives." It is not an easy time for teenagers, parents, or doctors.

The Parent's Role

In the very young child, the responsibility for control of diabetes lies mostly with the parents. Many parents feel guilty because of the hereditary aspect of diabetes, and they become overly protective. Children, whether diabetic or not, quickly learn that they can manipulate parents by eating or not eating, by eating the right foods or the wrong ones, or by behaving or misbehaving to get attention.

It helps, in the long run, to encourage the child to assume as much responsibility as possible for his or her own care. The doctor or nurse will help teach the child how to give his own insulin at the appropriate time.

Often parents, especially the mother, are particularly involved in the diet management. Even young children can be taught the basic exchanges. It is much like a board game. The child can help prepare meals, weigh and cut food portions, pack lunches, and so on. A dietitian can work with the child and parents; an ongoing relationship with a diet counselor is important.

You can teach the child that his or her diabetes is a fact, not a secret. Share the fact with others who will be supportive. Let the parents of the child's playmates know that the child has diabetes and send appropriate food and snacks to their home if necessary. Be sure that others don't misinterpret "I'm not allowed to have candy at home," to mean that the child deserves more treats when he comes over to play.

As the child gets older, more self-directed, and more accepting of his or her diabetes, there will be continued peaks and valleys. The adolescent, whether diabetic or not, will seek limits, defy authority, and test new behavior. Hormonal changes cause spurts of growth that change insulin and food needs. The diabetes may seem to be less in control. Often discussion groups will be useful for adolescents with diabetes as well as teens with other long-term medical problems.

Some parents have been able to create an emotional environment that makes their child, who happens to be diabetic, feel special rather than sick or odd. The emotional and physical needs of just being a child are far more important than those of being a diabetic. But don't forget Kermit, who said, "It's not easy. . . ."

Summer Camps

Very often a diabetic child thinks he or she is the only child in the whole world with diabetes. A summer camp for diabetic children helps many overcome this feeling of being different. There are more than 50 summer camps for children with diabetes in the United States. Most of them include all of the normal camping activities, such as swimming, boating, horseback riding, games, and physical exercises under instruction and supervision. The camps are staffed with complete health teams—doctors, dietitians, and nurses who supervise, teach, and help each child. The camps often have junior counselors who may or may not be diabetics or who have a family interest in diabetes.

One of the greatest experiences for the children is meeting other young diabetics—talking together, learning together, and finding out that they are not alone in their problems. Although there is a charge for each child, usually no child's application is refused because the parents cannot pay. The camp committee's main consideration is which of the applicants need camp the most. Write to the American Diabetes Association, Inc. (see address in the appendix), and ask for a list of summer camps for diabetic children in or near your state.

In addition to the physical benefits of summer camp, it is

often a good idea to get the child away from the parents for a few weeks. During this separation, the child can experience a great deal of personal growth and can develop independent behavior and self-confidence in a safe environment. Also, the parents may get a much-needed rest or vacation with other family members who may not have been getting their fair share of attention.

Handling Special Situations

If your child is diabetic, you probably have many questions about how to deal with certain situations that can pose problems for diabetics. In the following chapters you'll find information on traveling; eating out, including tips on brown-bagging school lunches; a list of fast-food exchanges; and exercise such as participating in gym classes and school sports.

8
Exercise and Sports

You may wonder why we have included this chapter in a book about the dietary control of diabetes. Well, calories come in through diet, but they need a bit of help from physical activity to be used.

From a simply caloric standpoint, all of us, whether we are diabetic or not, maintain our weight by balancing the calories we eat with the energy it takes to run our sophisticated motor of a body as well as support our physical activity. In other words, we can eat more without gaining weight if we are physically active, and we must eat less if we get little physical exercise. Maintaining reasonable weight is important to diabetics. Lean bodies use insulin more effectively, and if insulin therapy is necessary, less insulin is needed at ideal weight.

Regular exercise has benefits beyond weight control. Exercise that is strenuous and continued long enough (a minimum of 20 minutes per session) has cardiovascular benefits and produces hormones that lead to a feeling of well-being and satisfaction—a fine way of reducing stress. Do you know anybody who doesn't need to reduce his stress level? We don't.

Exercise also lowers serum cholesterol and triglyceride levels while increasing the production of HDL cholesterol, the type that is a protective factor for coronary heart disease. Even if you are not losing weight, exercise has great benefits, assuming, of course, that it is appropriate for your physical condition and ability.

The insulin-dependent diabetic must remember that exercise causes muscles to use blood sugar independent of insulin action. Exercise increases the need for carbohydrates both during and after physical activity. Those extra calories may be needed for up to 24 hours after strenuous or prolonged exercise. The extra carbohydrates replace muscle and liver glycogen stores to prevent hypoglycemic reactions after exercise.

The well-controlled insulin-dependent diabetic must either reduce his or her insulin dosage or consume some sugar prior to vigorous exercise. This is one of the rare instances when sweetened soft drinks, candy, honey, or fruit juice can be eaten between meals. Also, the insulin-dependent diabetic should carry additional sources of glucose in case more sugar is needed in the course of exercise. Your physician or dietitian will plan appropriate sugar sources with you and may alter the type, site, or timing of your insulin injections.

The positive effects of exercise will be maximized, and the potential for negative reactions will be minimized, if you exercise on a regular basis at approximately the same time. This consistency will allow you to make appropriate adjustments in your food intake and insulin. Frequent glucose self-monitoring and previous experience make adjustments for exercise easier.

After a meal is a good time to exercise because blood sugar levels are ample. Monitoring blood sugar levels before and after exercise will tell you how much extra carbohydrate you need. Mild exercise, like walking for 15 minutes, may not require any extra food, but an hour of bicycle riding may require 15 to 50 grams of carbohydrate, depending upon the intensity of the activity and how your body reacts to the exercise.

The non-insulin-dependent diabetic also can improve blood sugar control by exercising. It seems that exercise increases the ability of insulin to bind to its receptor sites on the cell membrane, thus helping the body use available insulin.

Many great athletes have been and are insulin-dependent diabetics. Children with diabetes should be encouraged to participate in active sports as well as other school programs. The gym teacher, classroom teacher, school nurse, lunchroom personnel and school bus drivers should be informed that a stu dent has diabetes and should be given a list of symptoms of hypoglycemia. Send some packets of sugar or glucose tablets to the teachers to keep available. Ask them to be especially watchful just before lunchtime. Before strenuous activity, such as football practice or tennis, be sure that the child takes extra sugar or less insulin.

Full participation in sports and school activities is very important to all children, whether they happen to have diabetes or not. The child with diabetes can do everything a nondiabetic child can—with planning and care and encouragement.

9
Eating Out

Everyone likes to eat out. Many of us eat out at least four times a week. The National Restaurant Association estimates that one out of every three meals in the United States is eaten away from home and predicts that this trend will continue. Fast-food restaurants are found everywhere, and 56 percent of Americans buy take-out food at least twice each week. Many workers eat out every workday because it is not possible for them to carry lunch with them. For the diabetic who has done some homework and knows the foods and portion sizes of his or her meal plan, choosing from menus is not too difficult.

Here are some basic ground rules:

- Don't be tempted by the gorgeous goodies on menus unless you have the willpower to eat very small portions and you include the estimated values in your meal.
- Make up your own pocket- or purse-sized cards of the number of exchanges allowed at each meal. These cards will help you select from menus.
- The fact that the restaurant serves large portions doesn't mean you must clean the plate. Eat only the amount your diabetic diet will allow—share with someone, leave the rest, or ask for a doggie bag to take home for another meal.
- Tell the waiter or waitress that you are a diabetic and ask him or her to tell the chef to "go easy on the fats." Ask for all sauces on the side so you can control portions.

- Always try to eat within one hour of your regular meal-time. Make a reservation earlier than your mealtime to allow time for your food to be prepared.

The local affiliate of the American Heart Association can tell you which restaurants in your area have heart-saver menus. These approved menu offerings are low in fats, cholesterol, saturated fats, and sodium. So if you choose from heart-saver items, you have a head start in choosing foods that are good for you. These menus do not reduce sugar, however, so choose the appropriate high-carbohydrate foods.

Restaurant Courses

And now, to guide you along the menu route from beginning to end:

Appetizers

Skip all cream soups, creamed herring, and cream cheese spreads. If you choose seafood, count it as part of your total meal's Meat Exchange. Crudités, the French word for raw vegetables, are free, but go easy on the dip. Clear beef or chicken soup and vegetable soups, including Manhattan clam chowder, are fine. Tomato juice, vegetable juice, or vegetable soup is allowed if you count a Vegetable Exchange. Or use a Fruit Exchange for a small fresh fruit cup or melon wedge.

Bread

Limit your choice to one small, plain roll, a slice of bread, half a large roll, melba toast, or bread sticks. Count them as an allowed bread exchange. Breads add up fast, so be sure to count them! If you use butter or margarine, count fat exchanges. Avoid fried doughnuts, sweet rolls, and rich fruit muffins. Remember to count potatoes and starchy vegetables as Starch Exchanges.

Salads and Dressing

Choose a mixed green salad garnished with a wedge of lemon or sliced tomato and count it as a Vegetable Exchange. Ask if a diet dressing is available. Order dressing on the side so that you can control the amount. If you are a regular patron of a certain restaurant, ask the staff to keep a jar of your favorite homemade dressing for you. Mark it with your name and give it to the staff to refrigerate. After all, in France restaurants save partial bottles of wine for customers!

Main Course for Lunch

Depending upon your bread allowance, consider an open-faced sandwich (one slice), a regular sandwich (two slices), or a club sandwich (three slices). The best fillings are lean meat, sliced chicken, turkey, and cheese. Avoid fried foods. Other main lunch choices might include cottage cheese and fresh fruit plate, tuna salad, hearty soup, stew or chili, julienne salad, thin-crust pizza, chicken, turkey, or fish. Gravies, sauces, cream cheese fillings, and salad fillings with lots of mayonnaise as a binder all require extra Fat Exchanges. Review the meat categories and choose a meat or meat alternative at the appropriate fat level. Hearty pea or lentil soups can be used if you count them as two Starch Exchanges plus one Lean Meat Exchange per bowl.

Main Course for Dinner

Choose lean meat, fish, or poultry—roasted, barbecued, baked, grilled, broiled, or poached. Trim off extra fats from chops, steaks, and sliced meats. Avoid thickened gravies and cream sauces. Eat only the portion you are allowed and take home the rest.

Vegetables

Ask if the restaurant has a fresh vegetable of the day. Avoid cream sauces, cheese sauces, and fried vegetables. Have you already used the allowed vegetables in your salad or appetizers?

Potatoes

Boiled, roasted, and mashed potatoes are fine. Consider rice, corn, peas, or pasta alternatives as Starch Exchanges. Skip french fries, potato chips, and butter or sour cream on potatoes, unless you have Fat Exchanges to use.

Desserts

Fresh fruit is by far the best choice. But if you have been careful about your other exchanges and your doctor permits you to have ice cream once in a while, ask for one small scoop (½ cup) of ice cream and count it as one Bread Exchange plus two Fat Exchanges—skip the fudge sauce. Restaurant cakes, pies, pastries, puddings, sherbets, and water ices are definitely not for diabetics. They have far too much sugar!

Beverages

If you have Milk Exchanges to use, milk is the best choice. If not, order tea or coffee (hot or cold, unsweetened); or drink water, mineral water, or club soda with lime. Half of all soft drinks sold are the diet variety, so you will have the company of many nondiabetics when you order a sugar-free soft drink. Choose caffeine-free types if you want to avoid caffeine. If fresh fruit is not available, use your Fruit Exchange for a small glass of unsweetened fruit juice.

Food Exchanges for Fast Foods

If you are a typical American man, woman, or child, you spent about $200 last year on fast foods. The hamburger remains the most popular overall seller, with fried chicken items gaining in popularity. The fast-food business is also booming with fast-food breakfasts, the fastest-growing segment of the industry.

Fortunately for diabetics, and everyone else trying to control weight, it is possible, but not easy, to select a prudent diet at a fast-food restaurant. The problem is usually calories, as many popular fast-food items—fries, shakes, chicken nuggets, croissants, and extra-large sandwiches—are rich in calories from sugars and/or saturated fats.

Unless you have lots of exchanges to use at a meal, which is sometimes true for teenage boys and athletes, look for lower-calorie options—single burgers, diet soft drinks, unsweetened juices, low-fat milk, a small order of fries, the salad bar with low-calorie dressing, chili, or a roast beef sandwich. Everybody knows that a bigger sandwich or "super" anything means more calories, fat, and salt. People with diabetes should choose the smaller sandwiches, chicken dinners, and such. If it says "double" or "triple," believe it!

Enjoy fast foods occasionally but choose them wisely. Good choices take self-discipline. Shakes, freezes, turnovers, pancakes with syrup, and pies are not for you. Don't be fooled into thinking that chicken and fish sandwiches are low in calories. Anything breaded and fried is highly caloric, and chicken nuggets contain ground chicken skin that adds fat and cholesterol. To limit fat, hold the sauces and avoid fried foods.

If you are trying to limit sodium, skip fried chicken and onion rings; there is lots of salt in the batter or breading. A large burger with cheese and special sauce often contains more than 1,000 milligrams of sodium—and that's before you eat anything else! Breakfast items and pizza that contain ham or sausage are also very high in sodium. To limit sodium, order sandwiches with lettuce and tomato but no sauces and ask for unsalted french fries. Have it *your* way!

The nutrition information provided by many fast-food chains can be converted into exchanges. Ask the manager if he or she has nutritional information at the restaurant or write the company headquarters for it.

If you eat at fast-food restaurants on a regular basis, you will want to own a copy of *Fast Food Facts*, a book published by the International Diabetes Center in Minneapolis. The section titled "Sources of Information" includes company addresses. This wonderful and inexpensive little book contains exchanges for virtually all fast-food chains from A to Z, Arby's to Zantigo. Here is a small sampling of some of the better fast-food choices, printed with permission of the authors.

	Calories	Fat (g)	Sodium (mg)	Exchanges
Arby's				
Roasted chicken breast	254	7	930	6 Lean Meat
Rice pilaf	123	2	438	1½ Starch
Tossed salad with low-calorie dressing	57	1	465	1 Vegetable
Reg. roast beef	353	15	590	2 Starch, 2 Medium-Fat Meat, 1 Fat
Baked potato, plain	290	1	12	4 Starch
Burger King				
Hamburger	275	12	509	2 Starch, 2 Medium-Fat Meat
Chicken tenders	204	10	636	1 Starch, 2 Medium-Fat Meat
Salad with reduced-calorie dressing	42	—	—	1 Vegetable
Dairy Queen				
Hamburger, single	360	16	630	2 Starch, 2 Medium-Fat Meat, 1 Fat
Frozen dessert	180	6	65	2 Starch, 1 Fat
Cone, small	140	4	45	1½ Starch, 1 Fat

	Calories	Fat (g)	Sodium (mg)	Exchanges
Hardee's				
Hamburger	276	15	589	1½ Starch, 1½ Medium-Fat Meat, 1 Fat
Roast beef sandwich	312	12	826	2 Starch, 2 Medium-Fat Meat
Hot ham 'n cheese	376	15	1067	2½ Starch, 2 Medium-Fat Meat, 1 Fat
Chef salad	277	16	517	2 Vegetable, 3 Medium-Fat Meat
Kentucky Fried Chicken				
Breast, original recipe	257	14	532	1½ Starch, 3 Medium-Fat Meat
Mashed potatoes with gravy	62	1	297	1 Starch
Corn-on-the-cob	176	3	21	2 Starch
Baked beans	105	1	387	1 Starch
McDonald's				
Hamburger	263	11	506	2 Starch, 1 Medium-Fat Meat, 1 Fat
Cheeseburger	318	16	743	2 Starch, 1½ Medium-Fat Meat, 1 Fat
Egg McMuffin	340	16	885	2 Starch, 2 Medium-Fat Meat, 1 Fat
English muffin with butter	186	5	5	2 Starch, 1 Fat

Long John Silver			
Baked fish dinner	387	19	1298	1 Starch, 4 Medium-Fat Meat
Ocean chef salad	222	8	983	1 Starch (or 2 Vegetable), 3 Lean Meat
Shrimp salad	183	3	658	1 Starch, 3 Lean Meat
Pizza Hut				
Thin-n-crispy cheese pizza (3 slices—10-inch)	450	15	NA*	3½ Starch (or 3 Starch, 1 Vegetable), 2 Medium-Fat Meat, 1 Fat
Wendy's				
Hamburger patty on bun	350	16	360	2 Starch, 3 Medium-Fat Meat
Plain baked potato	250	2	60	3½ Starch
Chili, regular	240	8	990	1½ Starch, 2 Medium-Fat Meat
Chicken breast fillet on bun	320	10	500	2 Starch, 3 Lean Meat
Pickup window side salad	110	6	540	1 Vegetable, 1 Fat
Zantigo				
Taco	198	12	318	1 Starch, 1 Medium-Fat Meat, 1 Fat
Beef enchilada	315	15	904	1½ Starch, 2 Medium-Fat Meat, 1 Fat
Cheese chilito	330	15	505	2 Starch, 1 Medium-Fat Meat, 2 Fat

*NA = information not available

Brown-Bag Foods

Frequently, it's easier for a diabetic child or adult to carry lunch in a brown bag than to choose food in a cafeteria or restaurant. Preparing lunches at home, you have both the food and the time to make sure that the correct food exchanges are included. But brown baggers get tired of the roast beef sandwich and canned soup routine! And who blames them?

As with any meal, look at the meal plan and choose a combination of foods to equal the allowed number of exchanges. If you are choosing a stew with two Meat Exchanges and one Starch Exchange, and you are allowed three Meat Exchanges and two Starch Exchanges, fill in the meal with a piece of bread and two ounces of cheese. Check the lunch to make sure that you have used all of the allotted exchanges.

One of the big problems, of course, is storage. When a refrigerator is not available, avoid foods that spoil quickly. If you are willing to carry a wide-mouthed thermos, the problem is more than half solved. Many recipes in this book can be packed into the wide-mouthed thermos and kept hot for lunch: all of the soups and most of the casseroles are perfect. When you have leftovers at mealtimes, save them in the refrigerator or freezer and reheat them as you pack your brown bag or pack them well chilled or frozen if a microwave oven is available for reheating.

Pack chicken, sliced meat loaf, cold meats, or cheese in foil or plastic bags. If you choose one of the meat dishes, add some cut vegetables wrapped in plastic wrap. If you select one of the hearty soups, add a protein-type sandwich or cheese and a roll. Some of our breads and sandwich fillings are delicious for brown-bag or picnic lunches.

Children can buy milk at most schools, and low-fat milk is available in cafeterias or from vending machines at many work sites. Adults often use their Milk Exchanges at other times during the day. V-8, tomato juice, fruit juice, coffee, and tea are alternate beverages that may be available at work. If you have a Milk Exchange available, carry a thermos of Hot Milk Chocolate (*see* Index) in cold weather.

10
Alcohol for Diabetics

Adult diabetics frequently ask whether they can have a drink before dinner. There is no standard answer to this question. So much depends upon the severity of the diabetes condition, the individual, and the diet counselor's knowledge as to whether the diabetic fully understands (1) what the permissive *occasionally* means, (2) that whatever alcoholic beverage is taken is counted along with the food, and (3) that other sources of calories must be omitted at the same meal.

It just makes good sense that, because your calories are restricted, every calorie should carry nutrients for good health. Also, for the diabetic whose medication is insulin and whose meal schedule must be regular, there is a real danger. The relaxing effect of a before-dinner drink just might relax you right past your regular mealtime and put you in danger of an insulin reaction. Or you may eat far too much or the wrong foods after a drink or two.

Even small amounts of alcohol can cause hypoglycemia and make a person appear very drunk so that appropriate treatment for diabetes may be delayed or denied. In addition, pure alcohol is quickly absorbed and contributes seven calories per gram. Although it is not converted into sugar or acetone, its caloric content can be responsible for gain in weight.

Non-insulin-dependent diabetics who take certain oral hypoglycemia agents may become ill when they drink alcohol. Ten to 30 percent of people on oral agents become nauseated, have flushed skin, impaired speech, and a quickened heart beat.

These symptoms make ordering Perrier with lime very appealing.

Early in 1987, the American Diabetes Association, Inc. issued a position paper on alcohol use by those with diabetes. They advised everyone, whether diabetic or not, to use alcohol in moderation and only with food. Alcohol in any form is discouraged in people with diabetes who risk alcohol abuse.

Moderation is defined as two drinks, once or twice a week. One drink (alcohol equivalent) is a 1.5 ounce shot of distilled liquor, 4 ounces of wine or 12 ounces of beer. Light beers and dry wines have less carbohydrates and are preferable to regular beer and sweet wines.

The statement points out that for diabetics, alcohol poses potential problems of blood sugar control and elevation of blood fats. Those who take insulin may have up to two alcohol equivalents in addition to the regularly planned meal. While alcohol does not require insulin for metabolism, it's important to eat a full meal to avoid alcohol induced hypoglycemia.

In addition, all diabetics must limit alcohol because it is high in calories and can easily lead to weight gain and impair the ability to make good food choices.

If you do drink alcohol on a daily basis, it can be worked into your regular meal plan. Because alcohol is metabolized to two-carbon fragments and handled by the body as fat, it may be calculated as a substitute for an appropriate number of Fat Exchanges. One Fat Exchange should be removed for every 45 calories contained in the alcoholic beverage being used. If, however, you are at ideal body weight, you may wish to use alcohol as extra calories without subtracting Fat Exchanges. The following formula can be applied to calculate the number of calories: $0.8 \times$ proof $\times$ ounces = calories. Labels on distilled liquor indicate the proof—50 percent of the stated proof is equal to the percentage of alcohol content.

Those with diabetes should reduce both the calorie and simple sugar content of mixed drinks to avoid extra calories and carbohydrate. Both of these excesses will influence blood glucose levels. If a mixer is needed, plan it as part of your meal.

For example, count orange juice as a Fruit Exchange. Whenever possible, use calorie-free mixes instead of those with sugar. If you want two drinks instead of one, add lots of club soda to dry wine to make spritzers that are lower in calories.

The following lists of very low-carbohydrate wines and mixers were originally published in *Handbook of Diabetes Nutritional Management* (1987) edited by Margaret A. Powers, R.D., M.S., and are reprinted with permission:

Wines with Less Than 2 Percent Carbohydrate Content

White

Chablis	Dry Riesling
Dry Chenin Blanc	Dry Sauterne
Chardonnay	Dry Sauvignon Blanc
French Colombard	White Burgundy

Red

Burgundy	Claret
Cabernet Sauvignon	Gamay Beaujolais

Other

Dry Rosé	Dry Sherry
Dry Champagne	

Mixers

Calorie-Free Beverages and Mixers

Water	Diet tonic
Club soda	Perrier water
Diet carbonated beverages	Mineral water (unsweetened)
Lemon juice	

Mixers

Calorie-Dense Beverages and Mixers

Regular carbonated beverages	Tonic
Fruit juice	Premade mixes

Some of the new flavored mineral waters are made with sugars, fruits, and sugar syrups. We calculated one of the peach-flavored waters to contain 120 calories and about 30 grams of carbohydrate from the added syrups and peach nectar. Other fruit-flavored waters have few or no calories. Read the label!

Keep in mind the five considerations for the use of alcoholic beverages by anyone with diabetes:

1. Use alcohol only when the diabetes is under control.
2. Because alcohol has blood-sugar-lowering ability under some circumstances, use alcohol only with meals and snacks and only in moderation.
3. Avoid sweet wines, liqueurs, beer, ale, wine coolers, and sweetened mixed drinks because of their high sugar contents.
4. Avoid alcohol if on a weight reduction diet; alcohol provides calories and stimulates the appetite.
5. Don't jeopardize your health by bowing to social pressures to drink.

11
Traveling Safely

By all means, don't stay at home just because you are a diabetic. Many insulin-dependent diabetics have traveled all over the world. Professional athletes such as Kurt Frazier and Bobby Clarke (hockey), Ron Santo (baseball), Mike Pyle (football), and Bill Talbert (tennis) have dealt with their insulin-dependent diabetes successfully while playing vigorously and traveling endlessly. One of our favorite Hollywood stars, Mary Tyler Moore, never has allowed her diabetes to prevent her from dancing, acting, and traveling. ("If they can do it, why not you and me?" said Kay!) Here are a few reminders:

- In your purse or pocket carry a letter from your physician stating your diabetes condition, your medication, and your doctor's name, address, and telephone number (including area code). For international travel, if you take insulin, the letter should explain to the border customs agent why you have syringes and needles. In this age of drugs, they are suspicious, especially of the young.
- Wear an identification bracelet or insignia on a neck chain to indicate that you have diabetes. These are worldwide signals to medical personnel. Mary's cousin was an insulin-dependent diabetic who refused to wear identification, and several times she had emergencies and was thought to be drunk! Proper care would have been provided much faster if medical alert identification was worn.
- Get several diabetes identification wallet cards from your

state or local affiliate of the American Diabetes Association, Inc. Fill them out, put one in purse or pocket, and another in a suitcase, and give another to a friend who is traveling with you. Also, ask the American Diabetes Association for any pamphlets it may have about traveling.

• Carry your insulin or other medications with you. Luggage can be separated from you or even lost. What you carry on your person is surely with you.

• Always carry a brown-bag meal in case of emergency. A runway delay, circling over an airport, and weather problems cannot be predicted. Computer foulups may put your specially ordered meal in Salt Lake City when you are on a plane to Indianapolis. Avoid stress and emergencies by planning ahead.

• If the timing of your meals is strictly regulated and you expect to travel to areas in a different time zone, talk to your doctor or diet counselor for help in making your mealtime adjustments.

• When making air travel reservations, tell your travel agent or reservations clerk that you are a diabetic and will require diabetic menus on the flight. Other passengers will be envious of your attractive diabetic meals.

• Carry with you for emergencies a roll of mints or other hard candy or glucose tablets. Don't forget that sweetened soft drinks are sold all over the world and are ideal for certain diabetic emergencies. Mary saw "Coca-Cola" signs even in remote villages in Kenya!

• Take copies of your meal plans and food exchange lists with you and be guided by suggestions in Chapter 9, "Eating Out." If traveling to a foreign country, read about the common foods and have them translated into exchanges for you in advance of your trip.

• When you stay in a foreign country, register with the American embassy or consular office; they can assist you with medical help if you need it. Also, your doctor can provide you with a list of physicians in each country who assist foreign travelers, speak English, and charge standard fees.

- You may not need the doctor, packed meal, or medical identification—we hope you won't. But planning will avoid emergencies and give you, and those who travel with you, extra piece of mind. Think of these actions as travel insurance.

12
Supermarket Skills

Most of us are concerned about food costs. A well-planned diet for a diabetic can be the basis for economical, nutritionally adequate meals for the whole family. The recipes in this book will please your family and friends. If you live alone, the recipes can be reduced by half, or you can plan on freezing individual portions and save cooking time later.

Food shopping will be easier if you do some planning beforehand:

- Plan the diabetic's menus for several days in advance; then add additional items for the family.
- Make a list from your menus, grouping foods together that you will find in the same areas of the store. This step saves needless running around the store. Write your grocery list on the back of an envelope that holds clipped coupons.
- Keep your list flexible so that you can take advantage of any unadvertised suitable foods at bargain prices. For example, a sale on juice oranges might make them a better buy than the juice itself.

When you shop:

- Shop soon after a meal. Studies show we spend one-third more on groceries when we are hungry. Temptations jump into the market basket!
- Buy fresh, whole foods as much as possible. Fresh fruits, vegetables, whole grains, fish and poultry, and low-fat dairy products usually are more nutritious than processed foods and are generally lower in fat, sugar, and salt.

• Read labels very carefully. If sugar in any form is the first ingredient on the ingredients list, you may want to avoid this food. Since label reading is the most important shopping skill, let's look at it more carefully.

Looking at Labels

For years, consumers have been demanding more and more information about the nutritive values of the foods they eat. In answer to these demands, the Food and Drug Administration developed a standardized form of nutritional labeling in 1973. At present, this program is voluntary, which means that unless the food processor adds nutrients to the product or makes dietary claims on the label, it is not required to provide nutrition information on the package. Many of the most nutritious foods are labeled, while producers of foods with little nutrient value (except for calories) are less likely to provide the consumer with full information. The 300 foods that follow FDA's "Standard of Identity" do not list ingredients at all. These foods include mayonnaise and catsup.

Nutritional labeling is an important tool for diabetics and others on special diets. Knowing carbohydrate, protein, fat, and calorie levels facilitates translating processed foods into exchanges.

If a product does not have a nutritional label, you can write to the packer and ask for nutrition information. Most companies will be happy to send you the nutritive content of their products, and some companies even have their products translated into food exchanges for you.

But how do we interpret nutritional labeling when it is provided? First, let's look at a label for V-8 vegetable juice:

The first section of the label tells the serving size, number of servings in the container, calories per serving, the grams of carbohydrate, protein, and fat per serving. This information can be evaluated to determine into which Food Exchange List the product fits. Sometimes, the identified serving size suggested by the packer does not fit into an even amount for an

V-8 Vegetable Juice

Nutrition Information Per Serving

Serving Size	6 fl.oz (182 g)
Servings per container	2
Calories	35
Protein (g)	1
Carbohydrate (g)	8
Fat (g)	0
Sodium	620 mg/serving

Percentage of U.S. Recommended Daily Allowances (U.S. RDA)

Protein	2	Riboflavin	2
Vitamin A	45	Niacin	6
Vitamin C	45	Calcium	2
Thiamine	2	Iron	4
Dietary Fiber	1 g/serving		

Vitamin A in V-8 juice comes from beta-carotene, which is provided by the vegetables.

Ingredients: Tomato juice from concentrate (water, tomato concentrate), reconstituted juices of carrots, celery, beets, parsley, lettuce, watercress, spinach, with salt, vitamin C (ascorbic acid), natural flavoring, and citric acid.

Distributed by Campbell Soup Company, Camden, N.J., U.S.A. 08103-1701

exchange. We know from the Vegetable Exchange List that a ½-cup serving (4 ounces) would be one Vegetable Exchange. So the diabetic would get three Vegetable Exchanges, 4 ounces each, from the 12-ounce can instead of the suggested two servings at 6 ounces. The 4-ounce serving would yield 5 grams of carbohydrate, 1 gram protein, 0 fat, and 23 calories. Perfect!

The packer determines the portion size for each product. Sometimes far too generous servings are suggested by the packers; other times, tiny servings are set so the packer can claim very small caloric values per serving. We found a label on a 4½-ounce box of dietetic imitation-chocolate-covered raisins that claimed very low caloric and carbohydrate values. Then we discovered the reason for these values: the packer claimed that there were 20 servings in the box! We wonder how many diabetics and weight watchers eat a whole box of that "dietetic" candy! This product, in which the only modification was to substitute imitation chocolate for real chocolate, had even more calories and fat than the product that it was supposed to replace. Its only real use would be for cases where there is an allergy or intolerance to chocolate. The product was very deceiving as well as expensive.

The next section of the label lists percentages of the U.S. Recommended Dietary Allowances (U.S. RDA). The U.S. RDAs are our goals for good nutrition. You should derive 100 percent of each nutrient from the variety of foods eaten in a whole day. The percentages on the vegetable juice cocktail label indicate that this product is a very good source of vitamin C and vitamin A and provides small amounts of other vitamins and minerals. The smaller percentages (2, 4, 6 percent) do add up to contribute to your daily need. Most of us eat about 25 different foods in a single day, and each contributes to our nutrient totals.

Sodium is also listed on the label. Because V-8 has 620 milligrams of sodium in a 6-ounce serving, you know it is high in sodium. If you are on a low-sodium diet, this juice is a poor choice. Look elsewhere on the grocery store shelf and reach

for the no-salt-added V-8. Read that label, and you will find
the same nutrients but only 45 milligrams sodium in 6 ounces
of juice.

The third section of the label is the ingredient list. Even
products without complete nutritional labeling are required
by law to provide a complete list of ingredients. Ingredients are
listed in order of weight. So because it's listed first, you know
that there is more tomato juice than any other single ingredient in the can. You also learn that there is more carrot juice
than celery juice from the order in which they appear on the
ingredient list.

Always check the ingredient list for sources of sugar. See
Chapter 3, "The Great Sugar Masquerade," for the list of sugars you should watch for. The ingredient list also will include
any nutrient additions, additives, preservatives, or coloring
added to the food. Sometimes the specific type of fat is identified. Corn oil or the more general term *vegetable oil* may be
used. If you are on a fat-modified diet, look for sources of
polyunsaturated and monounsaturated fats and avoid saturated coconut and palm oils.

The last required item on nutritional labeling is the packer or
processor's name and address, which you can use to get
further information. The label also may include several optional items such as milligrams of fiber or cholesterol.

We have seen some pretty strange things on labels—for example, peanut butter with a label claiming "no cholesterol."
Since cholesterol is found only in animal foods, no peanut
butter ever has cholesterol. However, peanut butter is high in
fat.

The labels of many breakfast cereals have a special panel
that lists total carbohydrate from starch, sugar, and indigestible carbohydrate (fiber). It also tells the number of grams of
both starch and sugar (sucrose). Look at this panel carefully.
Some cereals are really candy, with more sugar than grain.
Each 4 grams of carbohydrate from sucrose equals 1 teaspoon
of sugar from the sugar bowl. Some cereals contain 8 to 16
grams of sucrose; that's 2 to 4 teaspoons of sugar per serving.

Cereals with 6 grams of sucrose or fewer per serving are suitable for those with diabetes. If you want a sweeter taste, add fresh fruit or a sugar substitute.

Don't be misled by labels that say "dietetic"; this designation does not guarantee that the food is suitable for you. A "dietetic" food may be reduced in sugar, salt, fat, or calories, but still may not be appropriate, and it certainly doesn't mean that there is a "free" food in the box. Fortunately, all "dietetic" foods carry nutritional labeling. Unfortunately, while all the information is there, some people don't read the labels carefully. Remember those raisins? Many "dietetic" ice creams, cookies, candies, and cakes are actually higher in calories than the products they are designed to replace. Often they are made with sorbitol (*see* Word Power); products containing sorbitol can cause diarrhea.

On the labels of some "dietetic" foods, nutritive values are marked according to a system based on percentage by volume. This system is confusing to many diabetics who think that, for example, the 20 percent of carbohydrate labeled equals 20 grams of carbohydrate. If there are products labeled in percentage by volume that you want to use, ask your diet counselor to translate the values into grams of carbohydrate, protein, and fat and into exchanges.

Labels are a manufacturer's way of telling us what the product contains. Formulations change from time to time, and printed material becomes inaccurate. Learning to read labels will keep you "in the know."

13
Kitchen Tips for Controlled Diets

So many times a newly diagnosed diabetic asks, "Do I have to buy special scales and weigh all of my food?" Well, some diabetics must do this because their physicians have put them on a weighed diabetic diet.

Most diabetics, however, are on the Food Exchange System, which uses both weights (for meats) and measures (for the other food groups). So you will need a scale that measures food in grams, a set of standard measuring spoons, a set of metal measuring cups for dry measures, and a glass measuring cup to measure liquids. Without these few pieces of equipment, accuracy and good dietary control are impossible.

In developing the recipes for this book, we have weighed and measured every single ingredient. Then we converted weights into household measures so that cooking will be faster and easier for you. But cooking for the diabetic can never be a handful of this and that, cook until it looks right, or eat until you are full! Ingredients must be carefully measured, then portions measured or weighed again before serving.

Any diabetic who has done this will agree with the reasons behind this advice. There is no other possible way for anyone to become eye-wise in judging how much is "X" amount of any given food. If you consistently and conscientiously measure and weigh your foods for a few weeks, you no longer go by "guesstimates" but achieve a skill in judging amounts. Once a month, weigh and measure again for a few days to check that your mental image of a three-ounce portion hasn't grown to four ounces or even five ounces. Being able to estimate correct portions is invaluable when eating out! It helps you to select a greater variety and gives you confidence in managing your diabetic diet.

If the diabetic in the family is not the cook, these words are still directed primarily to the diabetic. The diabetic needs to know and be responsible for what he or she eats.

If you are on a fat-controlled diet or a low-sodium diet, you can make your life a lot easier by having fat- and sodium-reduced items in your refrigerator or pantry. If you are on a low-cholesterol diet, have egg substitutes handy. Try fat and sodium-reduced cheeses to find ones that you like. Salt-free herb blends, fresh herbs, fresh lemon, and fresh garlic all give a welcome flavor boost when fat and salt must be limited.

Part III
Recipes

14
About Our Recipes

Every recipe in this book has been kitchen-tested and evaluated by critical tasters. Family members and friends have been willing, interested, and eager taste-testers. Many of the recipes were originally developed by Kay Middleton during her years of volunteer work with the Northern Affiliate of the American Diabetes Association, Inc. Other recipes were adapted from favorite recipes Mary serves to her family. More than 75 new recipes were created for this revised edition, to encourage you to eat more complex carbohydrates, fiber, legumes, seafoods, and poultry. A few recipes were donated by diabetics and diet counselors we know and love. We tested them again, making sure that each met our standards for taste, texture, and appearance. Finally, all the recipes were calculated using the newest food composition tables and nutrient data provided on labels and by food manufacturers. At this point, the computers took over for calculations. Finally, each recipe was converted to exchanges. In addition to the calorie counts and the calorie-containing nutrients (carbohydrate, protein, and fats), we included fiber, sodium, and cholesterol values to help you make wise food choices.

Because many diabetics are also on low-sodium diets, we have calculated the sodium value for each recipe. If you have been advised to limit your salt or sodium intake, follow the directions at the end of each recipe. In many cases, salt is omitted and unsalted margarine is substituted. If you are on a low-sodium diet you are probably omitting salt and using un-salted margarine already. We did not take out baking powder and baking soda from the recipes. Even though they contain some sodium, the amount is small when divided by the number of portions that the recipe provides. If you are on a fat-modified or a sodium-restricted diet, a dietitian should re-view this book for you. You will need additional information on your special diet, and the recipes will be in addition to those instructions. If you are on a fat-modified diet, your diet coun-selor can easily mark this book to omit the high-fat meats and saturated-fat foods that you should avoid.

For each recipe, a serving size is indicated. That portion is adequate for most diabetics, but nondiabetics, especially hearty eaters, will want more. Consider the appetites of your family members and guests when deciding how much of each recipe to prepare. The diabetic's portion should be measured. You can freeze leftovers in single portions for quick and easy future meals.

Because of the concern about dietary fats and the current emphasis on planning meals with more polyunsaturated fats and less saturated fat, we have used vegetable margarine or vegetable oil instead of butter in almost all of the recipes.

Margarines that you use should be made from polyunsatu-rated or monounsaturated fats (corn, safflower, or Canola oils). Soft margarines are less saturated than hard sticks and a better choice. Some of our recipes, especially the new bean soups, include 1 strip of bacon for flavor and to add a little fat to sauté onions. Because the strip of bacon and its fat are divided among six servings, the amount of fat, cholesterol, and sodium is still acceptable unless your diet is particularly re-strictive. We also offer you lots of delicious desserts, fruit yogurts, and sweet spreads that diabetics have been asking for.

Seeing sugar listed as an ingredient in some of our recipes may surprise you. If you read the chapter, "The Great Sugar Masquerade" you will know why it is there. The amount of sugar per portion is within the limits appropriate to most dia-betic diets and, quite frankly, those recipes could not be made successfully without sugar. We used the least amount possible o make a tasty and attractive food. And the sugar is calculated nto the carbohydrate, calorie, and exchange values. Most diet counselors now allow their patients to have small amounts of ugar if they use the appropriate exchange values for those oods. Again, if you remain concerned—ask your dietitian or doctor.

You will see that some of our recipes use wine as an ingredient. In each case, the carbohydrate values have been calculated into the total for the recipe. When the recipe is cooked, and the calories from the alcohol in the wine have been cooked away, only the calories from the carbohydrates and the carbohydrates themselves are included in the total nutritive values. n those few "no-cook" recipes using wine, the total calorie values of the wines, both from carbohydrate and alcohol, are included. Using wine to add flavor to cooked foods is a good rick, especially when cutting back on salt and fat.

15
Appetizers and Dips

Eggs à la Russe

Simple but so elegant! Mary's guests enjoy this one.

    4 large eggs, hard-cooked
    ¼ teaspoon coarsely ground pepper
    6 tablespoons Thousand Island Dressing (*see* Index)
    4 leaves Boston or Bibb lettuce
    1 rounded teaspoon caviar *or* 1 teaspoon chopped
      ripe olives
    4 sprigs parsley

Remove shells from hard-cooked eggs; cut eggs in half length-wise. Add pepper to Thousand Island Dressing. On serving plates arrange two egg halves (cut side down) on small lettuce leaf. Top with 1½ tablespoons Thousand Island Dressing. Garnish top of each with ¼ teaspoon of caviar and a sprig of parsley.

4 servings   *1 serving: 2 egg halves plus*
                                      1½ tablespoons dressing

Nutritive values per serving:

CHO (g)	PRO (g)	FAT (g)	CAL —	Fiber (g)	Sodium (mg)	Cho (mg)
3	7	6	99	0.3	280	300

Food Exchange per serving: 1 High-Fat Meat Exchange.

Low-sodium diets: Omit salt in Thousand Island Dressing recipe.

Eggplant Provençale

This very special dish of Mary's can be served as a first course or as a salad.

1 cup Real Italian Sauce (*see* Index) or prepared
    spaghetti sauce
¼ teaspoon coarsely ground pepper
1 pound (2 small) eggplants
2 tablespoons Low-Calorie Italian-Style Dressing
    (*see* Index)
4 lettuce leaves
1 tablespoon snipped fresh parsley
1 teaspoon drained capers (optional)

Preheat oven to 350°F. Mix Real Italian Sauce with pepper and chill. Slice hard top off eggplant but leave skin on and slice them in half lengthwise. Pierce eggplant top and through skin several times with a fork. Brush eggplant all over with the Low-Calorie Italian-Style Dressing; place in a baking pan. Bake 25 to 30 minutes, turning and basting after 15 minutes. Chill eggplant. When ready to serve, line plates with lettuce, add a piece of eggplant, top with ¼ cup chilled Real Italian Sauce, and sprinkle with snipped parsley and a few capers.

4 servings   1 serving: 1 piece of eggplant plus ¼ cup sauce

			Nutritive values per serving:			
CHO (g)	PRO (g)	FAT (g)	CAL —	Fiber (g)	Sodium (mg)	Chol (mg)
15	2	1	68	4	314	0

Food Exchanges per serving: 2 Vegetable Exchanges or 1 Bread Exchange.

Low-Sodium diets: Modify Real Italian Sauce recipe and Low-Calorie Italian-Style Dressing recipe as directed. Omit capers.

NEW Prosciutto with Papaya

1 large ripe papaya
4 leaf lettuce leaves
2 ounce paper-thin slices of prosciutto or smoked
    ham
8 ripe olives (optional)

Pare the ripe papaya and remove seeds. Slice lengthwise into
eight slices. Line 4 plates with lettuce leaves and arrange two
strips of papaya on each plate. Gently wrap center of each
piece of papaya with prosciutto. Garnish with olives.

4 servings   *1 serving: 2 papaya strips*

			Nutritive values per serving:			
CHO (g)	PRO (g)	FAT (g)	CAL —	Fiber (g)	Sodium (mg)	Chol (mg)
12	4	2	79	1.5	214	8

Food Exchanges per serving: 1 Fruit Exchange plus ½ Lean
                Meat Exchange.

Low-sodium diets: This recipe is not suitable. Papaya may be
                served with thin slices of chicken or turkey
                breast.

Soused Scallops

12 ounces fresh or frozen sea scallops
½ cup cider vinegar
¼ cup water
1½ teaspoons mixed pickling spices
1 tablespoon finely chopped onion
½ teaspoon salt
Lettuce leaves to line plates

Preheat oven to 350°F. Separate defrosted scallops and spread in small baking dish. Cut large scallops in half. Combine all remaining ingredients except lettuce and pour over scallops. Cover and bake 15-20 minutes. Chill in liquid. Drain and serve on lettuce leaves.

8 servings   *1 serving: 3–4 pieces*

Nutritive values per serving:

CHO (g)	PRO (g)	FAT (g)	CAL —	Fiber (g)	Sodium (mg)	Chol (mg)
2	10	1	52	0.2	236	23

Food Exchange per serving: 1 Lean Meat Exchange.

Low-sodium diets: Omit salt.

Eggplant Caviar

2 medium (¾ pound each) eggplants
½ cup finely chopped onion
3 cloves garlic, minced
1 tablespoon fresh lemon juice
2 tablespoons olive oil
½ cup chopped fresh parsley
1 teaspoon salt
¾ teaspoon coarsely ground pepper

Preheat oven to 350°F. Bake whole eggplants for 1 hour or until tender, turning them occasionally. Peel off dark skin; mince the pulp. Stir in all other ingredients; mix well. Chill in covered bowl for several hours before using. Serve on crisp lettuce as a first course or mounded on melba toast as an hors d'oeuvre. Be sure to add the value of the melba toast (8 rounds = 1 Starch Exchange).

9 servings (yield: 2¼ cups)   *1 serving: ¼ cup*

Nutritive values per serving:

CHO (g)	PRO (g)	FAT (g)	CAL —	Fiber (g)	Sodium (mg)	Chol (mg)
7	1	3	54	2.4	222	0

Food Exchanges per serving: 1 Vegetable Exchange plus ½ Fat Exchange. Up to 1½ tablespoons may be considered "free."

Low-sodium diets: Omit salt. Serve on lettuce or unsalted melba toast.

Cocktail Meatballs

1 pound very lean ground beef
1 large egg, beaten
¼ cup condensed beef broth
¼ teaspoon ground nutmeg
¼ teaspoon ground allspice
¼ teaspoon grated lemon rind
4 teaspoons fresh lemon juice
1 teaspoon salt
1 slice fresh bread, finely crumbled
2 tablespoons finely chopped onion

Preheat oven to 400°F. Prepare a shallow baking pan with vegetable pan-coating; set it aside. Combine all ingredients; mix well. Form into tiny balls, each measuring 1 level teaspoonful. Place balls 1 inch apart in pan. Bake 10 minutes.

20 servings (yield: 80 meatballs)   *1 serving: 4 tiny balls*

Nutritive values per serving:

CHO (g)	PRO (g)	FAT (g)	CAL —	Fiber (g)	Sodium (mg)	Chol (mg)
1	6	4	66	0	153	33

Food Exchange per serving: 1 Lean Meat Exchange.
Low-sodium diets: Omit salt.

Stuffed Cherry Tomatoes

1 pound (about 32) cherry tomatoes, 1 inch in
  diameter
¾ cup Cheddar Cheese Dip or Curry Dressing
  (*see* Index)
2 tablespoons minced fresh parsley

Slice tops off cherry tomatoes; gently scoop seed centers from
tomatoes. Fill each with about 1 teaspoon of dip or dressing.
Sprinkle tops with parsley.

8 servings (yield: 32 tomatoes)   1 serving: 4 stuffed tomatoes

Nutritive values per serving with Cheddar Cheese Dip:						
CHO (g)	PRO (g)	FAT (g)	CAL —	Fiber (g)	Sodium (mg)	Chol (mg)
4	2	2	40	1.0	117	6

Food Exchange per serving: 1 Vegetable Exchange.

Low-sodium diets: Omit salt from Cheddar Cheese Dip.

Nutritive values per serving with Curry Dressing:						
CHO (g)	PRO (g)	FAT (g)	CAL —	Fiber (g)	Sodium (mg)	Chol (mg)
4	2	0	26	1.0	67	1

Food Exchange per serving: 1 Vegetable Exchange.

Low-sodium diets: Omit salt from Curry Dressing.

NEW Vegetable Dip for Crudités

Serve this dish with an assortment of fresh vegetables: celery sticks, carrot sticks, green onions, cauliflower pieces, kohlrabi coins, mushrooms, broccoli florets, red pepper strips, summer squash strips.

1 cup low-fat (2% milk fat) cottage cheese
1 cup shredded carrot
½ cup seeded, chopped green pepper
¼ cup minced onion
¼ cup plain low-fat yogurt
2 tablespoons catsup
1 teaspoon fresh lemon juice
½ teaspoon salt
½ teaspoon freshly ground pepper
½ teaspoon celery seed

Combine all ingredients in a food processor fitted with steel blade or in a blender; process until smooth. Place in bowl, cover, and refrigerate at least 2 hours before serving.

10 servings (yield: 2½ cups)   *1 serving: ¼ cup*

Nutritive values per serving:						
CHO (g)	PRO (g)	FAT (g)	CAL —	Fiber (g)	Sodium (mg)	Chol (mg)
4	4	0	36	0.4	253	2

Food Exchange per serving: ½ Skim Milk Exchange.

Low-sodium diets: Omit salt.

Whipped Cottage Cheese

This is a base for many of our dips, but it is also delicious atop a baked potato.

  1 cup creamed (4% milk fat) cottage cheese
  ¼ cup water
  ⅛ teaspoon salt
  1 tablespoon white vinegar

Place all ingredients in a blender, cover tightly, and whip at low speed for 30 seconds or until smooth. Chill at least 2 hours before serving. If using this as a dip base, add other ingredients before chilling.

9 servings   *1 serving: 2 tablespoons*
(yield: 1 cup plus 2 tablespoons)

Nutritive values per serving:

CHO (g)	PRO (g)	FAT (g)	CAL —	Fiber (g)	Sodium (mg)	Chol (mg)
1	3	3	24	0	121	3

Food Exchange per serving: ½ Lean Meat Exchange.

Low-sodium diets: Omit salt.

NEW Refried Bean Dip

This tasty high-fiber dip can be served with whole-grain crackers or tortillas.

  1 16-ounce can red kidney beans, including liquid
  ¼ cup finely chopped green onion with tops
  ½ cup low-fat (2% milk fat) cottage cheese
  1 4-ounce can chopped mild green chilies, drained
  ½ teaspoon ground cumin

Puree beans and bean liquid in a blender or food processor fitted with steel blade. Sauté pureed beans and onions in a nonstick pan over medium heat until hot, stirring often. Stir in cottage cheese, chilies, and cumin. Cover and refrigerate until cold.

10 servings (yield: 2½ cups)   *1 serving: ¼ cup*

Nutritive values per serving:

CHO (g)	PRO (g)	FAT (g)	CAL —	Fiber (g)	Sodium (mg)	Chol (mg)
9	4	0	54	4.9	84	1

Food Exchanges per serving: 1 Vegetable Exchange plus ½ Bread Exchange.

Low-sodium diets: This recipe is suitable.

Cheddar Cheese Dip

2 ounces sharp cheddar cheese, grated
   (about ½ cup)
1 cup (8 ounces) plain low-fat yogurt
1 tablespoon minced fresh parsley
½ teaspoon salt·

Combine all ingredients; chill in a covered container at least 2 hours before serving.

10 servings (yield: 1¼ cups)   *1 serving: 2 tablespoons*

Nutritive values per serving:

CHO (g)	PRO (g)	FAT (g)	CAL —	Fiber (g)	Sodium (mg)	Chol (mg)
2	3	2	37	0	149	7

Food Exchange per serving: ½ Medium-Fat Meat Exchange. One tablespoon may be considered "free."

Low-sodium diets: Omit salt.

Cheese and Onion Dip

1 cup plus 2 tablespoons Whipped Cottage Cheese
   (*see* Index)
4 tablespoons finely chopped green onion
5 tablespoons grated Parmesan cheese
Dash of cayenne pepper

Combine all ingredients, mix well, and chill at least 2 hours
before serving.

12 servings (yield: 1¼ cups)   1 serving: 2 tablespoons

CHO (g)	PRO (g)	FAT (g)	CAL —	Fiber (g)	Sodium (mg)	Chol (mg)
1	3	1	29	0	129	4

Nutritive values per serving:

Food Exchange per serving: ½ Lean Meat Exchange.

Low-sodium diets: This recipe is suitable.

Harlequin Dip

Zesty dip for chunks of cooked meat, fish, or raw vegetables.

1 cup (8 ounces) plain low-fat yogurt
¼ cup prepared chili sauce
1 tablespoon prepared horseradish, drained
1 teaspoon grated lemon rind
2 tablespoons finely chopped celery
1 tablespoon finely chopped green pepper
1 tablespoon finely chopped green onion
½ teaspoon salt

Combine all ingredients well. Chill in a covered container at
least 2 hours before serving.

10 servings (yield: 1¼ cups)   1 serving: 2 tablespoons

			Nutritive values per serving:			
CHO (g)	PRO (g)	FAT (g)	CAL —	Fiber (g)	Sodium (mg)	Chol (mg)
3	1	0	22	0	212	1

Food Exchange per serving: Up to 2 tablespoons may be considered "free."

Low-sodium diets: Omit salt. Substitute dietetic, low-sodium catsup for chili sauce.

West Indies Dip

Delightful as a dressing for a fresh fruit plate or with sliced apples, oranges, or bananas.

1 cup plus 2 tablespoons Whipped Cottage Cheese
 (*see* Index)
1 tablespoon chopped onion
3 tablespoons prepared chutney
1 teaspoon curry powder
⅛ teaspoon ground nutmeg

Combine all ingredients in a blender and cover tightly. Blend at low speed about 30 seconds or until smooth. Chill at least 2 hours before serving.

10 servings (yield: 1¼ cups)   *1 serving: 2 tablespoons*

			Nutritive values per serving:			
CHO (g)	PRO (g)	FAT (g)	CAL —	Fiber (g)	Sodium (mg)	Chol (mg)
2	4	1	38	0	212	3

Food Exchange per serving: ½ Lean Meat Exchange.

Low-sodium diets: Prepare using apple chutney instead of English chutney, such as Major Grey's.

A Dip with Zip

1 cup (8 ounces) plain low-fat yogurt
1 tablespoon prepared horseradish
1 tablespoon prepared mustard
¼ teaspoon salt
Few drops hot pepper sauce
Finely minced fresh parsley (optional)

Combine all ingredients except parsley; blend well. Chill in a covered bowl for a few hours. To serve, garnish with a sprinkle of finely minced parsley.

8 servings (yield: 1 cup)   *1 serving: 2 tablespoons*

Nutritive values per serving:

CHO (g)	PRO (g)	FAT (g)	CAL —	Fiber (g)	Sodium (mg)	Chol (mg)
2	2	1	20	0	127	2

Food Exchange per serving: Up to 2 tablespoons may be considered "free."

Low-sodium diets: Omit salt.

Tangy Dill Dip

1 cup (8 ounces) plain low-fat yogurt
¼ teaspoon dried dill weed *or* 1 teaspoon chopped
    fresh dill
¼ teaspoon salt
¼ teaspoon freshly ground pepper

Combine all ingredients and chill in covered container at least
2 hours before serving.

6–8 servings (yield: 1 cup)   *1 serving: 3 tablespoons*

Nutritive values per serving of dip only:						
CHO (g)	PRO (g)	FAT (g)	CAL —	Fiber (g)	Sodium (mg)	Chol (mg)
2	2	0	18	0	81	2

Food Exchange per serving: Up to 3 tablespoons may be
                           considered "free."

Low-sodium diets: Omit salt.

Horseradish Dip

Serve as a dip for raw vegetables or cooked ham cubes on toothpicks.

1 cup plus 2 tablespoons Whipped Cottage Cheese
(*see* Index)
2 tablespoons prepared horseradish
2 tablespoons finely chopped green pepper
¼ teaspoon dried basil
¼ teaspoon crushed dried marjoram
¼ teaspoon salt
Dash cayenne pepper

Combine all ingredients, mix well, and chill at least 2 hours before serving.

10 servings (yield: 1¼ cups)   *1 serving: 2 tablespoons*

Nutritive values per serving:						
CHO (g)	PRO (g)	FAT (g)	CAL —	Fiber (g)	Sodium (mg)	Chol (mg)
1	3	1	24	0	190	3

Food Exchange per serving: ½ Lean Meat Exchange.

Low-sodium diets: Omit salt. Do not use ham cubes.

16
Soups

Hearty Vegetable Soup

3½ cups boiling water
2 chicken bouillon cubes
2 beef bouillon cubes
1 16-ounce can tomatoes
½ cup chopped onion
½ cup thinly sliced carrot
½ cup diagonally sliced celery
½ cup coarsely chopped green pepper
½ teaspoon salt
1 tablespoon lemon juice
5 whole peppercorns
½ teaspoon crushed dried sage
½ teaspoon hot pepper sauce

Combine all ingredients in a 3- to 4-quart pot. Bring to a boil, stirring to dissolve bouillon cubes. Cover and simmer gently for 1 hour. Stir occasionally to break up tomatoes into bite-sized pieces.

4 servings (yield: 4 cups)   *1 serving: 1 cup*

Nutritive values per serving:						
CHO (g)	PRO (g)	FAT (g)	CAL —	Fiber (g)	Sodium (mg)	Chol (mg)
12	2	1	54	2.2	1313	0

Food Exchanges per serving: 2 Vegetable Exchanges.

Low-sodium diets: Omit salt. Substitute low-sodium bouillon cubes and unsalted canned tomatoes. Add 1 teaspoon dried basil.

NEW Split Pea Soup

This is one of the most fiber-vitamin-and-mineral-rich recipes in the book. Delicious, too!

1 pound dry split peas, washed
1½ quarts water
½ cup chopped onion
2 cups sliced celery
1 cup sliced carrot
½ teaspoon ground white pepper
½ teaspoon salt
1 teaspoon minced garlic
1 16-ounce can stewed tomatoes, including juice
1 10¾-ounce can chicken broth
1 tomato, diced fine

Combine the washed peas, water, onion, celery, and carrot in a large pot. Bring mixture to a boil and reduce heat to simmer; cover and continue cooking for 2 hours, stirring occasionally. Add more water if necessary. Season soup with pepper, salt, and garlic; continue cooking for 15 minutes or until peas are tender. Add canned tomatoes with liquid and chicken broth; allow to cool. Puree the soup in a blender or in a food processor fitted with steel blade. Return pureed soup to pot; reheat over moderate heat, stirring. Garnish with diced tomato at serving time.

10 servings (yield: 10 cups)   *1 serving: 1 cup*

			Nutritive values per serving:			
CHO (g)	PRO (g)	FAT (g)	CAL —	Fiber (g)	Sodium (mg)	Chol (mg)
33	12	1	178	7.7	362	0

Food Exchanges per serving: 2 Starch Exchanges plus ½ Lean Meat Exchange.

Low-sodium diets: Omit salt. Substitute unsalted canned tomatoes and broth.

NEW Tuscany White Bean Soup

¼ cup chopped onion
½ teaspoon minced garlic
3 tablespoons olive oil, divided
½ pound dry great northern beans, washed
2 quarts water
2 large bay leaves
1 teaspoon crumbled dried basil
½ teaspoon salt
½ teaspoon ground white pepper
2 tablespoons chopped fresh parsley
2 green onions, chopped

Sauté onion and garlic in 2 tablespoons olive oil until soft, stirring often. Add beans, water, bay leaves, and basil. Bring mixture to a boil, reduce to a simmer, and cover. Continue cooking until beans are tender, about 2 hours, adding more liquid if necessary and stirring occasionally. Season with salt and pepper. Cool soup; puree beans in a blender or food processor fitted with steel blade. Return pureed soup to pot; reheat over moderate heat, stirring often. Blend in remaining olive oil. Serve soup hot, garnished with chopped parsley and green onions. If soup is too thick, add water or chicken broth.

4 servings (yield: 4 cups)   *1 serving: 1 cup*

CHO (g)	PRO (g)	FAT (g)	CAL —	Fiber (g)	Sodium (mg)	Chol (mg)
37	13	11	293	9.7	256	0

Nutritive values per serving:

Food Exchanges per serving: 2½ Starch Exchanges plus
1 Lean Meat Exchange plus
1 Fat Exchange.

Low-sodium diets: Omit salt.

NEW Rio Grande Kidney Bean Soup

1 strip bacon
1 teaspoon minced garlic
½ cup chopped onion
2½ cups canned kidney beans with liquid
3 cups beef broth
3 bay leaves
½ teaspoon salt
⅛ teaspoon freshly ground pepper
¼ teaspoon crumbled dried basil

Fry bacon over medium heat in heavy frying pan; crumble bacon and set aside. Reheat bacon drippings over medium heat; sauté garlic and onion until tender, stirring occasionally. Puree beans in blender or food processor fitted with steel blade and stir into onion mixture. Blend in crumbled bacon and remaining ingredients, stirring occasionally until soup is hot. Remove and discard bay leaves. Soup will thicken as it stands and can be thinned with water or additional beef broth.

6 servings (yield: 6 cups)   *1 serving: 1 cup*

Nutritive values per serving:						
CHO (g)	PRO (g)	FAT (g)	CAL —	Fiber (g)	Sodium (mg)	Chol (mg)
19	8	3	136	5.4	927	22

Food Exchanges per serving: 1 Vegetable Exchange plus 1 Starch Exchange plus ½ Fat Exchange.

Low-sodium diets: This recipe is not suitable.

NEW **Tex-Mex Corn Soup**

Do try this one; our taste testers loved it and it is very quick and easy to prepare.

 1 tablespoon margarine
 ½ cup chopped onion
 1 cup chopped sweet red pepper
 1 teaspoon red pepper flakes
 4 cups chicken broth
 1 17-ounce can creamed corn, including liquid
 1 16-ounce can whole kernel corn, including liquid
 ¼ teaspoon salt
 ¼ teaspoon freshly ground white pepper

Melt margarine in a large saucepan; sauté onion and sweet pepper with red pepper flakes until tender, stirring occasionally, about 2 minutes. Stir in chicken broth and both cans of corn. Continue cooking until the soup is very hot. Add salt and pepper and serve immediately.

8 servings (yield: 8 cups)   *1 serving: 1 cup*

Nutritive values per serving:

CHO (g)	PRO (g)	FAT (g)	CAL —	Fiber (g)	Sodium (mg)	Chol (mg)
31	6	8	205	3.1	928	14

Food Exchanges per serving: 2 Starch Exchanges plus 1 Fat Exchange.

Low-sodium diets: Omit salt and substitute unsalted broth and canned vegetables.

$\boxed{NEW}$ Chinese Chicken Corn Soup

3 cups canned chicken broth
1 8¾-ounce can creamed corn
1 cup diced cooked skinned chicken
1 tablespoon cornstarch
2 tablespoons cold water
2 egg whites
2 tablespoons finely minced fresh parsley

Combine chicken broth, corn, and chicken pieces in a large saucepan. Bring mixture to a boil over medium heat, stirring occasionally. Blend cornstarch with cold water and add to soup. Continue cooking, uncovered, for 3 minutes. Beat egg whites until foamy; stir into soup. Reduce heat to a simmer and cook until foamy. Ladle soup into individual bowls and garnish with parsley. Serve hot.

4 servings (yield: 4 cups)   *1 serving: 1 cup*

Nutritive values per serving:						
CHO (g)	PRO (g)	FAT (g)	CAL —	Fiber (g)	Sodium (mg)	Chol (mg)
14	16	4	156	0.3	814	31

Food Exchanges per serving: 2 Lean Meat Exchanges plus 1 Starch Exchange.

Low-sodium diets: Substitute unsalted broth.

$\boxed{NEW}$ Black Bean Soup

1 strip bacon
½ cup chopped onion
1 cup chopped celery
2½ cups cooked black beans, drained
2½ cups water
½ teaspoon ground cumin
½ teaspoon salt
½ teaspoon freshly ground pepper

Fry bacon over medium heat in small heavy frying pan; crumble bacon and set aside. Heat bacon drippings over medium heat; sauté onion and celery until tender, stirring occasionally. Puree beans in blender or food processor fitted with steel blade and stir into vegetables. Mix in crumbled bacon and remaining ingredients, stirring occasionally until soup is hot. Soup will thicken as it stands and can be thinned with additional water. Serve hot.

6 servings (yield: 6 cups)   *1 serving: 1 cup*

Nutritive values per serving:

CHO (g)	PRO (g)	FAT (g)	CAL —	Fiber (g)	Sodium (mg)	Chol (mg)
18	6	3	124	6.9	205	21

Food Exchanges per serving: 1 Starch Exchange plus ½ Fat Exchange.

Low-sodium diets: Omit salt.

Fish Chowder

Because bacon burns easily, be sure to cook it over low or moderate heat.

1 pound fresh or frozen fish fillets
4 thin slices bacon
¾ cup chopped onion
1 16-ounce can tomatoes
2 cups boiling water
1 cup diced raw potato
½ cup diced carrot
½ cup finely chopped celery with leaves
⅓ cup catsup
2 teaspoons Worcestershire sauce
1 teaspoon salt
¼ teaspoon coarsely ground pepper
⅛ teaspoon dried thyme
⅛ teaspoon dried marjoram
1 tablespoon minced fresh parsley

Thaw fish fillets if frozen. Remove bones and skin from fish; cut fish into 1-inch pieces. Cut bacon into ½-inch pieces. In a large saucepan over moderate heat, fry bacon until crisp, turning frequently. Add onion, and cook and stir over moderate heat until tender and translucent. Cut tomatoes into bite-sized pieces. Add tomatoes, tomato liquid from can, and all remaining ingredients except the fish and the parsley to the onions. Bring to a boil; reduce heat to low, cover, and simmer for about 45 minutes. Add fish; cover and simmer for another 10–12 minutes, until fish flakes and is tender. Garnish each serving with a sprinkle of parsley.

6 servings (yield: 6 cups)   *1 serving: 1 cup*

Nutritive values per serving:

CHO (g)	PRO (g)	FAT (g)	CAL —	Fiber (g)	Sodium (mg)	Chol (mg)
14	22	8	213	1.9	786	49

Food Exchanges per serving: 2 Lean Meat Exchanges plus 1 Starch Exchange.

Low-sodium diets: Omit salt. Omit bacon. Use unsalted canned tomatoes and low-sodium catsup.

Quick French Onion Soup

6 beef bouillon cubes
5 cups boiling water
3 tablespoons Worcestershire sauce
2 cups sliced onion rings
6 small rounds melba toast
3 tablespoons grated Parmesan cheese

Dissolve bouillon cubes in boiling water. Add Worcestershire sauce and onion rings. Cover and simmer gently for 25–30 minutes. Serve in warmed bowls with 1 melba toast round plus 1½ teaspoons Parmesan cheese sprinkled on top of each.

6 servings (yield: 6 cups)   *1 serving: 1 cup*

Nutritive values per serving:

CHO (g)	PRO (g)	FAT (g)	CAL —	Fiber (g)	Sodium (mg)	Chol (mg)
7	3	1	47	0.7	1004	2

Food Exchange per serving: 1 Vegetable Exchange.

Low-sodium diets: Substitute unsalted beef bouillon cubes and unsalted melba toast.

Greek Egg-Lemon Soup

4 chicken bouillon cubes
4 cups boiling water
2 tablespoons raw rice
2 medium eggs, beaten
2 tablespoons fresh lemon juice
¼ teaspoon mixed herb seasoning
Dash coarsely ground pepper
Parsley sprigs

Dissolve bouillon cubes in boiling water; add rice slowly so as
not to stop the boiling. Cover, reduce heat to low, and let
simmer gently for 15 minutes or until rice is tender but firm.
Combine eggs and lemon juice. Slowly pour half of hot mixture into egg mixture, stirring quickly. Return to remaining
soup and cook over very low heat 3–4 minutes, stirring constantly, until mixture is smooth and coats the spoon. (Avoid
boiling or high heat to prevent curdling.) Stir in herb seasoning and pepper. Spoon into bowls, garnish with parsley, and
serve immediately.

4 servings (yield: 2⅔ cups)   *1 serving: ⅔ cup*

Nutritive values per serving:

CHO (g)	PRO (g)	FAT (g)	CAL —	Fiber (g)	Sodium (mg)	Chol (mg)
6	4	3	69	0.1	899	137

Food Exchanges per serving: ½ Starch Exchange plus
½ Medium-Fat Exchange.

Low-sodium diets: Substitute 4 cups unsalted chicken broth for
bouillon cubes and water.

Zucchini Soup

1 pound small zucchini, cleaned and sliced thin
1 tablespoon margarine
2 tablespoons finely chopped onion
1 clove garlic, crushed
2 tablespoons water
½ teaspoon curry powder
½ teaspoon salt
½ cup skim milk
1¾ cups chicken broth

Set aside a few slices of zucchini for garnish. Heat margarine in a heavy, deep skillet. Add onion, garlic, remaining zucchini, and water. Cover and simmer gently for 10 minutes; stir with a wooden spoon while cooking. Remove from heat; add all remaining ingredients and mix well. Turn into blender or food processor fitted with steel blade and blend for 30 seconds. Serve hot or well chilled. Garnish each bowl with thin slices of zucchini.

4 servings (yield: 4 cups)   *1 serving: 1 cup*

Nutritive values per serving:

CHO (g)	PRO (g)	FAT (g)	CAL —	Fiber (g)	Sodium (mg)	Chol (mg)
6	3	4	64	1.8	408	1

Food Exchanges per serving: 1 Vegetable Exchange plus 1 Fat Exchange.

Low-sodium diets: Omit salt. Substitute unsalted chicken broth.

| NEW | **Sunday Italian Vegetable Soup**

½ cup dry navy beans
Water
4 cups chicken broth
¾ cup sliced peeled carrot
½ cup sliced potato, with peel
1 tablespoon corn oil
½ cup sliced onion
1 16-ounce can Italian tomatoes, including liquid
2 cups thinly sliced cabbage
1 cup sliced zucchini
½ cup sliced celery
½ cup drained canned chick-peas (garbanzo beans)
½ cup uncooked rotini or other pasta
1 tablespoon finely minced fresh parsley
2 teaspoons crumbled dried basil
¼ teaspoon salt
¼ teaspoon freshly ground pepper

Cover navy beans with water in a large pot. Over medium heat, bring just to the boiling point. Remove pan from the heat, cover, and let stand for 1 hour. Drain. Add chicken broth, carrot, and potato. Cover and cook over medium heat until vegetables are almost tender, about 35 minutes. Heat oil in a small skillet and sauté onion until tender. Add onion and all remaining ingredients to soup pot. Cook 15 minutes or until pasta is cooked. Serve hot.

6 servings (yield: 6 cups)   *1 serving: 1 cup*

Nutritive values per serving:						
CHO (g)	PRO (g)	FAT (g)	CAL —	Fiber (g)	Sodium (mg)	Chol (mg)
34	12	4	216	6.4	764	0

Food Exchanges per serving: 2 Starch Exchanges plus
                              1 Vegetable Exchange plus 1 Fat
                              Exchange.

Low-sodium diets: Omit salt. Substitute unsalted canned
                    vegetables and broth.

Mushroom Vegetable Soup

A mushroom-picker's delight! Served with cheese and fruit, this hearty and delicious soup will make a full meal.

1 pound fresh mushrooms
2 tablespoons margarine, divided
1 cup finely chopped carrot
1 cup finely chopped celery
1 cup finely chopped onion
1 clove garlic, minced
1 13¾-ounce can condensed beef broth
2 cups water
¼ cup tomato paste
2 tablespoons parsley flakes *or* ¼ cup minced fresh
   parsley
1 bay leaf
½ teaspoon salt
¼ teaspoon freshly ground pepper
2 tablespoons dry sherry

Wash mushrooms; slice half of them and set aside. Chop remaining mushrooms and sauté them in 1 tablespoon margarine in a large pot. Add all the vegetables (except the sliced mushrooms) and cook 6–7 minutes, stirring often. Stir in all other ingredients except the mushrooms, the remaining margarine, and the sherry. Simmer, covered, for 1 hour. Puree soup in a blender or food processor fitted with steel blade. Sauté the sliced mushrooms in the remaining 1 tablespoon margarine. Return pureed soup to pot; add sautéed mushrooms and sherry. Reheat over moderate heat, stirring.

6 servings (yield: 6 cups)   *1 serving: 1 cup*

			Nutritive values per serving:			
CHO (g)	PRO (g)	FAT (g)	CAL —	Fiber (g)	Sodium (mg)	Chol (mg)
12	5	5	108	2.6	953	0

Food Exchanges per serving: 2 Vegetable Exchanges plus 1 Fat Exchange.

Low-sodium diets: Omit salt. Substitute unsalted beef broth and unsalted margarine.

Chicken Giblet Vegetable Soup

Leftover chicken giblets (heart, liver, gizzard) make a great soup. Chicken heart and gizzard should always be cooked until tender before combining with other ingredients.

Uncooked giblets of 1 or 2 chickens
4½ cups cold water
1 teaspoon salt
⅛ teaspoon freshly ground pepper
½ cup finely diced carrot
½ cup finely chopped onion
½ cup finely chopped celery with leaves
1 6-ounce can tomato juice
1 tablespoon parsley flakes or 2 tablespoons
    minced fresh parsley
¼ teaspoon paprika
2 tablespoons quick-cooking oatmeal

Wash giblets and discard all fat pieces. Place in a large cooking pot with water and salt. Bring to a boil and simmer about 25 minutes. Add all other ingredients except the oatmeal; simmer soup gently about 30 minutes more. Remove giblets and chop into small pieces. Return giblets to soup; add oatmeal, stir, and simmer 5 minutes.

4 servings (yield: 4 cups)   *1 serving: 1 cup*

			Nutritive values per serving:			
CHO (g)	PRO (g)	FAT (g)	CAL —	Fiber (g)	Sodium (mg)	Chol (mg)
7	5	1	56	1.6	683	56

Food Exchanges per serving: 1 Vegetable Exchange plus ½ Lean Meat Exchange.

Low-sodium diets: Omit salt. Substitute unsalted tomato juice.

Cream of Tomato Soup

1 16-ounce can tomatoes
½ cup chopped onion
2 tablespoons tomato paste
1½ cups chicken broth
1 bay leaf
½ teaspoon salt
⅛ teaspoon freshly ground pepper
¾ cup (6 ounces) evaporated low-fat (2% milk fat)
    milk
1 tablespoon finely chopped fresh parsley for
    garnish

Cut tomatoes in bite-sized pieces and place with tomato liquid in a saucepan; add onions, tomato paste, chicken broth, bay leaf, salt, and pepper. Bring to a boil; simmer, uncovered, for 5 minutes. Cool about 15 minutes, then turn into blender or food processor fitted with steel blade. Cover; blend at low speed until well mixed. Meanwhile, heat milk but do not allow it to boil or burn. Combine tomato mixture and hot milk. Simmer, uncovered, stirring constantly only until hot enough to serve. Garnish with parsley.

4 servings (yield: 3 cups)　　　　　　　　*1 serving: ¾ cup*

Nutritive values per serving:						
CHO (g)	PRO (g)	FAT (g)	CAL —	Fiber (g)	Sodium (mg)	Chol (mg)
13	5	2	89	1.3	636	7

Food Exchanges per serving: 1 Vegetable Exchange plus
                                ½ Low-Fat Milk Exchange.

Low-sodium diets: Omit salt. Substitute unsalted canned
                    tomatoes and unsalted broth.

Crème Vichyssoise

This soup is delicious either hot or chilled but is usually served chilled.

1 tablespoon vegetable oil
¼ cup finely chopped onion
1¾ cups chicken broth
1 cup skim milk
½ cup half-and-half
½ teaspoon salt
¼ teaspoon coarsely ground pepper
1 cup dehydrated potato flakes, firmly packed
1 tablespoon finely chopped fresh parsley for
    garnish

Heat vegetable oil in a large saucepan. Add onion and stir over medium heat until soft and tender but translucent. Add chicken broth; simmer 3–4 minutes. Add skim milk and half-and-half and bring just to a low boil, stirring constantly. Remove from heat. Add salt, pepper, and potato flakes. Stir vigorously until dissolved and blended. Turn into a quart jar, cover, and chill a few hours before serving. Stir well before serving and garnish servings with finely chopped parsley.

4 servings (yield: 3 cups)   *1 serving: ¾ cup*

Nutritive values per serving:						
CHO (g)	PRO (g)	FAT (g)	CAL —	Fiber (g)	Sodium (mg)	Chol (mg)
13	4	10	159	0.2	403	22

Food Exchanges per serving: 2 Fat Exchanges plus 1 Starch Exchange.

Low-sodium diets: Omit salt. Substitute unsalted chicken broth.

Gazpacho

1 clove garlic
1 pound ripe tomatoes
1½ pounds (about 2 large) cucumbers
1 cup finely diced green pepper
¾ cup finely diced celery
½ cup finely diced onion
2 cups tomato juice or V-8 Juice
1 tablespoon corn oil
1 cup cold water
3 dashes Tabasco sauce
1 teaspoon salt
½ teaspoon coarsely ground pepper
½ cup seasoned croutons
Chopped fresh parsley for garnish

Crush peeled garlic into the bottom of a 2½-quart bowl. Core tomatoes and discard cores and seeds; finely dice tomatoes. Pare cucumbers, cut lengthwise into eighths, discard centers and seeds; finely dice remaining cucumber. Measure all ingredients except croutons and parsley into the large bowl on top of garlic. Mix thoroughly. Cover bowl tightly and chill for 2 hours or longer. Serve soup in chilled bowls garnished with croutons and parsley.

9 servings (yield: 6¾ cups)   *1 serving: ¾ cup*

Nutritive values per serving:

CHO (g)	PRO (g)	FAT (g)	CAL —	Fiber (g)	Sodium (mg)	Chol (mg)
8	1	2	50	2.0	435	0

Food Exchanges per serving: 1 Vegetable Exchange plus ½ Fat Exchange.

Low-sodium diets: Omit salt. Substitute unsalted tomato juice or V-8.

Chilled Tomato Madrilene

1½ tablespoons granulated gelatin
½ cup cold water
2 cups tomato juice
¾ cup beef broth
1 teaspoon Worcestershire sauce
2 tablespoons fresh lemon juice
6 teaspoons plain low-fat yogurt
3 paper-thin lemon slices, halved
1 tablespoon finely minced fresh parsley

Soak gelatin in cold water. Combine tomato juice, beef broth, Worcestershire sauce, and lemon juice in a heavy saucepan. Heat until very hot; stir in gelatin until completely dissolved. Pour into a 9-inch square pan rinsed in cold water. Cool, cover pan, and chill in the refrigerator for several hours. Cut into ½-inch cubes. To serve, pile cubes carefully into wine or parfait glasses. Top each with 1 level teaspoon yogurt, garnish with ½ slice lemon, and sprinkle with minced parsley.

6 servings (yield: 3 cups)   *1 serving: ½ cup*

Nutritive values per serving:						
CHO (g)	PRO (g)	FAT (g)	CAL —	Fiber (g)	Sodium (mg)	Chol (mg)
5	3	0	28	1.0	404	0

Food Exchange per serving: 1 Vegetable Exchange.

Low-sodium diets: Substitute unsalted tomato juice and unsalted beef broth.

Beet Borscht

Save the beets for another meal.

1¼ cups beet liquid (drained from canned beets)
¾ cup tomato juice
¼ teaspoon onion powder
¼ teaspoon salt
1 tablespoon fresh lemon juice
¼ cup plain low-fat yogurt

Mix all ingredients except yogurt. Chill 2–3 hours in a covered jar. Serve in cocktail glasses or small glass bowls, topping each with 1 tablespoon yogurt.

4 servings (yield: 2 cups)   *1 serving: ½ cup*

			Nutritive values per serving:			
CHO (g)	PRO (g)	FAT (g)	CAL —	Fiber (g)	Sodium (mg)	Chol (mg)
6	2	0	36	0.6	464	1

Food Exchange per serving: 1 Vegetable Exchange.

Low-sodium diets: This recipe is not suitable.

Chilled Cucumber Soup

A delicious cold soup for hot weather.

> 1 pound (about 2) cucumbers, slender and firm
> 1¾ cups buttermilk, made from skim milk, divided
> 1 teaspoon salt
> 1 teaspoon fresh lemon juice
> 1 teaspoon finely minced onion
> Paprika or dill weed for garnish

Remove ends of cucumbers. Pare one, then slice into ¼-inch slices. If skins feel waxy, pare all cucumbers. Reserve four of the unpared slices for garnish, cut them again to yield eight very thin slices, wrap, and store in refrigerator. Pour ¼ cup buttermilk into blender or food processor; add half the cucumber slices. Blend at high speed for 30–40 seconds, until smooth. Add remaining cucumber slices, salt, lemon juice, and onion; blend about 1 minute. Stir in remaining buttermilk to mix thoroughly. Turn into a 1-quart jar, cover, and chill in refrigerator for at least 2 hours. (Do not keep longer than 48 hours before using.) Garnish each serving with thin slices of cucumber and a sprinkling of paprika or dill.

4 servings (yield: 3 cups)   *1 serving: ¾ cup*

			Nutritive values per serving:			
CHO (g)	PRO (g)	FAT (g)	CAL —	Fiber (g)	Sodium (mg)	Chol (mg)
9	4	1	59	1.6	603	4

Food Exchanges per serving: 1 Vegetable Exchange plus ½ Skim Milk Exchange.

Low-sodium diets: Omit salt. Substitute skim milk for buttermilk and increase lemon juice to 1 tablespoon. Add ½ teaspoon dried dill weed before blending.

17
Salads and Dressings

SALADS

NEW Asparagus Salad with Pecans

Water
24 medium-size fresh asparagus spears
6 crisp leaves red leaf lettuce
6 tablespoons Buttermilk Mayonnaise
    (*see* Index) or prepared light mayonnaise
2 tablespoons chopped pecans

Bring large pot of water to boil. Wash asparagus and snap off
tough bottoms of stems. When water is boiling, add asparagus
and let water return to a boil. Cook about 3 minutes, until
asparagus is crisp but tender. Remove asparagus, run it under
cold water, and refrigerate to chill. At serving time, line six
salad plates with lettuce and arrange four spears on each. Top
salads with 1 tablespoon Buttermilk Mayonnaise or commercial light mayonnaise and sprinkle with 1 teaspoon chopped
pecans.

6 servings   *1 serving: 4 spears plus 1 tablespoon dressing*

			Nutritive values per serving:			
CHO (g)	PRO (g)	FAT (g)	CAL —	Fiber (g)	Sodium (mg)	Chol (mg)
4	3	2	41	1.0	66	1

Food Exchange per serving: 1 Vegetable Exchange.

Low-sodium diets: This recipe is excellent.

NEW Indian Carrot Salad

This recipe is a vitamin A bonanza!

- 1 tablespoon corn oil
- 1 tablespoon lime juice
- ½ teaspoon ground cumin
- ½ teaspoon ground cinnamon
- ¼ teaspoon salt
- ½ teaspoon minced garlic
- 4 cups sliced cooked carrot
- ¼ cup wheat sprouts or cooked wheat berries for garnish

Whisk oil and lime juice together in large bowl. Whisk in cumin, cinnamon, salt, and garlic. Stir in carrot. Cover and refrigerate until cold. Serve chilled, garnished with wheat sprouts.

8 servings (yield: 4 cups)   *1 serving: ½ cup*

			Nutritive values per serving:				
CHO (g)	PRO (g)	FAT (g)	CAL —	Fiber (g)	Sodium (mg)	Chol (mg)
10	1	2	61	1.6	122	0

Food Exchanges per serving: 2 Vegetable Exchanges.

Low-sodium diets: This recipe is suitable.

Bright Bean Salad

- 1 9-ounce package frozen French-cut green beans
- 1 medium carrot, chopped fine
- 2 tablespoons finely chopped onion
- ⅛ teaspoon salt
- 3 tablespoons Lemon Shaker Dressing (*see* Index)

Cook green beans according to package directions, but reduce cooking time by 2 minutes so that beans are crisp. Drain beans and toss with chopped carrot, onion, salt, and dressing. Chill in a covered container for several hours.

4 servings (yield: 2 cups)   *1 serving: ½ cup*

Nutritive values per serving:

CHO (g)	PRO (g)	FAT (g)	CAL —	Fiber (g)	Sodium (mg)	Chol (mg)
7	1	0	28	1.5	113	0

Food Exchange per serving: 1 Vegetable Exchange.

Low-sodium diets: Omit salt in water in which beans are cooked
and also in the Lemon Shaker Dressing.

NEW Crisp and Cool Middle Eastern Salad

Try this salad served on Whole-Wheat Pita Bread (see Index).

1 green pepper, chopped
2 medium tomatoes, chopped
1 medium cucumber, peeled and chopped
3 green onions, with tops, chopped
1 cup plain low-fat yogurt
1 tablespoon fresh dill *or* 1½ teaspoons dried dill
    weed
½ teaspoon salt
½ teaspoon freshly ground pepper

Toss green pepper, tomatoes, cucumber, and green onions in a
medium-size bowl. In a small bowl combine yogurt, dill, salt,
and pepper. Spoon yogurt mixture over salad and toss.

6 servings (yield: 4½ cups)   *1 serving: ¾ cup*

Nutritive values per serving:

CHO (g)	PRO (g)	FAT (g)	CAL —	Fiber (g)	Sodium (mg)	Chol (mg)
7	3	1	44	1.2	229	2

Food Exchange per serving: 1 Vegetable Exchange.

Low-sodium diets: Omit salt.

Confetti Bean Salad

1 16-ounce can mixed cut green and wax beans
½ cup cider vinegar
1 teaspoon mixed pickling spices
½ cup finely diced celery
¼ cup chopped green pepper
¼ cup chopped onion
2 tablespoons chopped pimiento
Sugar substitute equivalent to 5 teaspoons sugar
Crisp lettuce leaves

Drain beans, saving liquid. Combine this liquid with vinegar in a saucepan. Add mixed pickling spices, either loose or in a small cheesecloth bag. Bring to a boil, cover, reduce heat to low, and simmer gently for 10 minutes. Meanwhile, mix all the vegetables in a bowl. Remove liquid from heat; add sweetener and stir until dissolved. Pour over vegetables and remove spice bag or loose spices. Chill several hours, stirring occasionally. Drain before serving on crisp lettuce.

6 servings (yield: 3 cups)   *1 serving: ½ cup*

		Nutritive values per serving:				
CHO (g)	PRO (g)	FAT (g)	CAL —	Fiber (g)	Sodium (mg)	Chol (mg)
7	1	0	28	1.6	110	0

Food Exchange per serving: 1 Vegetable Exchange.

Low-sodium diets: Substitute equal amounts of unsalted canned beans.

Brussels Sprouts and Carrot Salad

Colorful and attractive, this is an unusual salad for a buffet.

1 10-ounce package frozen brussels sprouts
1 16-ounce can sliced carrots or 5 medium carrots, sliced and cooked
½ cup Lemon Shaker Dressing (*see* Index)

Cook brussels sprouts according to package directions until they are crisp but tender; drain. Drain carrots and put them in a bowl; add brussels sprouts and Lemon Shaker Dressing; mix well. Cover and refrigerate 4–6 hours before using; stir occasionally.

5 servings (yield: 2½ cups)   1 serving: ½ cup

Nutritive values per serving:

CHO (g)	PRO (g)	FAT (g)	CAL —	Fiber (g)	Sodium (mg)	Chol (mg)
11	3	0	49	3.2	273	0

Food Exchanges per serving: 2 Vegetable Exchanges.

Low-sodium diets: Omit salt in cooking brussels sprouts and from Lemon Shaker Dressing.

Carrot and Raisin Salad

3 cups shredded carrot
½ cup Low-Calorie Cooked Dressing (*see* Index)
⅓ cup (1½-ounce box) seedless raisins
¼ teaspoon salt
Sugar substitute equivalent to 6 teaspoons sugar
Lettuce leaves

Combine all ingredients, except lettuce, thoroughly. Cover bowl. Chill 2 hours or longer before serving. Serve on crisp lettuce.

9 servings (yield: 3 cups)   1 serving: ⅓ cup lightly packed

Nutritive values per serving:

CHO (g)	PRO (g)	FAT (g)	CAL —	Fiber (g)	Sodium (mg)	Chol (mg)
9	1	1	47	1.7	153	10

Food Exchanges per serving: 2 Vegetable Exchanges.

Low-sodium diets: Omit salt and prepare the Low-Calorie Cooked Dressing without salt.

$\boxed{NEW}$ Romaine, Red Onion, and Fennel Salad with Tart Lime Dressing

6 ounces romaine lettuce
1½ cups shredded fennel bulb (about 1 large bulb)
1 cup cauliflowerets
½ cup sliced red onions
Tart Lime Dressing (recipe follows)

Wash, dry, and tear lettuce into bite-sized pieces. Arrange lettuce pieces in a salad bowl; toss with shredded fennel, cauliflowerets, and red onion. Prepare Tart Lime Dressing. Sprinkle dressing over salad and toss just before serving.

TART LIME DRESSING
¼ cup fresh lime juice
1 tablespoon olive oil
1 clove garlic, minced
¼ teaspoon salt
¼ teaspoon freshly ground pepper
¼ teaspoon paprika

Combine all ingredients and mix well.

4 servings   *1 serving: 1 cup salad with*
                                       1 tablespoon dressing

Nutritive values per serving:

CHO (g)	PRO (g)	FAT (g)	CAL —	Fiber (g)	Sodium (mg)	Chol (mg)
7	2	3	60	1.0	185	0

Food Exchanges per serving: 1 Vegetable Exchange plus 1 Fat Exchange.

Low-sodium diets: Omit salt from dressing.

NEW Tomato, Basil, and Mozzarella Salad

Make this only in the summer or when you can get very large, red, ripe tomatoes. It's one of our favorite summer salads and a great appetizer or part of an antipasto platter.

1 pound large, red, very ripe tomatoes
    (2–3 tomatoes)
2 ounces shredded mozzarella cheese
8 leaves fresh basil
2 teaspoons olive oil
Dash cracked pepper

Slice tomatoes crosswise into ½-inch-thick slices, 4 slices per tomato. Arrange 2–3 slices on each salad plate. Sprinkle the mozzarella on top of each tomato. Cut fresh basil leaves into strips and top each tomato with basil. Drizzle olive oil over the tops and add a dash of pepper. Enjoy!

4 servings   *1 serving: 2–3 slices tomato with topping*

Nutritive values per serving:

CHO (g)	PRO (g)	FAT (g)	CAL —	Fiber (g)	Sodium (mg)	Chol (mg)
6	5	4	70	1.9	76	8

Food Exchanges per serving: 1 Vegetable Exchange plus
                            ½ Medium-Fat Meat Exchange.

Low-sodium diets: This recipe is suitable.

Cucumber Salad

1 large cucumber, peeled
1 cup plain low-fat yogurt
2 tablespoons vinegar
1½ teaspoons dried dill weed *or* 1 tablespoon
    fresh dill
1 clove garlic, crushed, *or* ½ teaspoon garlic powder
½ teaspoon salt
¼ teaspoon freshly ground pepper

Slice cucumber lengthwise and remove seeds. Dice the cucumber and add remaining ingredients. Mix thoroughly and chill at least ½ hour before serving.

5 servings. (yield: 2½ cups)   *1 serving: ½ cup*

Nutritive values per serving:

CHO (g)	PRO (g)	FAT (g)	CAL —	Fiber (g)	Sodium (mg)	Chol (mg)
6	3	3	39	0.8	229	3

Food Exchange per serving: 1 Vegetable Exchange.

Low-sodium diets: Omit salt.

Jackstraw Salad

1 medium (about 4 ounces) red apple
½ cup thin green pepper strips
½ cup thin celery sticks
¾ cup shredded cabbage
¼ cup thinly sliced onion rings
⅓ cup Poppy Seed Dressing (*see* Index)
Crisp lettuce leaves

Remove core and stem of apple; leave skin on. Cut apple crosswise into ¼-inch rings; cut each ring into thin sticks about ⅛ inch wide. Combine all ingredients except lettuce in a large

bowl and toss lightly to mix Poppy Seed Dressing thoroughly.
Serve on crisp lettuce.

4 servings (yield: 3 cups)   *1 serving: ¾ cup*

Nutritive values per serving:						
CHO (g)	PRO (g)	FAT (g)	CAL —	Fiber (g)	Sodium (mg)	Chol (mg)
9	1	1	39	1.8	100	0

Food Exchange per serving: 1 Vegetable Exchange.

Low-sodium diets: Omit salt in dressing recipe.

Pickled Beets

1 8¼-ounce can whole very small beets
¾ cup cider vinegar
1 teaspoon mixed pickling spices
1 2-inch-long stick cinnamon
Sugar substitute equivalent to 3 teaspoons sugar

Drain beets, saving liquid. Combine liquid and vinegar in a 1-
quart pot. Add pickling spices (in a cheesecloth bag or small
tea ball) and cinnamon. Bring to a boil; simmer 5 minutes.
Discard spices. Pack beets into a pint jar. Dissolve sweetener in
hot liquid; pour on top of beets. Cover and store in refrigerator
a few days before serving.

4 servings   *1 serving: 3 small beets*

Nutritive values per serving:						
CHO (g)	PRO (g)	FAT (g)	CAL —	Fiber (g)	Sodium (mg)	Chol (mg)
7	0	0	30	0.4	154	0

Food Exchange per serving: 1 Vegetable Exchange. One small
beet served as a garnish on a salad
or cold meat plate may be
considered "free."

Low-sodium diets: Acceptable for occasional use unless the
sodium restriction is severe.

Mushroom Delight

1 tablespoon vegetable oil
1 tablespoon fresh lemon juice
1 tablespoon wine vinegar
¼ teaspoon salt
⅛ teaspoon coarsely ground pepper
½ teaspoon dry mustard
⅛ teaspoon garlic powder *or* 1 clove garlic, crushed
1–2 tablespoons finely chopped dill pickle
12 ounces fresh mushrooms, sliced thin (about 4½ cups)
6 lettuce leaves
2 tablespoons snipped fresh parsley

Place all ingredients except mushrooms, lettuce, and parsley in a small jar. Cover the jar and shake it well. Drizzle dressing over mushrooms and toss mushrooms gently so that dressing thoroughly coats them. Serve on lettuce leaves and garnish with snipped parsley.

6 servings (yield: 3 cups)   *1 serving: ½ cup*

			Nutritive values per serving:			
CHO (g)	PRO (g)	FAT (g)	CAL —	Fiber (g)	Sodium (mg)	Chol (mg)
4	1	3	40	1.3	121	0

Food Exchange per serving: 1 Vegetable Exchange.
Low-sodium diets: Omit salt.

Israeli Salad

2 medium cucumbers
½ cup chopped green pepper
2 cups shredded lettuce
2 tablespoons finely chopped green onion
¾ cup grated or shredded carrot
2 tablespoons finely chopped fresh parsley
1 cup diced fresh tomato (about 2 tomatoes)
¼ cup sliced radish
1 tablespoon vegetable oil
3 tablespoons fresh lemon juice
1 teaspoon salt
¾ teaspoon coarsely ground pepper

Pare cucumbers, halve lengthwise, and discard seeds and center pulp. Dice cucumber flesh and measure 2 cups. Combine all ingredients in a large bowl; toss until well mixed. Serve immediately.

6 servings (yield: 6 cups)   *1 serving: 1 cup*

Nutritive values per serving:

CHO (g)	PRO (g)	FAT (g)	CAL —	Fiber (g)	Sodium (mg)	Chol (mg)
7	1	3	51	2.3	340	0

Food Exchanges per serving: 1 Vegetable Exchange plus ½ Fat Exchange.

Low-sodium diets: Omit salt.

Red Cabbage Salad

¾ cup cider vinegar
¼ cup cold water
½ teaspoon salt
½ teaspoon crushed dried tarragon
Sugar substitute equivalent to 4 teaspoons sugar
2 cups shredded red cabbage
1 cup finely chopped celery
½ cup chopped onion

Combine vinegar, water, salt, and tarragon; heat almost to a boil. Remove from heat, add sweetener, and stir to dissolve. Mix vegetables, then pour vinegar mixture on top. Toss gently several times to mix well. Cover bowl and chill for a few hours. Just before serving, toss gently again.

5 servings (yield: about 4 cups)   *1 serving: ¾ cup*

			Nutritive values per serving:			
CHO (g)	PRO (g)	FAT (g)	CAL —	Fiber (g)	Sodium (mg)	Chol (mg)
7	1	0	21	1.3	220	0

Food Exchange per serving: 1 Vegetable Exchange.

Low-sodium diets: Omit salt.

Spinach Salad

¾ pound raw spinach
1 cup fresh or canned and drained bean sprouts
1 8½-ounce can water chestnuts, drained and sliced
2 medium eggs, hard-cooked
1 cup Miracle Red "French" Dressing (*see* Index)
Sugar substitute equivalent to 3 teaspoons sugar
1 tablespoon vegetable oil

Clean and wash spinach, remove and discard stems, and tear leaves into bite-sized pieces. Pat spinach dry with paper towels and put in a large salad bowl. Spread a layer of bean sprouts, then a layer of water chestnuts, over spinach. Slice eggs and distribute over salad. Cover salad with a damp paper towel and refrigerate to chill salad. Meanwhile, add sweetener and vegetable oil to Miracle Red "French" Dressing; mix well. Pour dressing over salad and toss immediately before serving.

10 servings (yield: 10 cups)   *1 serving: 1 cup*

Nutritive values per serving:

CHO (g)	PRO (g)	FAT (g)	CAL —	Fiber (g)	Sodium (mg)	Chol (mg)
6	3	3	56	1.4	188	55

Food Exchanges per serving: 1 Vegetable Exchange plus ½ Fat Exchange.

Low-sodium diets: Modify Miracle Red "French" Dressing as directed.

Christmas Vegetable Salad Mold

1 tablespoon granulated gelatin
½ cup cold water
1 cup chicken broth
¼ teaspoon salt
½ teaspoon dried dill weed
1 teaspoon sugar
1 cup plain low-fat yogurt
½ cup finely chopped green pepper
½ cup quartered and sliced radishes
¼ cup finely chopped green onion
2 tablespoons snipped fresh parsley
Crisp lettuce leaves

Combine gelatin and cold water in a heavy saucepan. Slowly heat over low heat, stirring constantly until gelatin is clear and liquid. Add chicken broth, salt, dill weed, and sugar; mix well. Add slowly to yogurt; mix well. Chill until it is of the consistency of unbeaten egg whites. Fold in remaining ingredients except lettuce; mix carefully. Turn into one 3-cup mold or six ½-cup molds. Cover lightly with clear plastic wrap. Chill until set. Unmold on crisp lettuce.

6 servings (yield: 3 cups)   *1 serving: ½ cup*

Nutritive values per serving:

CHO (g)	PRO (g)	FAT (g)	CAL —	Fiber (g)	Sodium (mg)	Chol (mg)
6	4	0	44	0.8	246	1

Food Exchange per serving: ½ Skim Milk Exchange.

Low-sodium diets: Omit salt. Substitute low-sodium chicken broth.

Waldorf Salad Mold

1 tablespoon granulated gelatin
¼ cup cold water
1 tablespoon grated lemon rind
1½ cups water
¼ cup fresh lemon juice
Sugar substitute equivalent to 7 teaspoons sugar
2 drops yellow food color
¼ teaspoon pure lemon extract
1 cup plain low-fat yogurt
¾ cup finely diced red-skinned apples
¼ cup finely diced celery
2 tablespoons finely chopped walnuts
Crisp lettuce leaves

Soak gelatin in ¼ cup cold water. Add lemon rind to another 1½ cups water; bring to a boil and simmer gently for 5 minutes. Strain, then measure only 1 cup to use; add gelatin mixture, lemon juice, sweetener, food color, and lemon extract, mix well. Chill until the consistency of unbeaten egg whites. Fold carefully into yogurt; then fold in diced apples, celery, and walnuts. Mix carefully but well. Turn into a 2½-cup salad mold or into five ½-cup molds. Cover and chill until firmly set. Serve as a salad on crisp lettuce.

5 servings (yield: 2½ cups)   *1 serving: ½ cup*

		Nutritive values per serving:				
CHO (g)	PRO (g)	FAT (g)	CAL —	Fiber (g)	Sodium (mg)	Chol (mg)
9	5	2	68	1.0	45	1

Food Exchange per serving: ½ Low-Fat Milk Exchange.

Low-sodium diets: This recipe is excellent.

Tomato Aspic Salad

½ cup cold water
1 tablespoon granulated gelatin
1½ cups tomato juice or V-8 Juice
1½ teaspoons fresh lemon juice or white vinegar
1–2 drops hot pepper sauce
½ teaspoon minced onion
Crisp lettuce
Green pepper strips

Measure cold water into a small saucepan; sprinkle gelatin on top. Stir over low heat 3–4 minutes, or until gelatin is completely dissolved. Remove from heat. Add tomato juice with other ingredients except lettuce and green pepper. Mix well. Chill until it is the consistency of unbeaten egg whites. Turn carefully into four ½-cup molds. Chill until firm. Unmold on crisp lettuce and garnish with green pepper strips.

4 servings (yield: 2 cups)   *1 serving: ½ cup*

			Nutritive values per serving:			
CHO (g)	PRO (g)	FAT (g)	CAL —	Fiber (g)	Sodium (mg)	Chol (mg)
4	2	0	25	1.3	332	0

Food Exchange per serving: 1 Vegetable Exchange.

Low-sodium diets: Substitute unsalted tomato juice.

Egg Salad

Mound on crisp lettuce, garnished with a dash of paprika, and serve as a salad. This may also be used as a spread for crackers or as a sandwich filling.

> 2 hard-cooked eggs, peeled and chilled
> 1 tablespoon finely chopped green onion
> 1 tablespoon finely chopped celery with leaves
> ¼ teaspoon salt
> Dash freshly ground pepper
> 3 tablespoons Lemon Mayonnaise (*see* Index)
> ½ teaspoon hot prepared mustard

Finely dice the eggs; mix thoroughly with all other ingredients. Cover and chill for at least 1 hour or until flavors are well blended.

2 servings (yield: ⅔ cup)   *1 serving: ⅓ cup*

Nutritive values per serving (filling only):						
CHO (g)	PRO (g)	FAT (g)	CAL —	Fiber (g)	Sodium (mg)	Chol (mg)
2	7	6	97	0.1	526	307

Food Exchange per serving (filling only): 1 Medium-Fat Meat Exchange.

Low-sodium diets: Omit salt from this recipe and from Lemon Mayonnaise.

Tuna Cheese Salad

1 7-ounce can tuna, packed in water
¼ pound American, cheddar, or Colby cheese
1½ tablespoons finely chopped sweet gherkins
½ cup finely chopped celery
½ cup Skim Milk Mayonnaise (*see* Index) or light
    mayonnaise
Crisp lettuce
Few strips green pepper

Drain tuna; flake with fork into small pieces. Cut cheese into ¼-inch cubes. Combine tuna, cheese, gherkins, celery, and Skim Milk Mayonnaise; mix well. Cover bowl and chill 1 hour or longer. Serve on crisp lettuce, garnished with thin strips of green pepper.

4 servings (yield: 2⅔ cups)   *1 serving: ⅔ cup*

Nutritive values per serving:

CHO (g)	PRO (g)	FAT (g)	CAL —	Fiber (g)	Sodium (mg)	Chol (mg)
5	23	15	251	0.4	552	113

Food Exchanges per serving: 3 Medium-Fat Meat Exchanges plus 1 Vegetable Exchange.

Low-sodium diets: Substitute low-sodium cheese. Omit salt from Skim Milk Mayonnaise.

Curried Tuna Salad

2 7-ounce cans tuna in oil
1 14½-ounce can asparagus pieces, drained
½ medium head lettuce, separated
¾ cup Curry Dressing or Dip (*see* Index)
3 hard-cooked eggs, sliced
Paprika

Chill canned tuna and asparagus. Drain tuna and flake lightly. Drain asparagus pieces well. Arrange lettuce on six salad plates. On each salad plate place ⅓ cup cut asparagus and ½ cup flaked tuna. Cover with 2 tablespoons Curry Dressing; top with 3 slices hard-cooked egg. Garnish with a sprinkle of paprika.

6 servings   *1 serving: ½ cup tuna plus*
                          2 tablespoons Curry Dressing

Nutritive values per serving:

CHO (g)	PRO (g)	FAT (g)	CAL —	Fiber (g)	Sodium (mg)	Chol (mg)
5	25	9	211	1.7	613	182

Food Exchanges per serving: 3 Lean Meat Exchanges plus 1 Vegetable Exchange.

Low-sodium diets: Substitute low-sodium canned tuna and low-sodium canned asparagus. Omit salt from Curry Dressing or Dip.

Chicken Salad Deluxe

2 cups firmly packed cubed cooked chicken
¼ cup chicken broth
1 cup diagonally sliced celery
2 tablespoons finely chopped green onion
¼ cup thinly sliced green pepper
1 2-ounce can mushroom stems and pieces,
    drained
24 small green or red seedless grapes
¼ cup slivered almonds
2 teaspoons margarine
¾ cup Low-Calorie Cooked Dressing (*see* Index) or
    light mayonnaise
Crisp lettuce leaves

In a large bowl combine chicken, chicken broth, celery, onion,
green pepper, mushrooms, and grapes; mix well. Cover and
chill several hours. Sauté the almonds in margarine, stirring
constantly, until they are browned; spread on paper towel to
cool. Immediately before serving stir the dressing into the
chicken salad. Arrange chicken salad on four plates, lined with
crisp lettuce leaves, and top each with 1 tablespoon of sautéed
almonds.

4 servings (yield: 4 cups)   *1 serving: 1 cup*

Nutritive values per serving:						
CHO (g)	PRO (g)	FAT (g)	CAL —	Fiber (g)	Sodium (mg)	Chol (mg)
13	24	15	278	1.8	441	97

Food Exchanges per serving: 3 Medium-Fat Meat Exchanges
                    plus 1 Fruit Exchange.

Low-sodium diets: Serve ½-cup portion (1½ Medium-Fat Meat
                    Exchanges plus ½ Fruit Exchange).

$\boxed{NEW}$ Chicken and Barley Salad

As a special treat, try serving the salad in a seeded red or green bell pepper.

2 cups water
⅔ cup uncooked quick-cooking barley
2 cups diced cooked chicken
½ cup diced celery
½ cup chopped tomatoes
½ cup chopped red onion
2 tablespoons fresh lemon juice
1 teaspoon Dijon mustard
5 lettuce leaves

Bring water to a vigorous boil in a medium saucepan over high heat. Stir in barley; return to a boil. Reduce heat, cover, and simmer 8–10 minutes or until barley is tender, stirring occasionally. Drain if necessary; cool. Toss barley with remaining ingredients except lettuce. Serve on lettuce leaves.

5 servings   *1 serving: 1 cup*

Nutritive values per serving:						
CHO (g)	PRO (g)	FAT (g)	CAL —	Fiber (g)	Sodium (mg)	Chol (mg)
24	19	4	213	3.1	75	50

Food Exchanges per serving: 2 Lean Meat Exchanges plus
1 Starch Exchange plus
1 Vegetable Exchange.

Low-sodium diets: This recipe is excellent.

DRESSINGS

Buttermilk Mayonnaise

This buttermilk dressing is delicious served on mixed greens or sliced tomatoes. It is also an excellent sauce for some cooked vegetables and for steamed or baked fish fillets.

½ teaspoon granulated gelatin
1 tablespoon cold water
½ teaspoon dry mustard
¼ teaspoon salt
Few grains freshly ground pepper
1 tablespoon water
1 cup buttermilk, made from skim milk
2 teaspoons finely chopped green onion
2 teaspoons minced fresh parsley

Soak gelatin in 1 tablespoon cold water. Dissolve over hot water. Mix together mustard, salt, pepper, and 1 tablespoon water until smooth. Combine all ingredients except parsley and blend well. Chill until it begins to thicken. Beat gently until smooth; stir in parsley. Turn into a jar and cover. Chill several hours.

8 servings (yield: 1 cup)   *1 serving: 2 tablespoons*

Nutritive values per serving:

CHO (g)	PRO (g)	FAT (g)	CAL —	Fiber (g)	Sodium (mg)	Chol (mg)
2	1	0	14	0	94	1

Food Exchange per serving: Up to 2 tablespoons may be considered "free."

Low-sodium diets: Omit salt.

Lemon Mayonnaise

For fruit, chicken, or seafood salads.

> 1 tablespoon cornstarch
> 2 teaspoons dry mustard
> 1½ teaspoons salt
> 1 cup water
> 2 medium eggs, beaten
> ⅓ cup fresh lemon juice
> 2 tablespoons white vinegar
> Sugar substitute equivalent to 6 teaspoons sugar

Combine cornstarch, mustard, and salt in the top of a double boiler. Combine water and beaten eggs. Slowly add to cornstarch mixture, stirring constantly, until smooth. Cook over simmering water for 5 minutes, stirring constantly. Very slowly stir in the lemon juice and vinegar. Continue cooking and stirring over simmering water for 10 more minutes. Remove from heat. Add the sweetener; mix well. Pour into a pint jar, cover, and store in refrigerator. Stir well before each use.

12 servings (yield: 1½ cups)   *1 serving: 2 tablespoons*

			Nutritive values per serving:			
CHO (g)	PRO (g)	FAT (g)	CAL —	Fiber (g)	Sodium (mg)	Chol (mg)
2	1	1	20	0	256	46

Food Exchange per serving: Up to 2 tablespoons may be considered "free."

Low-sodium diets: Omit salt.

Skim Milk Mayonnaise

Perfect as a sandwich spread or in mayonnaise-type salads. Only about 12 calories per tablespoonful.

1½ teaspoons granulated gelatin
¼ cup cold water
1½ cups skim milk
2 medium egg yolks, beaten
1½ teaspoons dry mustard
1 teaspoon salt
¼ teaspoon paprika
¼ cup white vinegar
Sugar substitute equivalent to 3 teaspoons sugar

Soak gelatin in cold water; set aside. Scald milk in the top of a double boiler. Slowly pour over beaten yolks, stirring constantly to prevent curdling. Return egg-milk mixture to the top of the double boiler and add mustard, salt, and paprika. Cook over simmering water, stirring constantly until mixture is thick enough to coat the spoon. Remove from heat. Add vinegar, sweetener, and gelatin; blend well. Pour into a pint jar, cover, and chill. Stir before using.

16 servings (yield: 2 cups)   *1 serving: 2 tablespoons*

			Nutritive values per serving:			
CHO (g)	PRO (g)	FAT (g)	CAL —	Fiber (g)	Sodium (mg)	Chol (mg)
2	1	1	2	0	136	50

Food Exchange per serving: Up to 2 tablespoons may be considered "free."

Low-sodium diets: Omit salt.

Miracle Red "French" Dressing

The miracle is that this delicious dressing is fat-free and will not use up your Fat Exchanges. Try it as a marinade for flank steak before grilling.

½ teaspoon granulated gelatin
1 tablespoon cold water
¼ cup boiling water
½ teaspoon salt
½ cup tomato juice
¼ cup white vinegar
⅛ teaspoon garlic powder *or* 1 clove fresh garlic,
    crushed
Dash freshly ground pepper
¼ teaspoon dry mustard
½ teaspoon Worcestershire sauce
Sugar substitute equivalent to 1 tablespoon sugar

Soften gelatin in cold water. Add boiling water; stir until dissolved. Turn into a pint jar with all the remaining ingredients. Cover tightly; shake thoroughly. Chill for a few hours before serving. Stir occasionally to prevent gelling at bottom. Shake gently before using.

8–16 servings (yield: 1 cup)   *1 serving: 1–2 tablespoons*

			Nutritive values per serving:			
CHO (g)	PRO (g)	FAT (g)	CAL —	Fiber (g)	Sodium (mg)	Chol (mg)
1	0	0	6	0.2	180	0

Food Exchange per serving: Up to ¼ cup may be considered "free."

Low-sodium diets: Omit salt. Substitute unsalted tomato juice.

Low-Calorie Cooked Dressing

⅓ cup instant nonfat dry milk
1¼ teaspoons dry mustard
1 teaspoon salt
⅛ teaspoon freshly ground pepper
1 tablespoon all-purpose flour
1 medium egg
1 cup water
2 tablespoons white vinegar
1 tablespoon margarine
Sugar substitute equivalent to 6 teaspoons sugar

Combine dry ingredients in the top of a double boiler. Beat egg slightly and combine with water and vinegar. Add to dry ingredients slowly, stirring to blend well. Cook over simmering water, stirring constantly until thick and smooth. Remove from heat. Add margarine and sweetener; blend well. Turn into a pint jar; cover. Store in refrigerator.

16 servings (yield: 1½ cups)   *1 serving: 1½ tablespoons*

CHO (g)	PRO (g)	FAT (g)	CAL —	Fiber (g)	Sodium (mg)	Chol (mg)
2	1	1	21	0	143	17

Nutritive values per serving:

Food Exchange per serving: Up to 1½ tablespoons may be considered "free."

Low-sodium diets: Omit salt.

Mustard Dressing

This dressing is excellent with seafood or when tangy mustard flavor is desired.

> 1½ teaspoons dry mustard
> 1 tablespoon water
> 2 tablespoons all-purpose flour
> 1 teaspoon salt
> Dash cayenne pepper
> 2 egg yolks, well beaten
> ¾ cup water
> 2 tablespoons white vinegar
> Sugar substitute equivalent to 3 teaspoons sugar

Mix mustard and 1 tablespoon water in a small container until smooth; let stand 5 minutes. Mix together flour, salt, and cayenne pepper in top of a double boiler. Combine beaten egg yolks, ¾ cup water, and mustard. Add to dry ingredients and mix well. Cook and stir over simmering water 10 minutes or until thick and smooth. Remove from heat. Add vinegar and sweetener; blend well. Pour into ½-pint jar, cover, and chill. Stir before using.

8 servings (yield: 1 cup)   *1 serving: 2 tablespoons*

CHO (g)	PRO (g)	FAT (g)	CAL —	Fiber (g)	Sodium (mg)	Chol (mg)
2	1	3	34	0.1	248	100

Nutritive values per serving:

Food Exchange per serving: ½ Fat Exchange.

Low-sodium diets: Omit salt.

Kay's Dressing

This is a variation of the old standard "Zero Dressing." Kay was especially proud of this one—her diabetic friends raved about it!

½ cup water
½ cup white vinegar
½ teaspoon salt
½ teaspoon dry mustard
⅛ teaspoon freshly ground pepper
1/16 teaspoon paprika
Sugar substitute equivalent to 4 teaspoons sugar

Combine all ingredients in a pint jar and cover tightly. Shake vigorously and store in refrigerator. Shake before using.

8–16 servings (yield: 1 cup)   1 serving: 1–2 tablespoons

			Nutritive values per serving:			
CHO (g)	PRO (g)	FAT (g)	CAL —	Fiber (g)	Sodium (mg)	Chol (mg)
1	0	0	4	0.1	122	0

Food Exchange per serving: This is a "free" food.

Low-sodium diets: Omit salt.

Variation: Poppy Seed Dressing Follow recipe for Kay's dressing, but use cider vinegar in place of white vinegar, omit paprika, and add 1 tablespoon poppy seeds. Delicious over fruit salads.

			Nutritive values per serving:			
CHO (g)	PRO (g)	FAT (g)	CAL —	Fiber (g)	Sodium (mg)	Chol (mg)
2	0	0	9	0.1	123	0

Food Exchange per serving: This is a "free" food.

Low-sodium diets: Omit salt.

Lemon Shaker Dressing

Tasty, very low-calorie dressing that can be used as a marinade for vegetables and meat.

½ cup fresh lemon juice
¾ cup water
¼ teaspoon salt
1 teaspoon grated lemon rind
½ teaspoon Worcestershire sauce
¼ teaspoon celery seed
⅛ teaspoon freshly ground pepper
¼ teaspoon dry mustard
Sugar substitute equivalent to 2 tablespoons sugar

Combine all ingredients in a pint jar; cover tightly and shake vigorously. Store in refrigerator. Shake before using.

14 servings (yield: 1¾ cups)   *1 serving: 2 tablespoons*

Nutritive values per serving:						
CHO (g)	PRO (g)	FAT (g)	CAL —	Fiber (g)	Sodium (mg)	Chol (mg)
1	0	0	5	0	52	0

Food Exchange per serving: Up to 3 tablespoons may be considered "free."

Low-sodium diets: Omit salt.

Thousand Island Dressing

For any green or protein salad. Try it on a julienne salad.

½ cup Skim Milk Mayonnaise (*see* Index)
1½ tablespoons catsup or chili sauce
¼ cup finely chopped dill pickle
2 tablespoons minced fresh parsley
1 tablespoon minced green onion

Combine all ingredients thoroughly. Chill before using.

12 servings (yield: ¾ cup)   1 serving: 1 tablespoon

| Nutritive values per serving: | | | | | | |
CHO (g)	PRO (g)	FAT (g)	CAL —	Fiber (g)	Sodium (mg)	Chol (mg)
1	0	0	11	0.1	136	17

Food Exchange per serving: This is a "free" food.

Low-sodium diets: Substitute sweet pickle relish for chopped dill pickle; substitute unsalted catsup.

Curry Dressing

This is easy and delicious as a dressing on chicken or fish salads or as a dip for assorted raw vegetables.

1 cup plain low-fat yogurt
½ teaspoon curry powder
⅛ teaspoon ground ginger
¼ teaspoon salt
Dash cayenne pepper

Blend all ingredients until smooth. Chill in a covered container at least 1 hour before serving.

8 servings (yield: 1 cup)   1 serving: 2 tablespoons

Nutritive values per serving:

CHO (g)	PRO (g)	FAT (g)	CAL —	Fiber (g)	Sodium (mg)	Chol (mg)
2	2	0	19	0	81	2

Food Exchange per serving: Up to 2 tablespoons may be considered "free."

Low-sodium diets: Omit salt.

Low-Calorie Italian-Style Dressing

⅔ cup tomato juice
1 tablespoon olive oil
⅓ cup wine vinegar
1 tablespoon Italian seasoning
2 small cloves garlic, crushed
¼ teaspoon salt

Measure all ingredients into a pint jar; cover. Shake vigorously. Store in refrigerator. Shake before using.

8 servings (yield: 1 cup)   *1 serving: 2 tablespoons*

Nutritive values per serving:

CHO (g)	PRO (g)	FAT (g)	CAL —	Fiber (g)	Sodium (mg)	Chol (mg)
1	0	2	20	0.2	134	0

Food Exchange per serving: Up to 2 tablespoons may be considered "free."

Low-sodium diets: Omit salt. Substitute unsalted tomato juice.

18
Breads, Crepes, and Sandwiches

Baking Powder Biscuits

2 cups sifted all-purpose flour
4 teaspoons baking powder
½ teaspoon salt
5 tablespoons margarine
¾ cup skim milk

Preheat oven to 425°F. Sift together flour, baking powder, and salt. Cut margarine in with a blending fork or dough blender until fat is the size of small peas. Add milk all at once. Stir until dough is all mixed and forms a ball. Roll out on a lightly floured board to a thickness of about ¼ inch. Cut with a 2½-inch round cutter or roll thicker and cut with a 2-inch cutter. Place 1 inch apart on a baking sheet. Bake 12 to 14 minutes.

12 biscuits   *1 serving: 1 biscuit*

Nutritive values per serving:

CHO (g)	PRO (g)	FAT (g)	CAL —	Fiber (g)	Sodium (mg)	Chol (mg)
16	3	5	119	0.5	254	0

Food Exchanges per serving: 1 Starch Exchange plus 1 Fat Exchange.

Low-sodium diets: Omit salt. Substitute unsalted margarine.

NEW Applesauce Cinnamon Muffins

Another favorite adapted with the permission of the Quaker Oats Company.

1¼ cups Oat Bran cereal, uncooked
1 cup whole wheat flour
2 teaspoons ground cinnamon
1 teaspoon baking powder
¾ teaspoon baking soda
½ teaspoon salt
¾ cup unsweetened applesauce
½ cup honey
¼ cup vegetable oil
1 egg
1 teaspoon pure vanilla extract
¼ cup chopped walnuts

Preheat oven to 375°F. Coat 12 medium-size cups with vegetable oil or line with paper baking cups. In medium bowl combine Oat Bran cereal, flour, cinnamon, baking powder, soda, and salt. In large bowl combine applesauce, honey, oil, egg, and vanilla. Stir in dry ingredients; mix well. Stir in nuts. Fill prepared muffin cups almost full. Bake 15–20 minutes or until golden brown. Serve warm.

12 muffins   *1 serving: 1 muffin*

			Nutritive values per serving:			
CHO (g)	PRO (g)	FAT (g)	CAL —	Fiber (g)	Sodium (mg)	Chol (mg)
23	3	7	159	2.8	185	23

Food Exchanges per serving: 1 Starch Exchange plus 1 Fat Exchange plus ½ Fruit Exchange.

Low-sodium diets: Omit salt.

Bran Muffins

1 cup All-Bran cereal
⅔ cup skim milk
½ cup sifted all-purpose flour
1½ teaspoons baking powder
½ teaspoon salt
¼ cup sugar
1 medium egg, beaten
2 tablespoons vegetable oil

Preheat oven to 400°F. Prepare nine 2-inch muffin cups with vegetable pan-coating or line with paper baking cups. Combine bran cereal and milk. Sift together flour, baking powder, salt, and sugar. Combine beaten egg and vegetable oil; add to bran and milk; mix well. Add dry ingredients all at once and stir (do not beat) just enough to mix. Measure 3 scant tablespoonfuls batter into each of the nine prepared muffin cups. Bake 25–30 minutes. Cool 5 minutes, then turn out of pans.

9 muffins   *1 serving: 1 muffin*

Nutritive values per serving:

CHO (g)	PRO (g)	FAT (g)	CAL —	Fiber (g)	Sodium (mg)	Chol (mg)
13	3	4	91	3.0	287	31

Food Exchanges per serving: 1 Starch Exchange plus ½ Fat Exchange.

Low-sodium diets: Omit salt. Substitute unsalted margarine.

Variation: Raisin Bran Muffins Add ¼ cup seedless raisins to the dry ingredients in the Bran Muffins recipe.

Nutritive values per serving:

CHO (g)	PRO (g)	FAT (g)	CAL —	Fiber (g)	Sodium (mg)	Chol (mg)
17	3	4	103	3.4	287	31

Food Exchanges per serving: 1 Starch Exchange plus ½ Fat Exchange.

Low-sodium diets: Omit salt. Substitute unsalted margarine.

$\boxed{NEW}$ Oat Bran Muffins

Oat bran is a terrific ingredient in foods for those with diabetes. (See Chapter 5, "Fantastic Fiber.") This recipe was provided courtesy of the Quaker Oats Company.

2¼ cups Oat Bran cereal, uncooked
¼ cup chopped nuts
¼ cup raisins
2 teaspoons baking powder
½ teaspoon salt
¾ cup skim milk
⅓ cup honey
2 eggs, beaten
2 tablespoons vegetable oil

Preheat oven to 425°F. Coat 12 medium-size muffin cups with vegetable oil or line with paper baking cups. In large bowl combine Oat Bran cereal, nuts, raisins, baking powder, and salt. Add remaining ingredients; mix just until dry ingredients are moistened. Fill prepared muffin cups almost full. Bake 15–17 minutes or until golden brown. Serve warm.

12 servings   *1 serving: 1 muffin*

			Nutritive values per serving:			
CHO (g)	PRO (g)	FAT (g)	CAL —	Fiber (g)	Sodium (mg)	Chol (mg)
14	3	5	114	2.6	188	46

Food Exchanges per serving: 1 Starch Exchange plus 1 Fat Exchange.

Low-sodium diets: Omit salt.

Corn Muffins

1 cup yellow cornmeal
¾ cup sifted all-purpose flour
½ teaspoon salt
1½ teaspoons baking powder
½ teaspoon baking soda
1 tablespoon sugar
1 medium egg, beaten
1 cup buttermilk, made from skim milk
2 tablespoons margarine, melted

Preheat oven to 400°F. Prepare 12 2½-inch muffin pans with vegetable pan-coating or line with paper baking cups. Sift together all dry ingredients and mix lightly with a fork. Combine beaten egg, buttermilk, and melted margarine; mix well. Add all at once to dry ingredients. Stir vigorously to mix well, then beat gently for 1–2 minutes. Fill prepared muffin pans half full (3 tablespoons of batter per muffin). Bake for 25–30 minutes. Serve hot.

12 muffins   *1 serving: 1 muffin*

Nutritive values per serving:

CHO (g)	PRO (g)	FAT (g)	CAL —	Fiber (g)	Sodium (mg)	Chol (mg)
17	3	3	104	0.2	206	24

Food Exchanges per serving: 1 Starch Exchange plus ½ Fat Exchange.

Low-sodium diets: Omit salt. Substitute unsalted margarine.

Buttermilk Corn Bread

1 cup sifted all-purpose flour
½ teaspoon baking soda
2 teaspoons baking powder
½ teaspoon salt
1 tablespoon sugar
1 cup yellow cornmeal
1 medium egg, beaten
1 cup buttermilk, made from skim milk
3 tablespoons margarine, melted

Preheat oven to 425°F. Prepare an 8″ × 8″ × 2″ pan with vegetable pan-coating. Sift together dry ingredients. Combine egg, buttermilk, and margarine and add to dry ingredients, stirring until well mixed. Beat with a mixer or rotary beater for 1 minute. Turn into the prepared pan. Bake 20–25 minutes. Cool slightly, then cut into 16 2-inch squares. Serve warm.

16 servings   *1 serving: a 2-inch square piece*

Nutritive values per serving:

CHO (g)	PRO (g)	FAT (g)	CAL —	Fiber (g)	Sodium (mg)	Chol (mg)
14	2	3	91	0.2	173	17

Food Exchanges per serving: 1 Starch Exchange plus ½ Fat Exchange.

Low-sodium diets: Omit salt. Substitute unsalted margarine.

Yankee Johnnycake

If you don't have buttermilk, substitute 1 cup skim milk mixed with 1 teaspoon lemon juice or vinegar.

1 cup sifted all-purpose flour
1 cup yellow cornmeal
1 teaspoon baking soda
½ teaspoon salt
Sugar substitute equivalent to 1 tablespoon sugar
1 medium egg, beaten
1 cup buttermilk, made from skim milk
3 tablespoons vegetable oil

Preheat oven to 400°F. Prepare an 8″ × 8″ × 2″ pan with vegetable pan coating. Sift together all dry ingredients. Combine egg and buttermilk and add to dry ingredients all at once; add oil. Stir (do not beat) just until dry ingredients are moistened. Pour into the prepared pan and bake 25–30 minutes. Cut into 16 2-inch squares.

16 squares   *1 serving: 2-inch square*

Nutritive values per serving:

CHO (g)	PRO (g)	FAT (g)	CAL —	Fiber (g)	Sodium (mg)	Chol (mg)
13	2	3	91	0.2	133	18

Food Exchanges per serving: 1 Starch Exchange plus ½ Fat Exchange.

Low-sodium diets: Omit salt.

NEW   Cracked Wheat Carrot Loaf

½ cup boiling water
¼ cup cracked wheat
1 package active dry yeast
¼ cup warm (110–115°F) water
⅓ cup warm (110–115°F) skim milk

¼ cup margarine
¼ cup firmly packed brown sugar
1 teaspoon salt
1 cup shredded carrot
1 egg
2⅓–2⅔ cups all-purpose flour
⅔ cup Oat Bran cereal

In small bowl pour boiling water over cracked wheat; let stand 15 minutes. Drain excess water; set aside. Dissolve yeast in warm water. In large bowl combine milk, margarine, brown sugar, salt, carrot, and egg. Add dissolved yeast and cracked wheat. The margarine may not melt completely. In small bowl, combine 1 cup of the all-purpose flour and Oat Bran cereal; add to yeast mixture. Beat at medium speed with an electric mixer for 1 minute. Add enough remaining all-purpose flour to make a moderately stiff dough.

Turn out onto lightly floured surface. Knead about 10 minutes or until dough is smooth and elastic. Shape into ball. Grease large bowl. Place dough in bowl, turning once to coat surface. Cover; let rise in warm place about 1½ hours or until nearly double in size.

Grease 9″ × 5″ loaf pan or coat with vegetable pan-coating. Punch dough down; shape into loaf. Place in prepared pan. Cover; let rise in warm place about 1 hour or until nearly double in size. Meanwhile, heat oven to 375°F. Bake 25–30 minutes, shielding crust with aluminum foil after 20 minutes of baking. Remove from pan; cool on wire rack.

12 servings (1 loaf)   *1 serving: 1 ¾-inch slice*

Nutritive values per serving:

CHO (g)	PRO (g)	FAT (g)	CAL —	Fiber (g)	Sodium (mg)	Chol (mg)
30	4	1	146	1.7	187	23

Food Exchanges per serving: 2 Starch Exchanges.

Low-sodium diets: Omit salt. Substitute unsalted margarine.

Dilly Bread

1 cup cream-style cottage cheese, at room
    temperature (70°F)
1 teaspoon salt
1½ tablespoons sugar (needed for yeast action)
2 tablespoons margarine, melted
1 tablespoon dried dill weed
1 teaspoon grated lemon rind
2 tablespoons finely minced green onion
½ cup lukewarm (110–115°F) water
1 package instant active dry yeast
2½ cups all-purpose flour
2 teaspoons margarine, at room temperature

When cottage cheese is warmed to room temperature, add salt, sugar, melted margarine, dill weed, grated lemon rind, and green onion; mix thoroughly, then set aside. Pour the lukewarm water into a large bowl. Sprinkle yeast on top; stir to dissolve. Stir in cottage cheese mixture; blend thoroughly. Add 1¼ cups flour gradually, beating until smooth. Stir (do not beat) in the remaining 1¼ cups flour gradually, mixing well.

Turn onto a lightly floured board; knead until smooth and elastic (about 7–8 minutes). Use 1 teaspoon softened margarine to grease a large bowl. Place dough in this bowl and turn it around to grease lightly on all sides. Cover bowl and place in a warm place, free from drafts, until dough doubles in bulk, about 1 hour. (The oven, turned off, works well for this.) Punch down in 4 or 5 places, turn out on a board, and let the dough rest for 15 minutes. Meanwhile, grease a 9″ × 5″ × 3″ loaf pan with remaining 1 teaspoon softened margarine. Shape dough into a loaf and place in the prepared pan. Cover; let rise in a warm place until center is slightly higher than edge of pan (about 1 hour). Preheat oven to 400°F 10 minutes before end of rising time. Bake loaf about 50 minutes.

22 slices (yield: 22-ounce loaf)   *1 serving: 1-ounce slice*

Nutritive values per serving:

CHO (g)	PRO (g)	FAT (g)	CAL —	Fiber (g)	Sodium (mg)	Chol (mg)
12	3	2	78	0.4	144	1

Food Exchange per serving: 1 Starch Exchange.

Low-sodium diets: Omit salt. Substitute unsalted margarine.

Bread Stuffing

This recipe may be made from any brand of dry herb stuffing mix. The amount here is for a 5- to 8-pound roasting chicken or capon. For a 12- to 16-pound turkey, double the recipe. It is an easy delicious dressing, and for many people the butter and eggs will never be missed!

    1 8-ounce package herb stuffing mix
    1 teaspoon grated lemon rind
    1½ cups (scant) chicken broth, boiling

Combine all ingredients; mix well. Stuff and roast prepared bird.

10 servings (yield: 5 cups)   *1 serving: ½ cup*

Nutritive values per serving:

CHO (g)	PRO (g)	FAT (g)	CAL —	Fiber (g)	Sodium (mg)	Chol (mg)
16	4	1	90	0	418	0

Food Exchange per serving: 1 Starch Exchange.

Low-sodium diets: This recipe is not suitable.

California Sunshine Bread

If the water or orange juice is very hot, the yeast will be destroyed. If the liquid is too cold, the yeast action will be too slow.

- ¼ cup lukewarm (110–115°F) water
- 3 tablespoons sugar (needed for yeast action)
- 1 package instant active dry yeast
- ⅔ cup fresh orange juice (warmed to room temperature)
- 2½ cups unsifted all-purpose flour
- 1 teaspoon salt
- 3 tablespoons margarine, melted
- 1 tablespoon finely grated fresh orange rind
- 1 teaspoon finely grated fresh lemon rind
- 2 teaspoons vegetable oil (to oil pans)

Combine lukewarm water, sugar, and dry yeast in a large bowl, stirring until completely dissolved. Add warm orange juice and beat until well blended. Add 1 cup of the flour gradually, beating gently until smooth. Cover bowl and set in a warm place until bubbly and light (30–40 minutes). Add salt, margarine, and grated orange and lemon rinds; beat gently to mix. Stir in remaining flour gradually, mixing well.

Turn onto a lightly floured board and knead until smooth and elastic (about 10 minutes). Place in a large, oiled bowl, turning dough around to coat all over. Cover bowl; place in a warm place until dough has doubled in size (1–2 hours). Punch dough down in several places. Knead on board for 5 minutes. Shape into a loaf and place in an oiled 8½″ × 4½″ × 2½″ loaf pan. Cover and let rise in a warm place about 1 hour. Preheat oven to 375°F. When bread has risen, bake 35–45 minutes. When done, remove bread from pan and cool on wire rack.

20 slices (yield: 1¼-pound loaf)   *1 serving: 1-ounce slice*

Nutritive values per serving:

CHO (g)	PRO (g)	FAT (g)	CAL —	Fiber (g)	Sodium (mg)	Chol (mg)
15	2	2	87	0.5	123	0

Food Exchange per serving: 1 Starch Exchange.

Low-sodium diets: Omit salt. Substitute unsalted margarine.

NEW Whole Wheat Pita Bread

1 package active dry yeast
1 teaspoon honey (needed for yeast action)
1 cup plus 2 tablespoons warm (110–115°F) water
2¼ cups all-purpose flour
½ cup whole wheat flour
1 teaspoon salt

Add yeast and honey to warm water in a medium-size bowl; let stand until foamy, about 5 minutes. Combine the flours and salt in a large mixing bowl. Pour yeast mixture into center and stir until dough can be gathered into a ball. Knead dough on floured board until smooth. Place dough in large, lightly oiled bowl. Cover with a damp towel and place in a dry, draft-free place until dough has doubled, 1 to 2 hours.

Punch down dough; place on lightly floured board. Divide dough into 12 equal pieces. Shape into circles and place on nonstick cookie sheets. Allow to rest, covered with damp towel, for 30 minutes. On lightly floured board, roll out each piece of dough to a circle, about 5 inches in diameter. Place on cookie sheets; let stand 30 minutes. Bake on middle rack of preheated 500°F oven for 5 minutes. Remove pitas from cookie sheets and let cool on rack. Store in airtight container in refrigerator. To serve, reheat wrapped in aluminum foil at 350°F for 10 minutes.

12 servings   *1 serving: 1 pita*

Nutritive values per serving:

CHO (g)	PRO (g)	FAT (g)	CAL —	Fiber (g)	Sodium (mg)	Chol (mg)
21	3	0	99	0.9	196	0

Food Exchanges per serving: 1½ Starch Exchanges.

Low-sodium diets: Omit salt.

Mustard Whole Wheat Bread

This bread, served with ham or roast beef, is a real treat for picnics.

2 packages instant active dry yeast
¾ cup lukewarm (110–115°F) water
2 teaspoons sugar (needed for yeast action)
1⅓ cups unsifted all-purpose flour
1 teaspoon salt
3 tablespoons margarine, melted
⅓ cup Dijon mustard
1⅓ cups whole wheat flour
2 teaspoons vegetable oil (to oil pans)

Combine yeast, lukewarm water, and sugar in a large bowl; stir until yeast is completely dissolved. Add the white flour gradually, beating until smooth. Cover bowl, set in a warm place, and let rise until surface is all bubbly and batter is light (30–40 minutes). Add salt, margarine, and mustard; mix well. Add whole wheat flour gradually, mixing thoroughly.

Turn onto a lightly floured board and knead for 10 minutes or until light and elastic. Place in a large oiled bowl, turning dough over several times to form a ball that is well coated. Cover bowl and set in a warm place until the dough is doubled in size, about 1–2 hours. Punch down in several places, turn onto a lightly floured board, and knead for 5 minutes. Let rest, covered, for 10 minutes. Shape into a loaf and place in an oiled 8½″ × 4½″ × 2½″ loaf pan. Cover and let rise until doubled in size. When almost ready, preheat oven to 375°F. Bake 40–45 minutes. When done, remove bread from pan and cool on wire rack.

20 slices (yield: 1¼-pound loaf)   *1 serving: 1-ounce slice*

Nutritive values per serving:						
CHO (g)	PRO (g)	FAT (g)	CAL —	Fiber (g)	Sodium (mg)	Chol (mg)
13	2	3	83	1.2	172	0

Food Exchange per serving: 1 Starch Exchange.

Low-sodium diets: Omit salt. Substitute unsalted margarine.

[NEW] Sesame Seed Sandwich Buns

1 cup skim milk
2 tablespoons margarine
2 tablespoons light molasses (needed for yeast
    action)
1 package active dry yeast
¼ cup lukewarm (110–115°F) water
2½ cups whole wheat flour
1 cup all-purpose flour
1 teaspoon salt
3 tablespoons sesame seeds, divided
1 egg white

Heat milk with margarine and molasses in small saucepan until hot but not boiling; cool. Combine yeast and lukewarm water in a large bowl; stir until yeast is completely dissolved. Let stand until foamy, about 5 minutes. Add flours, salt, and half the sesame seeds. Stir in cooled milk mixture; mix well.

Turn onto a floured board and knead until smooth and elastic, about 10 minutes. Place dough in a large, lightly oiled bowl. Cover bowl and set in a warm draft-free place until the dough is doubled, 1–2 hours. Punch down dough. Turn onto a lightly floured board and knead for 5 minutes. Divide dough into 12 medium pieces. Shape into smooth rounds. Place on a nonstick cookie sheet. Let rest, covered with a towel, for 45 minutes. Brush with egg white and sprinkle with remaining sesame seeds. Bake in preheated 375°F oven for 35–40 minutes. When done, remove buns from cookie sheet and cool on wire rack.

12 servings   *1 serving: 1 bun*

Nutritive values per serving:

CHO (g)	PRO (g)	FAT (g)	CAL —	Fiber (g)	Sodium (mg)	Chol (mg)
29	6	4	165	2.5	237	0

Food Exchanges per serving: 2 Starch Exchanges plus 1 Fat
                              Exchange.

Low-sodium diets: Omit salt. Substitute unsalted margarine.

Hotsy Totsy Buns

¾ cup skim milk
2 tablespoons sugar (needed for yeast action)
1½ teaspoons salt
4 tablespoons margarine
2 packages instant active dry yeast
¾ cup lukewarm (110–115°F) water
4½ cups sifted all-purpose flour
1 egg, beaten
¼ cup prepared mild mustard
¾ cup finely chopped onion
1 tablespoon vegetable oil (to oil pans)

Heat milk in the top of a double boiler until skin begins to form on surface. Stir in sugar, salt, and margarine; mix well, then let stand to cool until lukewarm. Add yeast to lukewarm water in a large bowl; stir until dissolved. Stir in the lukewarm milk mixture; mix well. Gently stir in 1 cup of the flour, then the beaten egg, mustard, and onion. Stir in another 1¼ cups flour, beating until smooth. Gradually stir in about another 2¼ cups flour, working it in carefully.

Turn onto a lightly floured board and knead until smooth and elastic. Place in a large bowl oiled with 1 teaspoon of the vegetable oil; turn ball of dough around so it will be well oiled.

Cover bowl lightly. Let rise in a warm place, free from drafts, about 40 minutes or until doubled in bulk. Punch down and let rest for 10 minutes. Turn out onto a lightly floured board. Shape into 2½-inch balls and place ½ inch apart on oiled baking sheets. With palm of hand pat down gently to flatten slightly. Preheat oven to 375°F. Cover buns lightly and let rise until oven is heated. Brush lightly with remaining vegetable oil. Bake about 18–20 minutes. When done, remove buns from cookie sheet and cool on wire rack.

18 buns   *1 serving: 1 bun*

Nutritive values per serving:						
CHO (g)	PRO (g)	FAT (g)	CAL —	Fiber (g)	Sodium (mg)	Chol (mg)
26	4	4	164	0.9	246	15

Food Exchanges per serving: 2 Starch Exchanges plus ½ Fat Exchange.

Low-sodium diets: This recipe is not suitable.

Popovers

If you want really puffed up, high popovers, heat the custard cups or muffin pans before you pour the batter in.

    1 teaspoon vegetable oil (to oil pans)
    2 medium eggs, beaten slightly
    1 cup whole milk
    1 cup sifted all-purpose flour
    ½ teaspoon salt
    2 teaspoons vegetable oil

Preheat oven to 475°F. Oil eight custard cups or 2½-inch muffin pans with vegetable oil and set aside. Combine eggs, milk, flour, and salt and beat until frothy, about 1½ minutes. Add 2 teaspoons vegetable oil; beat only 30 seconds, no more. Pour batter into the custard cups or muffin pans. Bake 15 minutes; then reduce heat to 350°F and bake for another 30 minutes or until firm and browned. A few minutes before popovers are completely cooked, pierce top or side of each with a sharp knife to let the steam escape. If you prefer drier popovers, leave them in the oven with the oven door wide open for 20 minutes after the heat has been turned off.

8 popovers   *1 serving: 1 popover*

Nutritive values per serving:

CHO (g)	PRO (g)	FAT (g)	CAL —	Fiber (g)	Sodium (mg)	Chol (mg)
13	4	4	106	0.4	155	73

Food Exchanges per serving: 1 Starch Exchange plus 1 Fat Exchange.

Low-sodium diets: Omit salt.

NEW Leningrad Special Buckwheat Pancakes

These blinis can be served many ways. Try them with fruited yogurt, one of our sweet spreads (see Index), or pear butter.

½ cup all-purpose flour
¾ cup buckwheat flour
1 teaspoon baking powder
Sugar substitute equivalent to 2 teaspoons sugar
1 egg, beaten slightly
1 cup water
1 tablespoon margarine, melted
1 teaspoon margarine (for cooking)

Blend flours, baking powder, and sugar substitute in a bowl. Mix in egg, water, and melted margarine. Let batter stand for 10 minutes. Melt 1 teaspoon margarine in a 10-inch nonstick skillet over medium heat. Drop batter by the tablespoonful onto hot skillet. Allow pancakes to cook until bubbles form around the edge of the pancakes. Thin remaining batter with additional water if necessary. Turn pancakes over with a spatula. Continue cooking until pancakes are done. Place on a heated dish and continue cooking until all the pancakes have been prepared.

6 servings (24 pancakes)   *1 serving: 4 pancakes*

Nutritive values per serving:

CHO (g)	PRO (g)	FAT (g)	CAL —	Fiber (g)	Sodium (mg)	Chol (mg)
18	3	4	118	0.3	98	46

Food Exchanges per serving: 1 Starch Exchange plus 1 Fat Exchange.

Low-sodium diets: This recipe is suitable.

$\boxed{NEW}$ Basic Crepes

Use the crepes as a wrapper for the Crabmeat Mushroom Crepes (see Index) or fill them with one of our fruit spreads (see Index).

⅔ cup all-purpose flour
⅛ teaspoon salt
2 eggs, beaten
1 cup skim milk
1 tablespoon margarine, melted
½ teaspoon vegetable oil

Combine flour and salt. Gradually add eggs, milk, and margarine, beating until smooth. Refrigerate crepe batter for several hours. Brush the bottom of an 8-inch crepe pan or heavy skillet with oil; place pan over medium heat until oil is hot but not smoking. Pour 3 tablespoons batter into pan; quickly tilt pan in all directions so batter covers pan in a thin film. Cook crepe 1 minute or until edge of crepe lifts easily from pan. Crepe is ready for flipping when it can be shaken loose from pan. Flip crepe and cook about 30 seconds on other side. Place on a towel to cool. Stack between layers of waxed paper to prevent sticking. Repeat procedure with remaining batter.

8 crepes   *1 serving: 2 crepes*

Nutritive values per serving:

CHO (g)	PRO (g)	FAT (g)	CAL —	Fiber (g)	Sodium (mg)	Chol (mg)
19	7	6	163	0.6	158	138

Food Exchanges per serving: 1 Starch Exchange plus 1 Fat Exchange plus ½ Lean Meat Exchange.

Low-sodium diets: Omit salt.

$\boxed{NEW}$ Buckwheat Crepes

Serve these crepes with Sautéed Vegetable Filling (see Index).

1½ cups buckwheat flour
½ cup all-purpose flour
¼ teaspoon salt
3 eggs, beaten slightly
2 cups skim milk
2 teaspoons margarine, melted
½ teaspoon vegetable oil (to oil frying pan)

In a medium-size mixing bowl combine the flours and salt. Blend in eggs, milk, and melted margarine. Whisk until smooth. Let batter stand at room temperature for 30 minutes. If batter is too thick, add water by the tablespoonful until batter is a pouring consistency.

Brush an 8-inch nonstick frying pan with vegetable oil and place over medium heat until warm. Pour 3 tablespoons of the batter into pan; rotate pan to cover pan with a thin coating of batter. Cook about 45 seconds or until crepe is cooked and beginning to brown on the bottom. Turn crepe using a spatula coated with vegetable spray and continue cooking for about 20–30 seconds or until crepe is cooked. Place cooked crepe on a clean dish towel or paper towel on the kitchen counter to absorb excess moisture. Repeat procedure until all the batter has been used. Crepes can be placed between sheets of waxed paper or aluminum foil for easy handling and refrigerated for 3 days or frozen until ready to use.

8 servings (yield: 16 crepes)   *1 serving: 2 crepes*

			Nutritive values per serving:			
CHO (g)	PRO (g)	FAT (g)	CAL —	Fiber (g)	Sodium (mg)	Chol (mg)
24	6	4	154	0.2	130	104

Food Exchanges per serving: 1½ Starch Exchanges plus
½ Medium-Fat Meat Exchange.

Low-sodium diets: Omit salt.

NEW Maine Applesauce Crepes

1½ cups all-purpose flour
¼ teaspoon salt
3 eggs, beaten slightly
2 cups skim milk
2 tablespoons margarine, melted and cooled
1 teaspoon vegetable oil (to grease crepe pan)
2⅔ cups Granny Smith Applesauce (*see* Index)
1 tablespoon margarine, melted
1 cup grated cheddar cheese

Combine flour and salt in a medium-size mixing bowl. Blend in eggs, milk, and the cooled melted margarine. Whisk until smooth. Let batter stand at room temperature for 30 minutes; stir. Brush an 8-inch nonstick crepe pan with vegetable oil and place over medium heat until warm. Pour 3 tablespoons of the batter into pan; rotate pan to cover pan with a thin coating of batter. Cook about 45 seconds or until crepe is dry. Place cooked crepe on a clean dish towel or paper towel on the kitchen counter to absorb excess moisture. Repeat procedure until all the batter has been used. Crepes can be placed between sheets of waxed paper or aluminum foil for easy handling. Refrigerate or freeze crepes no longer than 3 days or until ready to use. After the first few crepes have been cooked it is not necessary to brush pan with oil if it is a well-seasoned pan and crepes are easy to remove.

To assemble: Preheat oven to 325°F. Fill each crepe with ⅓ cup of the applesauce. Roll crepes and arrange seam side down on a 7″ × 11″ glass casserole that has been coated with the melted margarine. Sprinkle crepes with cheese and bake for 8–10 minutes or until crepes have warmed and cheese has melted. Serve hot.

8 servings (yield: 16 crepes)   *1 serving: 2 crepes*

Nutritive values per serving:						
CHO (g)	PRO (g)	FAT (g)	CAL —	Fiber (g)	Sodium (mg)	Chol (mg)
40	11	12	307	3.4	257	119

Food Exchanges per serving: 1½ Starch Exchanges plus 1 Fruit
Exchange plus 1 High-Fat Meat
Exchange plus 1 Fat Exchange.

Low-sodium diets: Omit salt. Substitute unsalted margarine.

Corn Toasties

1 cup sifted all-purpose flour
2 tablespoons sugar
1½ teaspoons baking powder
½ teaspoon salt
½ teaspoon baking soda
2 cups yellow cornmeal
¾ cup buttermilk, made from skim milk
1 medium egg, beaten
2 tablespoons margarine, melted

Sift together flour, sugar, baking powder, salt, and baking
soda. Stir dry ingredients into cornmeal. In another bowl, combine remaining ingredients and beat until frothy and well
blended. Add all at once to dry ingredients; stir until well
mixed. Turn onto a lightly floured board and knead only 10
times. Roll out to a thickness of ¼ inch; cut with a 3-inch-
diameter cutter. Bake on a warm ungreased griddle or frying
pan about 10 minutes on each side.

18 toasties   *1 serving: 1 toastie*

			Nutritive values per serving:			
CHO (g)	PRO (g)	FAT (g)	CAL —	Fiber (g)	Sodium (mg)	Chol (mg)
19	2	2	104	0.2	134	16

Food Exchanges per serving: 1 Starch Exchange plus ½ Fat
Exchange.

Low-sodium diets: Omit salt. Substitute unsalted margarine.

SANDWICHES

Baked Cheese Toastwiches

4 slices bread
1 egg, beaten with fork
2 tablespoons skim milk
¼ teaspoon salt
2 dashes paprika
4 1-ounce slices American cheese

Preheat oven to 400°F. Prepare shallow baking pan with vegetable pan-coating. Toast bread on one side only. Combine beaten egg, milk, salt, and paprika; mix well and pour into a pie plate. Dip bread in this mixture quickly until all is absorbed. Place 2 slices bread toasted side down in prepared pan and cover each with 1 slice cheese. Place remaining 2 slices bread toasted side up on top, then cover with remaining 2 slices cheese. Bake 10–12 minutes.

2 sandwiches   *1 serving: 1 sandwich*

			Nutritive values per serving:			
CHO (g)	PRO (g)	FAT (g)	CAL —	Fiber (g)	Sodium (mg)	Chol (mg)
29	18	19	362	1.4	1219	174

Food Exchanges per serving: 2 Starch Exchanges plus
2 High-Fat Meat Exchanges plus
½ Fat Exchange.

Low-sodium diets: Omit salt. Substitute low-sodium cheese.

Tuna Danish

2 7-ounce cans tuna, packed in oil
1 cup coarsely grated cabbage
⅔ cup grated carrot
½ cup plain low-fat yogurt
3 tablespoons catsup
1½ tablespoons vinegar
½ teaspoon salt
Few grains freshly ground pepper
6 slices bread, toasted
½ head lettuce
18 thin slices pared cucumber
⅛ teaspoon paprika

Drain tuna, then flake lightly. Combine tuna, cabbage, and carrot; set aside. Combine yogurt, catsup, vinegar, salt, and pepper; mix well. Add to tuna mixture and blend. Put 1 piece of toast on each plate; add several lettuce leaves. Add ⅔ cup of tuna mixture. Arrange 3 slices of cucumber across top. Sprinkle lightly with paprika.

6 servings (yield of   *1 serving: ⅔ cup tuna*
tuna mixture: 4 cups)   *mixture plus 1 slice toast*

Nutritive values per serving:

CHO (g)	PRO (g)	FAT (g)	CAL —	Fiber (g)	Sodium (mg)	Chol (mg)
19	23	7	236	2	630	44

Food Exchanges per serving: 2½ Lean Meat Exchanges plus
1 Starch Exchange plus
1 Vegetable Exchange.

Low-sodium diets: Omit salt. Use unsalted canned tuna and catsup.

Tuna Salad Sandwich

Use ¼ cup to spread on one slice of bread for an open-face sandwich or between two slices of bread for a regular sandwich, or mound on crisp lettuce.

1 3½-ounce can tuna, packed in oil
¼ cup finely chopped celery
1 tablespoon finely chopped green pepper
⅛ teaspoon salt
Few grains freshly ground pepper
1 tablespoon finely chopped green onion
¼ cup plain low-fat yogurt
1 teaspoon fresh lemon juice or vinegar
1 tablespoon grated American cheese

Drain tuna well, then flake it into a bowl. Add remaining ingredients and mix well.

3 servings (yield: ¾ cup)   *1 serving: ¼ cup*

CHO (g)	PRO (g)	FAT (g)	CAL —	Fiber (g)	Sodium (mg)	Chol (mg)
2	11	4	98	0.2	279	26

Nutritive values per serving:

Food Exchanges per serving: 1½ Lean Meat Exchanges.

Low-sodium diets: Omit salt. Substitute unsalted canned tuna.

Pizza Snacks

3 slices fresh bread
2 tablespoons catsup or tomato paste
1 tablespoon finely chopped green pepper
1 tablespoon finely chopped mushrooms
Dash dried oregano or basil
¼ cup shredded mozzarella cheese

Roll bread slices flat and thin with a rolling pin or an empty quart jar. Place on a flat pan 3 inches under the broiler; heat

until lightly toasted on one side, then remove from oven. Turn slices over and spread untoasted sides with a layer of each of the remaining ingredients, in the order listed, ending with a sprinkling of cheese. Broil until cheese melts and browns slightly. To serve, cut each pizza into quarters.

3 servings *1 serving: 1 pizza*

Nutritive values per serving:

CHO (g)	PRO (g)	FAT (g)	CAL —	Fiber (g)	Sodium (mg)	Chol (mg)
16	7	4	123	0.8	278	5

Food Exchanges per serving: 1 Starch Exchange plus ½ Lean Meat Exchange.

Low-sodium diets: Substitute tomato paste for catsup.

NEW Cold Turkey Reuben Sandwich

    4 teaspoons plain low-fat yogurt
    8 slices rye bread
    8 ounces thinly sliced cooked turkey breast
    1⅓ cups Sweet and Sour Red Cabbage, drained
       (*see* Index)

Spread 1 teaspoon yogurt on each of 4 slices of rye bread. Divide the sliced turkey among tops of the bread slices. Spoon ⅓ cup Sweet and Sour Red Cabbage on each sandwich; top with remaining bread.

4 servings *1 serving: 1 sandwich*

Nutritive values per serving:

CHO (g)	PRO (g)	FAT (g)	CAL —	Fiber (g)	Sodium (mg)	Chol (mg)
31	22	5	254	2.3	351	40

Food Exchanges per serving: 2 Starch Exchanges plus 2 Lean Meat Exchanges.

Low-sodium diets: Omit salt from Sweet and Sour Red Cabbage.

Chicken Salad Baked in Nests

Students at Mundelein College tested this recipe, and they judged it a prizewinner.

4 hard rolls
½ cup Lemon Mayonnaise (*see* Index)
1½ teaspoons curry powder
1½ cups lightly packed diced cooked chicken
½ cup diced tomato
¼ cup finely chopped green onion
2 1-ounce slices American cheese, halved

Preheat oven to 350°F. Cut top off rolls and scoop out soft bread from inside. Discard scooped-out portions. Mix Lemon Mayonnaise and curry powder; add chicken, tomato, and onion and mix again. Spoon mixture into the nests (each nest will hold ½ cup of the mixture). Place nests in a shallow baking pan and cover with foil. Bake 20 minutes; remove foil and put ½ slice of American cheese on top of each; continue baking, uncovered, 8–10 minutes, until cheese melts.

4 servings   *1 serving: 1 nest*

Nutritive values per serving:

CHO (g)	PRO (g)	FAT (g)	CAL —	Fiber (g)	Sodium (mg)	Chol (mg)
35	20	8	290	0.6	767	85

Food Exchanges per serving: 2 Starch Exchanges plus 2 Lean Meat Exchanges.

Low-sodium diets: Omit salt from Lemon Mayonnaise. Use low-sodium cheese.

19
Meats

BEEF

Berna's Round Steak

2 pounds round steak
2 tablespoons vegetable oil
½ teaspoon ground ginger
¼ teaspoon garlic powder
½ teaspoon salt
2 cups beef broth
1 tablespoon cornstarch
2 tablespoons water
1 tablespoon soy sauce
1 green pepper, cut into thin strips

Cut off separable fat and discard. Cut lean meat into ½- by 3-inch strips. Brown meat in oil. Add ginger, garlic powder, salt, and broth. Bring to a boil, lower heat, and cover pan. Cook for 1 hour or until tender. Blend cornstarch, water, and soy sauce and stir this mixture into the pan. Add green pepper and cook a few minutes until sauce is thickened and clear.

6 servings (yield: 4 cups)   *1 serving: ⅔ cup*

Nutritive values per serving:

CHO (g)	PRO (g)	FAT (g)	CAL —	Fiber (g)	Sodium (mg)	Chol (mg)
2	28	12	235	0.2	647	72

Food Exchanges per serving: 4 Lean Meat Exchanges.

Low-sodium diets: Omit salt. Substitute unsalted broth and sodium-reduced (light) soy sauce.

Flank Steak Swiss Style

Unless you marinate it or are able to get prime-quality (top, fancy-grade) flank steak, do not attempt to just broil it for it will be tough. The best method to cook this very lean cut is by braising, and here is a simple, delicious recipe that follows the basic braising directions of professional meat experts.

1½ pounds flank steak
2 tablespoons all-purpose flour
1 teaspoon salt
¼ teaspoon coarsely ground pepper
1 teaspoon dry mustard
2 tablespoons vegetable oil
2 cups hot water
2 beef bouillon cubes
½ cup chopped onion
½ cup chopped celery
¼ cup catsup

Preheat oven to 325°F. Cut meat into six equal individual serving pieces. Combine flour, salt, pepper, and mustard; mix well and place in a paper bag. Shake each piece of meat in the bag to coat evenly with seasoned flour; place floured pieces aside. Heat vegetable oil in large frying pan over medium heat. Brown meat pieces in hot oil, turning frequently. Place browned meat in a large shallow casserole; set aside. Put hot water, bouillon cubes, vegetables, and catsup into the frying pan. Stir over medium heat until bouillon cubes are dissolved. Spread vegetable mixture evenly on top of meat. Cover and cook in oven for 2½ hours or until meat is fork-tender. Or prepare this recipe on top of the stove in a 12-inch frying pan. After browning meat, spread vegetables on top, combine remaining ingredients until bouillon cubes are dissolved, pour on top of meat, cover pan tightly, and simmer gently 2–2½ hours.

6 servings   *1 serving: ⅙ of meat plus*
                                ⅓ cup gravy and vegetables

Nutritive values per serving:

CHO (g)	PRO (g)	FAT (g)	CAL —	Fiber (g)	Sodium (mg)	Chol (mg)
6	25	11	234	0.4	813	79

Food Exchanges per serving: 3½ Lean Meat Exchanges plus 1 Vegetable Exchange.

Low-sodium diets: Omit salt. Use low-sodium catsup and low-sodium beef bouillon cubes.

Roast Beef with Anchovies

4 pounds eye of round of beef, well trimmed
2 tablespoons olive oil
1 2-ounce can flat anchovies, packed in oil
2 teaspoons coarsely ground pepper

Preheat oven to 300°F. Rub beef with olive oil and oil from anchovy can. Cut slits into beef and insert half the anchovies inside the slits; spread remaining anchovies on top of meat. Sprinkle roast with pepper. Put roast in a shallow roasting pan; cover tightly with foil. For medium-rare, roast 1 hour. Meat thermometer should read 150°F. Cook longer if you prefer your meat more well done.

12 servings   1 serving: 4 ounces lean mean. (Hearty eaters may have larger portions, so plan accordingly.)

Nutritive values per serving:

CHO (g)	PRO (g)	FAT (g)	CAL —	Fiber (g)	Sodium (mg)	Chol (mg)
0	29	12	223	0	292	91

Food Exchanges per serving: 4 Lean Meat Exchanges.

Low-sodium diets: This recipe is not suitable.

Peppered Rib Eye

Start early or the day before—this must be marinated for at least 12 hours.

6 pounds boneless rib eye roast, well trimmed
⅓ cup peppercorns (more or less to taste)
1 teaspoon ground cardamom
1 cup soy sauce
¾ cup vinegar
1 tablespoon tomato paste
1 teaspoon paprika
½ teaspoon garlic powder *or* 2 cloves garlic, minced

Wipe roast with dampened paper towel. Put peppercorns in a small paper or plastic bag and pound them with a rolling pin or meat mallet until well cracked. Mix cracked peppercorns and cardamom and press into meat. Mix remaining ingredients to make a marinade. Pour marinade over meat and store in the refrigerator for 12 hours or longer, turning meat in marinade occasionally. Wrap beef in foil and roast at 300°F for 2 hours for medium-rare or longer if you prefer.

About 12 servings   *1 serving: 4 ounces lean meat.*
(yield: 45 ounces   *(Hearty eaters may have larger*
lean meat)   *portions, so plan accordingly.)*

Nutritive values per serving:

CHO (g)	PRO (g)	FAT (g)	CAL —	Fiber (g)	Sodium (mg)	Chol (mg)
2	30	15	264	0	770	85

Food Exchanges per serving: 4 Lean Meat Exchanges.

Low-sodium diets: Use sodium-reduced (light) soy sauce. Marinate meat in Miracle Red "French" Dressing (*see* Index), omitting the salt and adding extra garlic, instead of the marinade mixture above. Cook as directed.

Roast Beef with Caraway Seeds

¾ cup chopped onion
1 teaspoon salt
1 tablespoon caraway seeds
2½ pounds boneless rolled rump or chuck roast
1 tablespoon vegetable oil
⅓ cup vinegar
1 cup unsweetened apple juice
Water

Preheat oven to 325°F. Combine ¼ cup of the onions with salt and caraway seeds. Press this mixture into the roast. In a roasting pan heat the oil and add remaining onion; stir over medium heat for 5 minutes, until onions are translucent. Put roast in pan; add vinegar, apple juice, and enough water to cover the bottom of the pan with ½ inch liquid. Bake, uncovered, about 1½ hours for medium rare or longer if you prefer. Baste with liquid several times during cooking. Trim away extra fat and discard drippings.

7 servings (yield: 1¾ pounds cooked before final trimming; 22 ounces edible lean meat)

1 serving: 3-ounce slice of lean beef

Nutritive values per serving:

CHO (g)	PRO (g)	FAT (g)	CAL —	Fiber (g)	Sodium (mg)	Chol (mg)
5	30	12	249	0.3	340	90

Food Exchanges per serving: 4 Lean Meat Exchanges plus 1 Vegetable Exchange.

Low-sodium diets: Substitute 2 cloves garlic, crushed, for the salt.

Creole Steak

2 pounds lean round steak
¼ cup all-purpose flour
2 teaspoons salt
2 teaspoons paprika
½ teaspoon freshly ground pepper
3 tablespoons vegetable oil
1 cup chopped onion
⅓ cup chopped green pepper
1 16-ounce can tomatoes
½ cup raw rice
1 cup condensed beef broth
1 cup water

Cut steak into seven equal serving pieces. Mix flour, salt, paprika, and pepper; dredge meat in mixture. Heat oil in a large frying pan. Lightly brown onions and peppers and remove from oil. Brown meat in remaining oil. Cover meat with onion and green pepper. Cut up tomatoes and add with their liquid to meat. Sprinkle rice into pan; add broth and water. Mix thoroughly. Bring to a boil, lower heat, and cover tightly. Simmer 1½ hours or until meat is tender, stirring occasionally.

7 servings   1 serving: 3 ounces meat plus ½ cup rice mixture

Nutritive values per serving:

CHO (g)	PRO (g)	FAT (g)	CAL —	Fiber (g)	Sodium (mg)	Chol (mg)
19	26	13	300	1.3	933	62

Food Exchanges per serving: 3 Lean Meat Exchanges plus
1 Starch Exchange plus
1 Vegetable Exchange.

Low-sodium diets: Omit salt. Use unsalted canned tomatoes and beef broth.

Swiss Steak

1 2-pound round steak, ¾ inch thick
2 tablespoons all-purpose flour
1 teaspoon salt
½ teaspoon freshly ground pepper, divided
1 tablespoon vegetable oil
1 16-ounce can tomatoes, cut up, with liquid
1 cup chopped onion
1 medium green pepper, sliced
1 2½-ounce can sliced mushrooms
1 tablespoon cornstarch
¼ cup cold water

Trim fat and bone from meat and divide meat into six portions. Mix flour, salt, and ¼ teaspoon pepper together and sprinkle over both sides of meat; pound flour mixture into meat with a meat mallet or the side of a heavy plate. Brown meat in vegetable oil in a heavy frying pan. Add tomatoes, tomato liquid, and onion; cover and bring to boil. Reduce heat and simmer about 2 hours or until meat is tender. Add green pepper and mushrooms during last 10 minutes of cooking. Put meat on heated platter, leaving tomato mixture in frying pan. Blend cornstarch into cold water, blend into pan liquids and add remaining ¼ teaspoon pepper. Cook, stirring constantly, until gravy is thickened.

6 servings   1 serving: 4 ounces steak plus ½ cup sauce

			Nutritive values per serving:			
CHO (g)	PRO (g)	FAT (g)	CAL —	Fiber (g)	Sodium (mg)	Chol (mg)
10	28	10	244	1.5	500	72

Food Exchanges per serving: 3½ Lean Meat Exchanges plus 2 Vegetable Exchanges.

Low-sodium diets: Omit salt. Use unsalted canned tomatoes.

Old-Fashioned Beef Stew

This recipe may be simmered in a large covered pot on top of the stove. The oven method saves pot watching.

¼ cup all-purpose flour
1¼ teaspoons salt
⅛ teaspoon freshly ground black pepper
¼ teaspoon dry mustard
1¼ pounds top round steak, 1 inch thick
1 tablespoon vegetable oil
2½ cups water
1 teaspoon Worcestershire sauce
2 cups pared, quartered, and sliced potato
1 cup sliced onion
1 cup sliced carrot
½ teaspoon dill weed (optional)

Preheat oven to 350°F. Combine flour, salt, pepper, and mustard in a paper bag. Trim off all fat around outside of round steak; cut meat into 1-inch cubes. Shake meat cubes in the paper bag with flour, a few at a time, until well coated. Heat oil in a large frying pan; brown meat cubes over medium heat, turning with tongs until meat is evenly browned. Transfer meat cubes to a 2½-quart casserole; set aside. Sprinkle seasoned flour remaining in paper bag into the fat remaining in the frying pan; stir vigorously until smooth and mixed. Add water very slowly and stir; add Worcestershire sauce. Cook and stir until smooth; pour on top of meat in casserole. Cover and cook in the oven for 2 hours. Mix vegetables and dill weed into meat, cover, and cook in oven for 1 more hour or until meat and vegetables are tender.

Variation: Old-Fashioned Lamb Stew Substitute lean lamb and add 1 teaspoon extra dill.

4 servings (yield: 4 cups)   *1 serving: 1 cup*

			Nutritive values per serving:			
CHO (g)	PRO (g)	FAT (g)	CAL —	Fiber (g)	Sodium (mg)	Chol (mg)
31	36	13	391	3.2	719	90

Food Exchanges per serving: 4 Lean Meat Exchanges plus
2 Starch Exchanges.

Low-sodium diets: Omit salt.

Spicy Meatballs with Tomato Sauce

1 pound 85% lean ground beef
1 large egg, beaten
¼ cup beef broth
¼ teaspoon dry mustard
1 teaspoon chili powder
½ teaspoon crushed dried marjoram
⅛ teaspoon garlic powder *or* 1 clove garlic, minced
½ teaspoon salt
1 slice fresh bread, crumbled fine
1 15-ounce can tomato sauce with tomato bits
¼ cup water

Preheat oven to 400°F. Prepare a shallow baking pan with
vegetable pan-coating; set aside. Combine all ingredients except tomato sauce and water. Mix meat ingredients well. Form
into 12 balls, allowing 3 level tablespoonfuls for each ball;
place in the pan about 2 inches apart. Bake 18–20 minutes.
Heat tomato sauce with tomato bits and water in saucepan.
Pour sauce over meatballs prior to serving.

4 servings (yield: 12 meatballs   *1 serving: 3 meatballs*
plus 2 cups sauce)   *plus ½ cup sauce*

Nutritive values per serving:

CHO (g)	PRO (g)	FAT (g)	CAL —	Fiber (g)	Sodium (mg)	Chol (mg)
11	26	20	326	0.2	1069	69

Food Exchanges per serving: 3 Medium-Fat Meat Exchanges
plus 2 Vegetable Exchanges.

Low-sodium diets: Omit salt. Substitute water for beef broth.
Substitute low-sodium catsup for tomato
sauce.

Beef and Zucchini Casserole

2 teaspoons vegetable oil
½ cup finely chopped onion
1 pound (3 small) zucchini
1 4-ounce can mushroom pieces
1 pound 85% lean ground beef
1 16-ounce can tomatoes
¼ teaspoon salt
2 cloves garlic, minced
½ teaspoon dried oregano
¼ cup grated Parmesan cheese

Preheat oven to 350°F. Heat oil in a frying pan; add onion and stir over medium heat until tender and light golden in color. Wash zucchini, discard ends, and cut crosswise into ¼-inch slices; add to onion; add mushrooms and liquid in can; cook and stir for 3–4 minutes over medium heat. Turn into a 2-quart casserole. Turn ground beef into the frying pan, stir over medium heat, and cook until color changes; drain well. Cut up canned tomatoes in their own liquid; add salt, garlic, and oregano to tomatoes. Add to meat and mix well. Add meat mixture to zucchini in casserole. Mix carefully. Sprinkle cheese on top. Bake 35–40 minutes.

6 servings (yield: 6 cups)   *1 serving: 1 cup*

Nutritive values per serving:

CHO (g)	PRO (g)	FAT (g)	CAL —	Fiber (g)	Sodium (mg)	Chol (mg)
8	23	16	262	2.3	336	66

Food Exchanges per serving: 3 Medium-Fat Meat Exchanges plus 1 Vegetable Exchange.

Low-sodium diets: Omit salt. Use unsalted canned tomatoes and substitute 1 cup sliced fresh mushrooms.

Beef Porcupines in Tomato Gravy

1 pound 85% lean ground beef
¼ cup raw long-grain rice
¼ cup dry bread crumbs
1 teaspoon salt
2 tablespoons minced fresh parsley
2 tablespoons water
1 tablespoon vegetable oil
1 10½-ounce can tomato soup
½ teaspoon garlic powder *or* 2 cloves garlic, minced
1 teaspoon Worcestershire sauce
2 cups water

Combine ground beef, rice, bread crumbs, salt, parsley, and 2 tablespoons water. Shape into an 8-inch square or pack evenly into an 8-inch square pan. Cut three lines on one side and four lines on the other side to make 20 equal sections; shape each section into a meatball. Heat oil in a large skillet; brown meatballs in hot oil over medium heat, turning frequently. Combine tomato soup, garlic powder, Worcestershire sauce, and 2 cups water. Add to meatballs; cover and simmer gently for 1 hour or until rice is tender. Serve meatballs with tomato gravy from pan.

4 servings (yield: 20 meatballs   *1 serving: 5 meatballs*
plus 1⅓ cups gravy)   *plus ⅓ cup gravy*

Nutritive values per serving:

CHO (g)	PRO (g)	FAT (g)	CAL —	Fiber (g)	Sodium (mg)	Chol (mg)
23	26	23	405	0.2	1158	78

Food Exchanges per serving: 3 Medium-Fat Meat Exchanges plus 1½ Starch Exchanges plus 1 Fat Exchange.

Low-sodium diets: Omit salt. Use unsalted tomato soup.

Kay's Favorite Meat Loaf

This meat loaf is great cold, served plain or in sandwiches. Good hot, too!

> 1 beef bouillon cube
> ½ cup boiling water
> 2 slices bread, crumbled fine
> 1½ pounds 85% lean ground beef
> 2 medium eggs, beaten slightly
> ½ cup finely chopped onion
> ¼ cup finely chopped celery
> 2 teaspoons Worcestershire sauce
> 1 tablespoon catsup

Preheat oven to 350°F. Line a shallow 8-inch baking pan with foil. Dissolve beef bouillon cube in boiling water in a large bowl. Add all other ingredients except the catsup and blend well with a fork. Turn onto foil in pan and, with hands, shape quickly into a 6 by 4½ by 2 inch loaf. With the dull edge of a knife make a crisscross pattern across the top; spread catsup on top. Cover loaf with a tent of foil that does not touch the top. Bake for 45 minutes. Remove foil; bake, uncovered, for another 45 minutes. Remove from oven and cool in pan for 2–3 minutes before serving. Using this molded method instead of loaf pan allows the fat to drain from the loaf, whereas a loaf pan retains fat.

6–8 servings   *1 serving: 1 large slice (4½ by 2 by 1 inch) or 1 medium slice (4½ by 2 by ¾ inch)*

Nutritive values per serving (1 large slice, ⅙ of loaf):

CHO (g)	PRO (g)	FAT (g)	CAL —	Fiber (g)	Sodium (mg)	Chol (mg)
7	25	15	267	0.5	334	91

Food Exchanges per serving: 3 Medium-Fat Meat Exchanges plus 1 Vegetable Exchange plus 1 Fat Exchange.

Low-sodium diets: Substitute a low-sodium bouillon cube.

Nutritive values per serving (1 medium slice, ⅛ of loaf):

CHO (g)	PRO (g)	FAT (g)	CAL —	Fiber (g)	Sodium (mg)	Chol (mg)
5	19	10	189	0.4	251	69

Food Exchanges per serving: 2 Medium-Fat Meat Exchanges plus 1 Vegetable Exchange.

Low-sodium diets: Substitute a low-sodium bouillon cube.

Ground Beef Patties

Americans consumed over one billion hamburgers last year! This is an excellent basic recipe with two different preparation methods.

1 teaspoon salt
½ teaspoon dry mustard
¼ teaspoon freshly ground pepper
1 tablespoon water
2 teaspoons Worcestershire sauce
1 pound 85% lean beef, ground once

Combine seasonings and liquid, sprinkle on top of meat, and mix together. To make four meat patties, measure ½ cup for each. To make six meat patties, measure ⅓ cup for each. Shape lightly into patties.

To *oven-broil* remove broiler rack from oven; preheat broiler for 10 minutes. Arrange patties on cold rack and place rack 3 inches below broiler heat. For thick patties broil 4–6 minutes on each side, turning once with a wide spatula. Thin patties will require 3–5 minutes on each side.

To *pan-broil* use a nonstick frying pan or a heavy regular metal frying pan prepared with vegetable pan coating. Heat pan over high heat for about 30 seconds. Add meat patties and brown on both sides, then turn heat to medium and cook 4–8 minutes. Do not press down on patties with spatula or "spank" them, or you will get dry patties.

4–6 servings   *1 serving: 1 large or 1 small patty*

Nutritive values per serving (1 large patty):

CHO (g)	PRO (g)	FAT (g)	CAL —	Fiber (g)	Sodium (mg)	Chol (mg)
1	22	18	257	0	590	78

Food Exchanges per serving: 3 Medium-Fat Meat Exchanges.

Low-sodium diets: Omit salt.

Nutritive values per serving (1 small patty)

CHO (g)	PRO (g)	FAT (g)	CAL —	Fiber (g)	Sodium (mg)	Chol (mg)
0	15	12	171	0	394	52

Food Exchanges per serving: 2 Medium-Fat Meat Exchanges.

Low-sodium diets: Omit salt.

Variation: Cheeseburgers After turning meat patties once, place on top of each patty a 1-ounce slice of American cheese. Finish cooking.

Nutritive values per serving (1 large patty with cheese):

CHO (g)	PRO (g)	FAT (g)	CAL —	Fiber (g)	Sodium (mg)	Chol (mg)
1	28	27	364	0	1001	27

Food Exchanges per serving: 4 Medium-Fat Meat Exchanges plus 1 Fat Exchange.

Low-sodium diets: Omit salt. Substitute low-sodium cheese.

Chili Con Carne

If you break crackers on top of chili, count 5 saltines or ½ cup oyster crackers as 68 more calories and add CHO 15 g, PRO 3 g, and 1 Bread Exchange.

1 pound 85% lean ground beef
1¼ teaspoons salt
1 cup chopped onion
1 cup finely chopped celery
½ cup finely cut green pepper
1 16-ounce can tomatoes, cut up, with liquid
¼ teaspoon garlic powder *or* 1 clove garlic, minced
½ teaspoon dried oregano
1 tablespoon chili powder (more if desired)
1 16-ounce can kidney beans
½ cup beef broth

Turn beef into a 2½-quart nonstick pot or coat pot with vegetable pan-coating; sprinkle with salt. Stir over medium heat with a blending fork (not a spoon) until all meat changes color. Add onion, celery, and green pepper; mix well. Cover and cook over medium heat 2–3 minutes. Add tomatoes and liquid and all seasonings, mixing well. Bring to a boil; cover, reduce heat to low, and simmer gently for 25 minutes, stirring occasionally. Add kidney beans and beef broth. Continue cooking over low heat 15–20 minutes.

6 servings (yield: 4½ cups)   *1 serving: ¾ cup*

CHO (g)	PRO (g)	FAT (g)	CAL —	Fiber (g)	Sodium (mg)	Chol (mg)
20	21	13	273	5.1	925	50

Nutritive values per serving:

Food Exchanges per serving: 2 Medium-Fat Meat Exchanges plus 1 Starch Exchange plus 1 Vegetable Exchange.

Low-sodium diets: Omit salt. Use unsalted canned vegetables and unsalted beef broth. Use unsalted crackers for topping.

Sloppy Joes

This is one of Kay's most famous recipes. Nondiabetic families with children make this frequently because they like it so much.

1 teaspoon salt
1 pound 85% lean beef, ground twice
¼ cup finely chopped onion
¾ cup finely chopped celery with leaves
¼ cup chopped green pepper
½ teaspoon grated lemon rind
¼ cup catsup
¾ cup beef broth
½ teaspoon dry mustard
1 teaspoon Worcestershire sauce

Add salt to meat. Turn into a large, dry, cold frying pan. Stir over medium heat with a large kitchen fork (not a spoon) until meat changes color all over, pouring off any liquid fat as it collects. Add onion, celery, and green pepper. Stir and cook 1–2 minutes. Combine all remaining ingredients; add to meat and mix well. Bring to a boil, cover, reduce heat to low, and let simmer gently for 15–20 minutes, stirring frequently, until cooked and well mixed.

6 servings (yield: 3 cups)   *1 serving: ½ cup*

Nutritive values per serving:

CHO (g)	PRO (g)	FAT (g)	CAL —	Fiber (g)	Sodium (mg)	Chol (mg)
4	15	9	165	0.3	589	47

Food Exchanges per serving: 2 Medium-Fat Meat Exchanges plus 1 Vegetable Exchange. When served on whole hamburger bun, add 2 Starch Exchanges.

Low-sodium diets: Omit salt. Use low-sodium catsup and unsalted beef broth.

Beef Crust Pizza

CRUST

1 pound 85% lean ground beef
1 slice bread, crumbled fine
1 medium egg, beaten
2 teaspoons onion powder
½ teaspoon garlic powder *or* 2 cloves garlic, minced
1 teaspoon salt
¼ teaspoon freshly ground pepper
½ teaspoon dried oregano

FILLING

1 6-ounce can tomato paste
½ teaspoon dried basil
1¼ cups thinly sliced green pepper
1 4-ounce can mushroom pieces, drained
4 ounces shredded mozzarella cheese

Preheat oven to 375°F. Combine all crust ingredients and mix thoroughly. Press into a 10-inch pie pan to form a crust. Bake 10 minutes. Leaving crust in the pie pan, drain off all liquid fat. Spread tomato paste on bottom and sides of crust, then sprinkle with basil. Spread on even layers of sliced green pepper, mushrooms, and cheese. Bake 15 minutes. Serve immediately, cutting pizza into six equal wedges.

6 servings (yield: 1 10-inch pizza)   *1 serving: ⅙ of pizza*

Nutritive values per serving:

CHO (g)	PRO (g)	FAT (g)	CAL —	Fiber (g)	Sodium (mg)	Chol (mg)
11	27	17	304	0.8	726	120

Food Exchanges per serving: 3 Medium-Fat Meat Exchanges
                                                  plus 2 Vegetable Exchanges.

Low-sodium diets: Omit salt. Substitute 1 cup sliced fresh
                             mushrooms and low-sodium cheese.

Meat-Stuffed Eggplant

2 eggplants (about 1 pound each)
1½ teaspoons salt
¼ teaspoon freshly ground pepper
1 pound 85% lean ground beef
1 cup chopped onion
1 tablespoon minced fresh parsley
½ teaspoon dried oregano
1 16-ounce can tomato paste
2 tablespoons Worcestershire sauce
1 tablespoon grated Parmesan cheese

Preheat oven to 350°F. Cut eggplants in half lengthwise; scoop out centers, leaving ½-inch walls. Sprinkle shells with salt and pepper and place cut side up in a large shallow baking dish. Chop scooped-out eggplant centers and set aside. In a large frying pan, brown the meat, stirring; pour off fat. Stir in chopped eggplant, onion, parsley, and oregano. Cook over medium heat about 10 minutes or until tender, stirring occasionally. Add tomato paste and Worcestershire sauce; mix well. Spoon about ¾ cup of the mixture into each eggplant shell. Sprinkle with cheese. Cover with foil and bake 45–50 minutes.

4 servings   *1 serving: ½ eggplant with stuffing*

Nutritive values per serving:

CHO (g)	PRO (g)	FAT (g)	CAL —	Fiber (g)	Sodium (mg)	Chol (mg)
28	34	20	418	7.1	1259	96

Food Exchanges per serving: 4 Lean Meat Exchanges plus
1 Starch Exchange plus
1 Vegetable Exchange.

Low-sodium diets: Omit salt. Use unsalted tomato paste.

Party Beef Tenderloin

A whole beef tenderloin, when trimmed, will be approximately 4 pounds (raw). Have your meat cutter trim a whole or a half tenderloin. He will lard it or put strips of fat across the top because it is a very lean cut.

    1 whole beef tenderloin, trimmed
    2 teaspoons minced fresh garlic
    1 teaspoon cracked pepper
    ½ teaspoon salt

Preheat oven to 450°F. Season roast with garlic, cracked pepper, and salt or your favorite seasonings. Put tenderloin on a rack in an uncovered roasting pan and roast 45–50 minutes for rare to medium-rare beef. A meat thermometer will register 140°F. This cut is also wonderful cooked on a barbecue but be careful not to overcook it. The diabetic should discard fat from around outside edges of meat. The diabetic's portion should be weighed as cooked lean meat; the number of ounces is approximately equal to the number of allowed Meat Exchanges for that meal.

10 servings   1 serving: 3 ounces (Hearty eaters will want more, so plan accordingly.)

Nutritive values per serving:

CHO (g)	PRO (g)	FAT (g)	CAL —	Fiber (g)	Sodium (mg)	Chol (mg)
0	26	8	186	0	138	76

Food Exchanges per serving: 3 Lean Meat Exchanges.

Low-sodium diets: Omit salt.

Joan's Beef Oriental

    1 pound lean round steak, ¼ inch thick
    2 tablespoons vegetable oil
    1½ cups hot water

1 beef bouillon cube
1 tablespoon soy sauce
1 clove garlic, crushed
⅛ teaspoon coarsely ground pepper
½ cup raw carrot strips (3 by ¼ inches)
½ cup diagonally sliced celery
1 cup firmly packed diagonally sliced green onion
1 cup chopped green pepper, 1-inch squares
2½ cups (about ½ pound) sliced fresh mushrooms
½ cup drained sliced water chestnuts
1–1½ cups boiling water
2 tablespoons cornstarch
¼ cup cold water

If time allows, partially freeze meat for easier slicing. Remove and discard fat around outside; cut meat into thin strips, 3–4 inches long and ⅛ inch thick. Heat oil in a large heavy frying pan. Brown meat strips, stirring with a wooden spoon to brown all over. Add 1½ cups hot water, beef bouillon cube, soy sauce, garlic, and black pepper. Cover and simmer very slowly for 40 minutes. Meanwhile, prepare vegetables. When meat is cooked, add vegetables in order listed, spreading evenly. If meat is cooked almost dry, add 1½ cups boiling water; otherwise, add 1 cup. Cover and let cook over low heat 10 minutes. Mix cornstarch into cold water. Add slowly to liquid in pan. Stir and cook over moderate heat until thick, smooth, and clear.

4 servings (yield: 4 cups)   *1 serving: 1 cup*

Nutritive values per serving:

CHO (g)	PRO (g)	FAT (g)	CAL —	Fiber (g)	Sodium (mg)	Chol (mg)
15	23	11	254	2.3	539	52

Food Exchanges per serving: 3 Lean Meat Exchanges plus 2 Vegetable Exchanges.

Low-sodium diets: Use low-sodium bouillon cube. Substitute sodium-reduced (light) soy sauce.

Sukiyaki

Sukiyaki can be arranged decoratively on a large platter and cooked at the table using an electric skillet, a wok, or a chafing dish. This dish is traditionally served with steamed rice.

1 pound boneless lean skirt steak, sirloin, or
    tenderloin, partially frozen
6 green onions, cut into 1½-inch slivers
1 cup sliced onion
1 cup sliced celery
1 cup sliced mushrooms
1 quart water
5 ounces bean threads or other transparent noodles
    suitable for sukiyaki
2 ounces soft tofu, cut into ½-inch cubes
½ pound fresh spinach, trimmed, washed, and
    dried with paper towels
4 tablespoons beef broth

SAUCE
¼ cup reduced-sodium (light) soy sauce
4 tablespoons dry white wine
¼ cup beef broth
Sugar substitute equivalent to 2 tablespoons sugar

Meat is partially frozen to aid in slicing; cut against the grain in paper-thin ($\frac{1}{16}$-inch) slices. Arrange meat on platter. Arrange onions, celery, and mushrooms on platter decoratively. Heat water to boiling point in a 2-quart saucepan over high heat. Add noodles. Continue cooking for 2 minutes. Drain. For easy handling, use kitchen scissors and cut noodles into 2- to 3-inch pieces; add to platter along with tofu and spinach. Combine sauce ingredients and place in a small bowl.

Heat wok to high. Add the 4 tablespoons of beef broth. Add beef slices and cook, stirring quickly with chopsticks until beef is beginning to brown. Add one-third of the sauce. Stir in onions, celery, and mushrooms; continue cooking and stirring as they cook. Stir in noodles and one-third of the sauce and mix well. Add tofu, spinach, and remaining sauce. Serve immediately.

6 servings   *1 serving: 1 cup*

Nutritive values per serving:

CHO (g)	PRO (g)	FAT (g)	CAL —	Fiber (g)	Sodium (mg)	Chol (mg)
24	27	8	282	2.6	782	64

Food Exchanges per serving: 3 Lean Meat Exchanges plus
1 Starch Exchange plus
1 Vegetable Exchange.

Low-sodium diets: This recipe is not suitable.

Japanese Steak and Pea Pods

If the steak is partially frozen, it will be much easier to slice. After cutting, thaw to room temperature before cooking. This is a stir-fry recipe.

1½ pounds sirloin with fat and bone
2 tablespoons soy sauce
2 tablespoons dry sherry
1 tablespoon vegetable oil
1 cup diagonally sliced celery
¾ cup diagonally sliced green onion with tops
1 6-ounce package frozen Chinese pea pods,
    thawed, or 6 ounces cleaned fresh snow peas
¾ cup tomato juice

Remove all fat and bone from meat and discard. Cut meat into strips 1 by 2 by ½ inch. Mix the soy sauce and sherry together and pour over the steak strips; allow to marinate 10 minutes. Meanwhile, prepare the vegetables. Heat oil in a 10- or 12-inch frying pan over high heat. Brown the meat quickly while stirring vigorously. Add the celery and onion; cover, lower heat to medium, and cook 3 minutes. Add snow peas and tomato juice and cook, stirring, until snow peas are hot but still crisp. The total cooking time is only about 7–8 minutes.

4 servings (yield: 4 cups)   *1 serving: 1 cup*

Nutritive values per serving:

CHO (g)	PRO (g)	FAT (g)	CAL —	Fiber (g)	Sodium (mg)	Chol (mg)
9	40	18	376	3.8	817	111

Food Exchanges per serving: 5 Lean Meat Exchanges plus
                                                  2 Vegetable Exchanges plus ½ Fat
                                                  Exchange.

Low-sodium diets: This recipe is not suitable.

|*NEW*| **Szechwan Bean Curd**

4 ounces 85% lean ground beef
1 cup chopped green onion with tops
1 clove garlic, minced
¾ cup chicken broth
2 tablespoons reduced-sodium (light) soy sauce
1 tablespoon chili sauce
1 teaspoon sesame oil (*see* note below)
¼ teaspoon hot oil (optional; *see* note below)
¼ teaspoon red pepper flakes
2 tablespoons cornstarch
2 tablespoons cold water
1 cup bean curd (tofu), cut into ½-inch cubes

Place ground beef, green onions, and garlic in a nonstick skillet and cook, stirring quickly, until beef is browned. Stir in chicken broth, soy sauce, chili sauce, oils, and red pepper flakes. Mix cornstarch with cold water. Add to skillet. Cook, stirring constantly, until sauce thickens. Gently stir in bean curd. Continue cooking over medium heat 3 minutes.

Note: Sesame oil and hot oil are available in Oriental sections of food markets and in specialty stores.

4 servings   *1 serving: 1 cup*

Nutritive values per serving:

CHO (g)	PRO (g)	FAT (g)	CAL —	Fiber (g)	Sodium (mg)	Chol (mg)
9	15	7	149	0.9	518	18

Food Exchanges per serving: 2 Lean Meat Exchanges plus
1 Vegetable Exchange.

Low-sodium diets: This recipe is not suitable.

NEW Hungarian Cabbage Rolls

2 quarts water
12 large green cabbage leaves (about 1 pound)
1 cup diced cooked carrot
¾ pound 85% lean ground beef
¼ cup raw brown rice
1 egg, beaten slightly
1½ cups tomato juice
1 16-ounce can stewed tomatoes, with liquid
1 medium onion, sliced
¼ teaspoon salt
¼ teaspoon freshly ground pepper
2 cloves garlic, crushed

Preheat oven to 325°F. Boil 2 quarts of water in a large sauce-pan or dutch oven. Arrange cabbage leaves loosely in pan. Cover and cook over medium heat until cabbage is limp but not soft, about 8 minutes. Drain and cool leaves. Puree carrot in blender or food processor fitted with steel blade; mix with ground beef, rice, and egg. Spoon 2 tablespoons of the meat mixture onto each leaf. Tuck ends in and roll up jelly roll style. Place seam side down in 9″ × 13″ baking pan. Pour tomato juice, tomatoes, onion slices, and seasonings over cabbage rolls. Cover and bake 1 hour; uncover and cook for an additional 30 minutes.

6 servings (yield: 12 rolls)   *1 serving: 2 cabbage rolls*

Nutritive values per serving:

CHO (g)	PRO (g)	FAT (g)	CAL —	Fiber (g)	Sodium (mg)	Chol (mg)
20	16	6	197	2.3	504	86

Food Exchanges per serving: 2 Lean Meat Exchanges plus
1 Starch Exchange plus
1 Vegetable Exchange.

Low-sodium diets: Omit salt. Substitute unsalted tomato juice
and unsalted canned tomatoes.

Veal Piccata

Veal scallops, which are used in this recipe of Mary's, are very thin slices of veal from the round or loin. They should have no visible fat or tendon, and are sometimes cut and sold frozen. Turkey breast slices may be substituted to make Turkey Piccata.

2 tablespoons all-purpose flour
½ teaspoon salt
¼ teaspoon freshly ground pepper
1¼ pounds veal scallops, sliced very thin
3 tablespoons margarine
1 lemon with rind, sliced very thin crosswise
⅓ cup dry white wine
⅓ cup fresh lemon juice
2 tablespoons chopped fresh parsley

Combine the flour, salt, and pepper: sprinkle on both sides of veal scallops. Heat half the margarine over medium heat in a very large frying pan and quickly sauté half the veal 2–3 minutes, until the edges brown slightly; repeat process with remaining margarine and veal. Remove meat from pan and set it aside. To the pan drippings add three-quarters of the lemon slices, the wine, and the lemon juice; scrape drippings into this liquid, mix well, and bring mixture to a boil. Return veal to pan and cook gently 2–3 minutes to blend flavors. Serve immediately on warmed platter. Garnish with remaining lemon slices and chopped parsley.

4 servings

1 serving: 3½ ounces cooked veal plus 2 tablespoons lemon sauce

Nutritive values per serving:

CHO (g)	PRO (g)	FAT (g)	CAL —	Fiber (g)	Sodium (mg)	Chol (mg)
6	27	22	350	0.3	411	101

Food Exchanges per serving: 4 Medium-Fat Meat Exchanges plus ½ Fruit Exchange.

Low-sodium diets: Omit salt. Use unsalted margarine.

Veal Marengo

1 pound fresh tomatoes
1 pound veal cutlets, about ¼ inch thick
2 tablespoons all-purpose flour, divided
½ teaspoon salt
¼ teaspoon freshly ground pepper
2 tablespoons vegetable oil
¼ cup chopped onion
1 clove garlic, crushed
1 chicken bouillon cube
1 cup boiling water
¼ teaspoon grated lemon rind
½ teaspoon dried thyme
½ teaspoon oil (to oil pan)
¼ pound fresh mushrooms, sliced

Preheat oven to 350°F. Dip tomatoes in boiling water for 10 seconds and remove skins; cut out cores; set tomatoes aside. Cut cutlets in four or eight equal-sized pieces. Measure into a small brown paper bag 1 tablespoon of the flour, salt, and pepper; shake well. Add pieces of veal. Hold top of bag closed tightly with one hand and place other hand at bottom of bag; turn bag upside down and back several times to coat all pieces evenly; set aside.

Heat 2 tablespoons vegetable oil in a large frying pan. Cook onion and garlic over medium heat, stirring until onion is a light golden color; remove carefully from oil and set aside. Brown meat in hot oil, turning with tongs frequently; remove meat from pan. Add remaining 1 tablespoon flour to pan and stir vigorously until browned. Dissolve bouillon cube in boiling water, then add slowly to flour in pan; continue stirring. Cook and stir over moderate heat until thickened and smooth. Add lemon rind, thyme, and onion; mix; remove from heat. Slice tomatoes; arrange in the bottom of a 1½-quart baking pan coated with ½ teaspoon oil. Arrange meat on top, then cover with brown sauce. Cover and bake 30 minutes. Add mushrooms to sauce. Bake, uncovered, 20 minutes more.

4 servings (yield: 12 ounces cooked veal plus 2 cups vegetable gravy)　　*1 serving: 3 ounces cooked veal plus ½ cup vegetable gravy*

Nutritive values per serving:

CHO (g)	PRO (g)	FAT (g)	CAL —	Fiber (g)	Sodium (mg)	Chol (mg)
11	33	20	363	2.7	562	116

Food Exchanges per serving: 4 Medium-Fat Meat Exchanges plus 2 Vegetable Exchanges.

Low-sodium diets: Omit salt. Use low-sodium chicken bouillon cube.

NEW Roast Veal with Mushrooms

1 3-pound boneless veal rump roast, boned and tied
1 teaspoon salt
½ teaspoon cracked pepper
½ teaspoon dried rosemary
8 slices bacon
½ pound fresh mushrooms, sliced

Preheat oven to 325°F. Select very light-colored veal, which is younger and will be more tender than dark-colored veal. Season roast with salt, pepper, and rosemary. Place bacon slices across top of roast. Insert a meat thermometer into the thickest part of the meat, not touching the bone. Roast the meat, uncovered, about 40 minutes per pound, until the meat thermometer registers 165°F, which is medium–well done. During last half hour of cooking, add sliced mushrooms to roasting pan.

8 servings   *1 serving: 3 ounces veal*
(fewer if larger portions)   *plus ½–1 slice bacon*

Nutritive values per serving:

CHO (g)	PRO (g)	FAT (g)	CAL —	Fiber (g)	Sodium (mg)	Chol (mg)
1	21	5	141	0.3	279	67

Food Exchanges per serving: 3 Lean Meat Exchanges.

Low-sodium diets: Omit salt. The bacon may be used because it contributes only 57 mg sodium per serving.

Baked Veal Chops

4 lean loin or shoulder veal chops (about
    1½ pounds)
⅓ cup skim milk
1 teaspoon salt
¼ teaspoon freshly ground pepper
Dash hot pepper sauce
½ cup crushed cornflakes
2 teaspoons dried basil
1 tablespoon vegetable oil
1 tablespoon fresh lemon juice
1 teaspoon chopped fresh parsley

Soak veal chops in a mixture of milk, salt, pepper, and hot
pepper sauce for 30 minutes. Mix cornflakes and basil. Lift
chops from milk mixture and dip in cornflake crumbs to coat
all over; place on a plate and chill in refrigerator for 1 hour.
Preheat oven to 375°F.

Use 1 teaspoon of the vegetable oil to coat inside of a shallow
baking pan. Place chops in this, then drizzle remaining oil on
top. Bake 1 hour or until tender. Drizzle lemon juice and sprinkle parsley on top during last 5 minutes of cooking.

4 servings   *1 serving: 1 chop*

Nutritive values per serving:

CHO (g)	PRO (g)	FAT (g)	CAL —	Fiber (g)	Sodium (mg)	Chol (mg)
8	30	18	317	0.1	721	156

Food Exchanges per serving: 4 Lean Meat Exchanges plus
                              1 Fat Exchange plus
                              ½ Starch Exchange.

Low-sodium diets: Omit salt. Use low-sodium cornflakes,
                    crushed.

Calves' Liver and Onions

4 tablespoons all-purpose flour
1 teaspoon salt
½ teaspoon freshly ground pepper
1 pound calves' liver, sliced ⅜ inch thick (6–8 slices)
3 tablespoons margarine, divided
1⅓ cups sliced onion

Mix together flour, salt, and pepper and dredge the liver in the flour mixture (*see* note below). Heat 2 tablespoons of the margarine in a large frying pan and sauté the onions until they begin to brown. Remove onions from pan; add remaining tablespoon of margarine to the pan and sauté the liver 2–3 minutes on each side, turning twice with tongs. Add onions and mix with liver. Cook 2 minutes more. Serve immediately.

Note: Only one-half the flour mixture will be used to dredge liver, and the nutritive values and exchanges are calculated on this basis. Discard the rest.

4 servings   1 serving: 3½ ounces liver plus ¼ cup onions

Nutritive values per serving:

CHO (g)	PRO (g)	FAT (g)	CAL —	Fiber (g)	Sodium (mg)	Chol (mg)
10	22	10	214	0.6	377	337

Food Exchanges per serving: 3 Lean Meat Exchanges plus 1 Vegetable Exchange.

Low-sodium diets: Omit salt. Use unsalted margarine.

LAMB

Roast Lamb

Roasting cuts of lamb include the leg, loin, and shoulder of lamb. All of these cuts may be boned at the market for easier carving. This method works best with roasts weighing at least 3 pounds.

Season lamb by inserting slivers of garlic into the meat with the tip of a sharp knife, sprinkle with coarsely ground pepper, and rub with soy sauce. Or use your favorite herb seasonings, such as mint or dill.

Roast lamb at 325°F, 25–30 minutes per pound, with the fat side up. Rolled cuts take longer, about 40 minutes per pound. A meat thermometer inserted into the thickest part of the meat should register 170°F when lamb is done.

Nutritive values per serving
(lamb rib roast or rib chop, 3 ounces lean, trimmed of fat):

CHO (g)	PRO (g)	FAT (g)	CAL —	Fiber (g)	Sodium (mg)	Chol (mg)
0	22	13	211	0	167	78

Food Exchanges per serving: 3 Medium-Fat Meat Exchanges.

Low-sodium diets: Do not use salt or soy sauce in seasoning meat.

Nutritive values per serving
(leg of lamb, 3 ounces lean, trimmed of fat):

CHO (g)	PRO (g)	FAT (g)	CAL —	Fiber (g)	Sodium (mg)	Chol (mg)
0	24	6	156	0	154	81

Food Exchanges per serving: 3 Lean Meat Exchanges.

Low-sodium diets: Do not use salt or soy sauce in seasoning meat.

Shashlik

The meat in this recipe must marinate for 24 hours, so you must begin preparations the day before you are to serve this dish. This is sometimes called shish kebab and may be prepared with lean beef cubes if you prefer.

3¾-pound lean leg of lamb, sirloin half
¼ cup olive oil
¼ cup wine vinegar
1 teaspoon dried basil
1 clove garlic, crushed
2 medium green peppers, cored and cut into 1-inch
  cubes
2 medium onions, each cut into 6 wedges
½ pound fresh mushrooms, cleaned
1 medium sweet red pepper, cleaned and cut into
  1-inch cubes

Have meat cutter remove bone, fat, and tendons and cut the lamb into 1-inch cubes. The yield will be about 2 pounds of lean lamb cubes. Place meat in medium size bowl. Combine the oil, vinegar, basil, and garlic. Pour over meat and mix well. Cover and place in the refrigerator for 24 hours, turning meat through marinade occasionally. Remove meat from refrigerator at least 1 hour before use; drain off all oil mixture. On 11-inch skewers thread alternating pieces of vegetables and meat (green pepper, meat, onion, red pepper, meat, mushroom, green pepper). Charcoal-broil or oven-broil kebabs for 5 minutes on each side or until meat is cooked but pink inside.

7–14 servings (yield: 14 skewers)   *1 serving: 1–2 skewers*

			Nutritive values per skewer:			
CHO (g)	PRO (g)	FAT (g)	CAL —	Fiber (g)	Sodium (mg)	Chol (mg)
3	19	9	169	1.5	47	59

Food Exchanges per serving: 2 Medium-Fat Meat Exchanges
                                        plus 1 Vegetable Exchange.

Low-sodium diets: This recipe is excellent.

Lamb Curry

If you serve this delicious, traditional Lamb Curry with rice, don't forget to add the nutritive values and food exchanges. Try it over Rizzi Bizzi (see Index).

    2 tablespoons margarine
    2 cups coarsely chopped onion
    1 large clove garlic, minced
    1½ pounds boneless lean lamb, cut into 1-inch
        cubes
    3 tablespoons all-purpose flour
    1 tablespoon curry powder (or more to taste)
    ¼ teaspoon ground ginger
    1 teaspoon salt
    1½ cups hot chicken broth
    1 16-ounce can tomatoes
    1 cup cubed pared apple

Melt margarine in a large deep frying pan. Add onion, garlic, and lamb and cook it over a medium heat until meat is browned all over. Remove lamb and onion with a slotted spoon and set aside. Combine flour, curry powder, ginger, and salt and stir into remaining fat in frying pan; blend well. Add hot chicken broth slowly, stirring constantly, until smooth and beginning to bubble. Cut tomatoes into bite-sized pieces; add tomatoes with tomato liquid, lamb, onion, and apple to mixture in pan. Stir to blend; bring to a simmer. Cover and cook over low heat about 45 minutes or until meat is tender, stirring occasionally.

6 servings (yield: 4½ cups)   *1 serving: ¾ cup*

Nutritive values per serving:

CHO (g)	PRO (g)	FAT (g)	CAL —	Fiber (g)	Sodium (mg)	Chol (mg)
14	36	13	316	2.0	768	42

Food Exchanges per serving: 4 Lean Meat Exchanges plus
                    1 Starch Exchange.

Low-sodium diets: Omit salt. Use unsalted chicken broth and
                    unsalted canned tomatoes.

PORK

Pork Roast

Lean pork from a young animal is a pale pink color. Meat from older animals is a darker pink. For roasting, choose a pork loin or shoulder or a fresh ham.

Season the roast with (1) ginger and garlic, (2) marjoram and salt, (3) Dijon mustard and pepper, or (4) any combination of your favorite seasonings.

Place the roast on a rack in a shallow roasting pan with the fat side up. Roast at 350°F until the meat is tender, about 35 minutes per pound. Insert a meat thermometer into the thickest part of the meat. Pork is done when the thermometer registers 170°F. Older cookbooks advise 185°F, but newer information suggests that temperature is too high and makes the meat less palatable. The 170°F temperature is perfectly safe.

If you want the roast to have slightly glazed appearance, baste it during the last 15–20 minutes of cooking time with ⅓ cup unsweetened pineapple juice or apple juice. Serve with Granny Smith Applesauce, Sweet Pickled Cherries, or Raisins Indienne (*see* Index).

Nutritive values per serving
(3 ounces cooked, boneless lean pork roast trimmed of fat,
seasoned with ginger and garlic):

CHO (g)	PRO (g)	FAT (g)	CAL	Fiber (g)	Sodium (mg)	Chol (mg)
0	23	11	—	0	53	77

Food exchanges per serving: 3 Medium-Fat Meat Exchanges.

Low-sodium diets: Omit salt. Also, choose an accompaniment low in sodium.

NEW Pork Chops with Apples

- 2 teaspoons margarine
- 1 cup sliced apples
- ½ teaspoon ground cinnamon
- 2 center-cut pork chops, ½ inch thick, well trimmed
- ¼ teaspoon salt
- ¼ teaspoon freshly ground pepper

Melt margarine in a large nonstick frying pan; sauté apples until tender but not mushy. Sprinkle with cinnamon. Push apples to one side or remove to serving plate. Fry pork chops in liquid from apples until almost cooked, turning to brown both sides. Sprinkle with salt and pepper. Cook until chops are done. Don't overcook as chops will become rubbery. Arrange a chop on each plate and serve apples over chops.

2 servings   *1 serving: 1 pork chop plus ½ cup apples*

Nutritive values per serving:

CHO (g)	PRO (g)	FAT (g)	CAL —	Fiber (g)	Sodium (mg)	Chol (mg)
9	18	14	236	1.2	338	63

Food Exchanges per serving: 2 High-Fat Meat Exchanges plus ½ Fruit Exchange.

Low-sodium diets: Omit salt.

Savory Loin Pork Chops

4 loin pork chops, bone in (2 pounds)
½ teaspoon salt
⅛ teaspoon dried marjoram
⅛ teaspoon dried thyme
⅛ teaspoon dried sage
¾ cup chicken broth
½ teaspoon grated orange rind
⅛ teaspoon ground ginger

Preheat oven to 300°F. Cut off fat around outside of all chops. Over medium heat partially cook some of the fat pieces in a heavy frying pan until there is about a tablespoon of liquid fat in pan. Discard all the rest of the fat. Combine salt, marjoram, thyme, and sage. Sprinkle on both sides of chops and press in with fingers. Brown chops on both sides in the frying pan, turning twice. Transfer to a shallow casserole. Combine chicken broth, orange rind, and ginger; pour over chops. Cover casserole. Bake 45 minutes, uncovering for last 5 minutes of cooking.

4 servings   *1 serving: 1 chop*

Nutritive values per serving:

CHO (g)	PRO (g)	FAT (g)	CAL —	Fiber (g)	Sodium (mg)	Chol (mg)
0	30	13	245	0	460	90

Food Exchanges per serving: 4 Medium-Fat Meat Exchanges. Purchase 1½ pounds of thinner chops to yield 3 Medium-Fat Meat Exchanges per serving.

Low-sodium diets: Omit salt. Use unsalted chicken broth.

Basil Pork Chops

4 lean center-cut pork chops (1¼ pounds)
1 cup V-8 Juice
1 teaspoon dried basil
½ teaspoon salt
¼ teaspoon coarsely ground pepper

Trim and discard excess fat from chops. In a large frying pan, brown chops without added fat. When chops are browned, add other ingredients. Cover tightly and simmer 40 minutes or until tender. Turn meat occasionally and add a few tablespoons of water if necessary to prevent burning.

4 servings   *1 serving: 1 chop plus 1 tablespoon sauce*

Nutritive values per serving:

CHO (g)	PRO (g)	FAT (g)	CAL —	Fiber (g)	Sodium (mg)	Chol (mg)
3	25	14	240	0.7	521	91

Food Exchanges per serving: 3 Medium-Fat Exchanges plus
1 Vegetable Exchange.

Low-sodium diets: Omit salt. Substitute unsalted V-8 Juice.

$\boxed{NEW}$ Stir-Fried Pork with Napa Cabbage

This spicy entree is delicious served with rice or noodles.

    4 tablespoons beef broth
    ½ teaspoon minced garlic
    ½ teaspoon minced fresh gingerroot
    8 green onions, chopped
    1 pound pork tenderloin, cut into 1½- by ½-inch
        strips
    4 cups shredded Napa cabbage
    ½ teaspoon salt
    ½ teaspoon red pepper flakes

Heat broth in a large nonstick frying pan or in a wok. Stir-fry the garlic, ginger, and green onions for 1 minute. Add pork and stir-fry until pink color is nearly gone, about 1 minute. Mix in cabbage, cover, and continue cooking for 3–5 minutes or until cabbage is tender, stirring once. Season with salt and red pepper flakes to taste.

6 servings   *1 serving: ¾ cup*

Nutritive values per serving:

CHO (g)	PRO (g)	FAT (g)	CAL —	Fiber (g)	Sodium (mg)	Chol (mg)
2	23	4	135	1.1	277	70

Food Exchanges per serving: 3 Lean Meat Exchanges.

Low-sodium diets: Omit salt.

HAM

Baked Ham

Precooked hams are widely available both in cans and in the meat display case of your local market. Place the ham on a rack in a shallow roasting pan. Score the surface of the ham and season with dry mustard powder and stud with whole cloves.

Heat precooked ham in a 325°F oven for 10–15 minutes per pound of ham. According to the National Live Stock and Meat Board, "fully cooked," or precooked, hams should reach a temperature of 140°F when they are heated for serving hot.

Trim ham of separable fat before serving. Serve with Mustard Sauce or Sweet and Sour Sauce (*see* Index). Add values of sauce to nutritive and exchange values below.

CHO (g)	PRO (g)	FAT (g)	CAL —	Fiber (g)	Sodium (mg)	Chol (mg)
0	18	7	142	0	908	34

Nutritive values per serving (3 ounces lean only):

Food Exchanges per serving: 3 Lean Meat Exchanges.
Low-sodium diets: This recipe is not suitable.

Broiled Ham Steak

Choose a precooked center-cut ham steak ½ inch thick. Cut ridges in the fat surrounding ham so that the edges will not curl. Brush each side with 1 teaspoon prepared mustard. Broil ham 3 inches from broiler heat for 3 minutes on each side. Trim fat from outside edges and discard.

If you are using fresh ham, broil ham slice 3 inches from broiler heat for 7–8 minutes on each side.

Nutritive values per serving *(3 ounces lean):*						
CHO (g)	PRO (g)	FAT (g)	CAL —	Fiber (g)	Sodium (mg)	Chol (mg)
0	19	7	140	0	1177	48

Food Exchanges per serving: 3 Lean Meat Exchanges.

Low-sodium diets: This recipe is not suitable.

Baked Ham Loaf

2 medium eggs, beaten
¼ cup catsup
1 tablespoon prepared mustard
½ cup skim milk
2¾ cups ground cooked ham
2 slices fresh bread, crumbled fine
2 tablespoons finely chopped onion
½ cup finely chopped celery
3 tablespoons minced fresh parsley

Preheat oven to 350°F. Prepare a 7½″ × 3½″ × 2″ loaf pan or four 6-ounce custard cups with vegetable pan-coating. Combine beaten eggs, catsup, mustard, and milk. Add all remaining ingredients; mix well. Turn into the loaf pan or custard cups. Bake 1 hour for loaf pan or 40 minutes for individual custard cups. Remove from oven and allow to stand for 5 minutes. Unmold on a serving platter. Cut loaf into four slices.

4 servings   *1 serving: a 1¾-inch-thick slice*

Nutritive values per serving:						
CHO (g)	PRO (g)	FAT (g)	CAL —	Fiber (g)	Sodium (mg)	Chol (mg)
13	24	8	225	0.7	1336	180

Food Exchanges per serving: 3 Lean Meat Exchanges plus 1 Starch Exchange.

Low-sodium diets: This recipe is not suitable.

Knockwurst and Sauerkraut

½ cup chopped onion
1 teaspoon margarine
1 16-ounce can sauerkraut
1½ teaspoons caraway seed (optional)
5 knockwursts (1 12-ounce package)

Preheat oven to 350°F. Brown onion in margarine in a large frying pan. Add sauerkraut with its liquid and caraway seeds; heat together 3–4 minutes to blend flavors. Transfer mixture to a large flat casserole and top with knockwursts. Bake 20–25 minutes, turning knockwursts several times so that they brown as they cook.

5 servings   1 serving: 1 knockwurst plus ¼ cup sauerkraut

Nutritive values per serving:

CHO (g)	PRO (g)	FAT (g)	CAL —	Fiber (g)	Sodium (mg)	Chol (mg)
7	9	21	250	2.8	1375	35

Food Exchanges per serving: 3 Fat Exchanges plus
1 High-Fat Meat Exchange plus
1 Vegetable Exchange.

Low-sodium diets: This recipe is not suitable.

20
Poultry

CHICKEN

Roast Chicken or Capon

Here is a basic roast capon recipe. Stuff it with our Bread Stuffing (see Index) if you like and add those exchanges. A stuffed bird will take about 20 minutes longer to cook. Garnish the bird with small bunches of grapes for an elegant presentation.

Select a plump meaty bird for roasting, either a young roasting chicken or a capon. Clean the bird. If bird is very fat, remove and discard separable fat in body cavity. Tie legs securely.

Place bird breast side up on a rack in an open roasting pan. Rub skin with margarine. Season with garlic and paprika if desired. Cover bird loosely with foil. Roast at 325°F until tender (about 2 hours for a 4-pound bird). Thirty minutes before the roasting time is up, remove foil and baste with drippings so that the skin will brown. When bird is done, the drumstick will twist easily. Let bird stand 15 minutes after removal from oven for easier carving.

			Nutritive values per serving:			
CHO (g)	PRO (g)	FAT (g)	CAL —	Fiber (g)	Sodium (mg)	Chol (mg)
0	29	12	229	0	49	86

Food Exchanges per serving: 4 Lean Meat Exchanges.

Low-sodium diets: This recipe is excellent.

Dijon Chicken

2 whole boneless skinned chicken breasts
2 tablespoons margarine
2 cloves garlic, crushed
½ cup dry white wine
¼ cup water
2 tablespoons Dijon mustard
½ teaspoon dried dill weed
½ teaspoon salt
¼ teaspoon coarsely ground pepper
⅓ cup chopped fresh parsley

Preheat oven to 325°F. Cut each boned breast into two pieces; put pieces on a wooden cutting board and pound them with a meat mallet or the side of a rolling pin until ½ inch thick. Heat margarine in a large frying pan; add garlic and cook 2 minutes over medium heat. Brown chicken pieces 3 minutes on each side. Transfer chicken to a 1½-quart shallow casserole. Put the wine, water, mustard, dill weed, salt, and pepper into the frying pan; stir to mix with the chicken drippings in the pan. Bring to a boil and cook 1 minute. Pour over chicken in casserole. Cover and bake 30 minutes. Add parsley; baste the chicken with the sauce and cook 5 more minutes.

4 servings   *1 serving: ½ breast plus 2 tablespoons sauce*

Nutritive values per serving:

CHO (g)	PRO (g)	FAT (g)	CAL —	Fiber (g)	Sodium (mg)	Chol (mg)
2	27	9	223	0.1	235	73

Food Exchanges per serving: 4 Lean Meat Exchanges.
Low-sodium diets: Omit salt.

Java Chicken

Serve mashed potatoes, cooked noodles, or Rizzi Bizzi (see Index) with this recipe (be sure to add the nutritive values and food exchanges for whichever you choose).

⅓ cup all-purpose flour
2 teaspoons coarsely ground pepper
1 teaspoon salt
1 2½-pound chicken, cut up
2 tablespoons margarine
1 tablespoon vegetable oil
1 cup skim milk

In a small brown bag combine flour, pepper, and salt. Coat chicken pieces, one at a time, by shaking in the bag. Fold the top of the bag to contain the flour mixture while shaking. Reserve remaining flour mixture. Heat margarine and oil in a large frying pan; brown the chicken. Cover pan, reduce heat, and cook 30–40 minutes, until done. Remove chicken from pan; stir remaining flour mixture (about 2 tablespoons) into pan drippings. Slowly add milk and stir until gravy is thickened. Pour gravy over chicken before serving.

4 servings   1 serving: ½ breast and wing or 1 leg and thigh

Nutritive values per serving:

CHO (g)	PRO (g)	FAT (g)	CAL —	Fiber (g)	Sodium (mg)	Chol (mg)
12	33	14	306	0.3	694	97

Food Exchanges per serving: 4 Lean Meat Exchanges plus 1 Starch Exchange.

Low-sodium diets: Omit salt. Substitute unsalted margarine.

Chicken Cacciatore

1 2½ pound chicken, cut into pieces
1 tablespoon vegetable oil
½ cup chopped onion
½ cup finely sliced strips of green pepper
1 16-ounce can tomatoes, cut up, with liquid
⅓ cup tomato paste
¾ teaspoon salt
⅛ teaspoon garlic powder *or* 1 clove garlic, crushed
½ teaspoon crushed dried oregano
⅛ teaspoon ground allspice
¼ cup fresh lemon juice
½ cup water

Preheat oven to 400°F. Prepare a large casserole with vegetable pan-coating. Wipe chicken pieces with damp cloth. Heat vegetable oil in a large frying pan. Brown chicken pieces on both sides; transfer to casserole. Cook onion and pepper strips in frying pan for 3–4 minutes, stirring frequently. Combine tomatoes with all remaining ingredients and mix well; add to onion and green pepper. Bring to a boil. Pour evenly on top of chicken. Bake 30 minutes. Turn chicken over and baste with sauce; bake 20–30 minutes more, until chicken is tender.

4 servings   *1 serving: ½ breast and wing plus*
½ cup tomato mixture or 1 leg and
1 thigh plus ½ cup tomato mixture

Nutritive values per serving:

CHO (g)	PRO (g)	FAT (g)	CAL —	Fiber (g)	Sodium (mg)	Chol (mg)
12	31	8	244	1.3	828	96

Food Exchanges per serving: 4 Lean Meat Exchanges plus 2 Vegetable Exchanges.

Low-sodium diets: Omit salt. Use unsalted canned tomatoes and unsalted tomato paste.

NEW **Chicken and Shrimp Paella**

6 chicken pieces (2 legs, 2 thighs, 2 breasts)
1 tablespoon corn oil
4 cloves garlic, minced
½ cup chopped green onion with tops
4 cups cooked brown rice
2 cups tomato wedges (3 medium tomatoes)
½ cup sliced red onion
12 large, raw shrimp (10 ounces), shelled and
    cleaned
2 cups frozen green peas, defrosted
1 2-ounce jar chopped pimiento with juice
½ teaspoon salt
½ teaspoon freshly ground pepper
3 large bay leaves

Preheat oven to 375°F. Arrange chicken in baking pan on a
rack; bake 45 minutes or until chicken is tender. Remove and
discard chicken skin. Set chicken pieces aside. Heat oil in a
large nonstick skillet or wok. Sauté garlic and green onion
until tender, stirring occasionally. Add reserved chicken pieces
and remaining ingredients. Cover and continue cooking until
shrimp are pink, about 5 minutes. Remove bay leaves. Serve
hot.

6 servings   *1 serving: 1 chicken piece plus*
                                 1 cup rice/vegetable mixture

---

Nutritive values per serving:

CHO (g)	PRO (g)	FAT (g)	CAL —	Fiber (g)	Sodium (mg)	Chol (mg)
45	33	7	383	4.0	368	124

Food Exchanges per serving: 3 Lean Meat Exchanges plus
                             3 Starch Exchanges.

Low-sodium diets: Omit salt. Substitute 1 chopped red sweet
                    pepper for pimiento.

Chicken à la King

This recipe can be served over toast, baking powder biscuits, or noodles, but remember to add the additional nutritive values and food exchanges.

2 tablespoons margarine
¼ cup all-purpose flour
1¼ cups chicken broth
1 cup skim milk
⅛ teaspoon freshly ground pepper
¼ teaspoon paprika
½ teaspoon salt
1 teaspoon minced onion
⅛ teaspoon ground ginger
1¾ cups diced cooked skinned chicken
1 3½- to 4-ounce can button mushrooms, drained
   or 1 cup fresh mushrooms, sliced
1½ tablespoons finely diced pimiento

Melt margarine in a large saucepan. Stir in flour, mixing until smooth. Add chicken broth and milk gradually, stirring constantly. Cook and stir over medium heat until thick and smooth. Add pepper, paprika, salt, onion, and ginger; stir to mix well. Add chicken and mushrooms and stir over low heat for 5 minutes. Add pimiento, stir over heat about 2–3 minutes, then serve.

4 servings (yield: 2⅔ cups)   *1 serving: ⅔ cup*

			Nutritive values per serving:			
CHO (g)	PRO (g)	FAT (g)	CAL —	Fiber (g)	Sodium (mg)	Chol (mg)
11	24	9	222	0.7	630	53

Food Exchanges per serving: 3 Lean Meat Exchanges plus
                          ½ Starch Exchange.

Low-sodium diets: Omit salt. Use unsalted chicken broth, and
                    substitute 6 ounces fresh mushrooms, sliced
                    for canned mushrooms. Use unsalted
                    margarine.

Chicken Paprika

1 chicken (2½ pounds), cut into pieces
2 tablespoons olive oil
1 clove garlic, crushed
1 cup chopped onion
1½ tablespoons paprika (more or less, as desired)
½ teaspoon ground cumin
2 cups chicken broth
½ teaspoon salt
1 cup sliced carrot
2 tablespoons tomato paste

Wipe chicken pieces with a damp paper towel and set aside. Heat oil in a deep 10- or 12-inch frying pan. Add garlic and onion and cook gently over low heat, stirring occasionally, until they are a very light golden color. Add paprika and cumin and continue cooking about 1 minute. Place chicken pieces in pan with skin side down. Add chicken broth, salt, and carrot; cover pan tightly and simmer over low heat for 25 minutes. Stir in tomato paste. Turn chicken pieces, cover again, and simmer over low heat for 25–30 minutes or until chicken is tender.

4 servings (yield 1⅓ cups vegetables and gravy plus chicken pieces)

1 serving: ½ breast and wing plus ⅓ cup vegetables and gravy or 1 leg and thigh plus ⅓ cup vegetables and gravy

Nutritive values per serving:

CHO (g)	PRO (g)	FAT (g)	CAL —	Fiber (g)	Sodium (mg)	Chol (mg)
11	33	12	289	1.8	820	97

Food Exchanges per serving: 4 Lean Meat Exchanges plus 2 Vegetable Exchanges.

Low-sodium diets: Omit salt. Use unsalted chicken broth and unsalted tomato paste.

Recipes

Lemon Chicken

Delicious cold for picnics or on a buffet.

  1 2½-pound frying chicken, cut into pieces
  1 teaspoon salt
  ¼ teaspoon freshly ground pepper
  ¼ teaspoon garlic powder *or* 1 clove fresh garlic, minced
  1 teaspoon dried basil
  ⅓ cup fresh lemon juice
  ¼ cup water
  1½ teaspoons grated lemon peel
  3–4 thin slices of lemon for garnish

Preheat oven to 400°F. Sprinkle chicken pieces with salt, pepper, and garlic powder. Place pieces in a shallow baking pan with skin side down. Combine remaining ingredients except lemon slices and pour over chicken. Bake, uncovered, for 20 minutes. Turn chicken and baste with pan drippings. Bake for 30–40 minutes more, until chicken is tender. Serve on a platter garnished with lemon slices.

4 servings   1 serving: 1 leg and thigh or ½ breast and wing

Nutritive values per serving:

CHO (g)	PRO (g)	FAT (g)	CAL —	Fiber (g)	Sodium (mg)	Chol (mg)
3	30	4	172	0.1	595	96

Food Exchanges per serving: 4 Lean Meat Exchanges.
Low-sodium diets: Omit salt.

Chicken Chow Mein

  1 tablespoon vegetable oil
  3 cups diagonally sliced celery
  ½ cup diagonally sliced green onion with tops
  2½ cups hot chicken broth

3 tablespoons cornstarch
½ teaspoon salt
⅛ teaspoon garlic powder *or* 1 clove garlic, minced
½ teaspoon ground ginger
½ cup cold water
1 tablespoon soy sauce
3¼ cups firmly packed chopped cooked chicken
    (bite-sized pieces)
1¼ cups chopped green pepper (1-inch cubes)
2 6-ounce cans mushroom stems and pieces,
    drained, or 8 ounces fresh mushrooms, sliced
1 8-ounce can water chestnuts, drained and sliced
1 3½-ounce can chow mein noodles
2 tablespoons finely chopped candied ginger

Heat vegetable oil in a deep heavy cooking pot; add celery and onion; stir-fry over moderate heat until onions are transparent but not brown. Add chicken broth, cover, and cook over low heat 4–5 minutes. Meanwhile, combine cornstarch, salt, garlic, ginger, cold water, and soy sauce and mix until smooth. Add slowly to hot mixture, stirring constantly. Cook and stir over medium heat until liquid thickens and is clear. Add chicken, green pepper, mushrooms, and water chestnuts; mix well. Cover and cook over low heat about 5 minutes, until heated through. To serve, turn into a 2-quart serving dish. Mix noodles and candied ginger and scatter on top of chicken mixture.

6 servings (yield: 6 cups)   *1 serving: 1 cup chicken-vegetable*
mixture plus about ⅓ cup
chow mein noodles

			Nutritive values per serving:			
CHO (g)	PRO (g)	FAT (g)	CAL —	Fiber (g)	Sodium (mg)	Chol (mg)
29	30	10	327	2.0	773	67

Food Exchanges per serving: 3 Lean Meat Exchanges plus
    2 Vegetable Exchanges plus
    1 Starch Exchange.

Low-sodium diets: This recipe is not suitable.

Ginger Chicken and Vegetables

3 tablespoons soy sauce
1 tablespoon cornstarch
⅓ cup water
1 tablespoon dry sherry
1 teaspoon grated fresh gingerroot
¾ pound boned chicken breasts
1 tablespoon vegetable oil
1 medium onion, cut into wedges
¾ cup diagonally sliced celery
¼ pound fresh mushrooms, sliced
¼ pound fresh spinach, cleaned and torn

Prepare a marinade of soy sauce, cornstarch, water, dry sherry, and ginger. Cut chicken into thin strips and soak in marinade 20 minutes. Meanwhile, clean and cut the vegetables. Heat oil in a very large frying pan. Drain the chicken and reserve the marinade; sauté chicken in oil 2 minutes. Add onion and celery and stir-fry for 3 more minutes. Stir in the mushrooms; mix well. Add the spinach and stir-fry 2 minutes. Add reserved marinade and heat through. Serve immediately.

4 servings (yield: 4 cups)   *1 serving: 1 cup*

Nutritive values per serving:

CHO (g)	PRO (g)	FAT (g)	CAL —	Fiber (g)	Sodium (mg)	Chol (mg)
8	30	7	218	2.1	878	72

Food Exchanges per serving: 3 Lean Meat Exchanges plus
2 Vegetable Exchanges.

Low-sodium diets: Substitute reduced-sodium (light) soy sauce.
Add 1 tablespoon dry sherry.

Chicken Cantonese

1½ pounds boneless skinned chicken breast
1 tablespoon vegetable oil
½ cup diagonally-sliced celery
½ cup sliced green onion
1 clove garlic, minced
1¼ cups chicken broth
1 teaspoon salt
½ teaspoon ground ginger
¹⁄₁₆ teaspoon freshly ground pepper
1 cup coarsely chopped green pepper (2-inch
    squares)
6 ounces frozen snow peas
1 tablespoon cornstarch
¼ cup cold water

Cut boned and skinned chicken breasts into 2- by ½-inch strips. Heat oil in a large deep skillet. Stir-fry celery, onion, garlic, and chicken strips over medium heat 3–4 minutes, turning the ingredients frequently with a large wooden spoon or fork. Add chicken broth, salt, ginger, and pepper; cover and bring to a boil. Add green pepper and snow peas; cover and cook over medium heat 6 minutes or until green pepper and pea pods are crisp-tender. Meanwhile, combine cornstarch and cold water; stir cornstarch mixture into skillet. Cook over medium heat until thick and clear, stirring constantly.

6 servings (yield: 4½ cups)   *1 serving: ¾ cup*

Nutritive values per serving:

CHO (g)	PRO (g)	FAT (g)	CAL —	Fiber (g)	Sodium (mg)	Chol (mg)
5	32	6	208	2.1	581	80

Food Exchanges per serving: 4 Lean Meat Exchanges plus
                                 1 Vegetable Exchange.

Low-sodium diets: Omit salt. Substitute unsalted chicken broth.

Mideast Chicken

This makes an attractive dinner when served with a bright green vegetable or salad.

2 tablespoons vegetable oil
¼ cup finely chopped onion
½ cup thinly sliced carrot
⅛ teaspoon dried dill weed
¼ teaspoon ground ginger
½ teaspoon curry powder
¹⁄₁₆ teaspoon ground cardamom
½ teaspoon ground cinnamon
1 teaspoon salt
1½ pounds chicken breasts (2 whole or 4 halves)
½ cup finely chopped green pepper
2 chicken bouillon cubes
2 cups boiling water
½ teaspoon paprika
⅓ cup bulgur

Heat oil in a large deep 12-inch frying pan. Add onion, carrot, dill, ginger, curry, cardamom, cinnamon, and salt; cook over moderate heat, stirring with a wooden spoon, until onion is tender. Meanwhile, split whole chicken breasts; add to cooking vegetable mixture and brown halves on both sides, turning with tongs. When lightly browned, add green pepper, chicken bouillon cubes, boiling water, and paprika; mix carefully. Simmer, covered, for 20 minutes. Add bulgur carefully; bring to a boil again, cover, and simmer gently for 20–25 minutes or until bulgur is tender. Check pan occasionally to prevent mixture from boiling dry; if necessary, add a little boiling water.

4 servings   *1 serving: ½ chicken breast plus*
                                          ⅓ cup cooked bulgur

			Nutritive values per serving:			
CHO (g)	PRO (g)	FAT (g)	CAL —	Fiber (g)	Sodium (mg)	Chol (mg)
16	20	10	233	1.0	993	58

Food Exchanges per serving: 3 Lean Meat Exchanges plus
1 Starch Exchange.

Low-sodium diets: Omit salt. Substitute 2 cups unsalted chicken
broth for bouillon cube and boiling water.

NEW Barbecued Chicken —Inside or Out

Great on the outdoor grill; delicious oven-baked, too!

1 whole chicken (2½ pounds), cut up
1 cup barbecue sauce, hickory or other flavor

Oven-baked: Preheat oven to 400°F. Line bottom and sides of a
shallow baking pan with foil or prepare pan with vegetable
pan-coating. Baste each chicken piece with sauce. Arrange
chicken pieces in pan with skin sides up; pour remaining sauce
evenly on top. Cover pan with foil; bake 45 minutes; uncover
pan and bake for another 20 minutes.

Outdoor grill: Prepare outdoor grill. When coals are hot and
ashen, baste chicken with sauce. Put chicken on grill and cook
about 30 minutes, turning and basting several times during
the cooking process.

4 servings

*1 serving: ½ breast and wing plus
2 tablespoons sauce or 1 leg and
1 thigh plus 2 tablespoons sauce*

Nutritive values per serving:

CHO (g)	PRO (g)	FAT (g)	CAL —	Fiber (g)	Sodium (mg)	Chol (mg)
4	30	5	187	0	360	96

Food Exchanges per serving: 4 Lean Meat Exchanges.

Low-sodium diets: Substitute the Barbecue Sauce recipe in this
book (*see* index). It is lower in sodium than
commercial brands of barbecue sauce.

Spicy Szechwan Chicken

This is one of our favorite recipes in the whole book! Be sure to have all ingredients sliced or diced and measured before you start the stir-fry cooking. Warning, this recipe is delicious but hot!

1 pound boneless skinned chicken breasts
4 teaspoons cornstarch, divided
1 egg white
2 tablespoons vegetable oil
¾ cup thinly sliced drained canned bamboo shoots
¼ cup diced drained green chilies
½ cup shelled, roasted, skinned peanuts
1 clove garlic, minced fine
1 teaspoon sugar
2 tablespoons soy sauce
3 tablespoons dry sherry
1 teaspoon grated peeled fresh gingerroot
2 tablespoons finely chopped green onion

Cut chicken into 2- by ½-inch strips. Place in a large pie plate. Sprinkle 2 teaspoons cornstarch over chicken and mix well to coat chicken. Add egg white and mix again. Heat oil in a 12-inch frying pan. Add chicken and bamboo shoots and stir-fry about 3 minutes (use a wooden spoon or wooden fork). Add chilies and peanuts; stir-fry 2 minutes. Combine all remaining ingredients except green onion with remaining 2 teaspoons cornstarch and add to the pan. Stir-fry and heat until sauce is thick and smooth and mixture is well blended. Add green onion. Stir-fry 30 seconds to warm onions. Serve immediately.

6 servings (yield: 4 cups)   *1 serving: ⅔ cup*

Nutritive values per serving:						
CHO (g)	PRO (g)	FAT (g)	CAL —	Fiber (g)	Sodium (mg)	Chol (mg)
7	28	13	266	1.4	493	64

Food Exchanges per serving: 4 Lean Meat Exchanges plus 1 Vegetable Exchange.

Low-sodium diets: Substitute reduced-sodium (light) soy sauce.

Chicken Breasts with Orange Sauce

2 tablespoons margarine
2 whole chicken breasts, halved *or* 1 2½ pound
    chicken cut into pieces
1 teaspoon salt
⅛ teaspoon paprika
⅛ teaspoon ground ginger
1 tablespoon all-purpose flour
1 cup chicken broth
¼ cup orange juice
2 thin slices orange with rind, cut crosswise
2 tablespoons finely chopped candied ginger
1½ teaspoons grated fresh orange rind

Preheat oven to 325°F. Melt margarine in a large skillet.
Brown chicken breasts in skillet over medium heat, turning
two or three times. Transfer chicken to a shallow casserole,
skin side up; set aside. Add seasonings and flour to hot fat in
the skillet and stir to blend until smooth and lightly browned.
Gradually add chicken broth and orange juice, stirring constantly. Cook and stir over low heat until smooth and thickened. Pour on top of chicken; bake 30 minutes. Cut each
orange slice into quarters and place two quarter slices on top
of each piece of chicken. Scatter ginger and grated orange
rind on top. Bake another 10–15 minutes.

4 servings (yield: 4 pieces   *1 serving: ½ breast plus*
chicken plus 1 cup sauce)   *¼ cup sauce*

Nutritive values per serving:

CHO (g)	PRO (g)	FAT (g)	CAL —	Fiber (g)	Sodium (mg)	Chol (mg)
5	17	14	210	0.2	794	48

Food Exchanges per serving: 2 Medium-Fat Meat Exchanges
                           plus ½ Fruit Exchange plus
                           ½ Fat Exchange.

Low-sodium diets: Omit salt. Substitute unsalted chicken broth.

NEW Chicken Breasts with Pickled Ginger

Pickled Ginger (*see* Index, use whole recipe, ¼ cup)
2 teaspoons sodium-reduced (light) soy sauce
1 clove garlic, crushed
2 whole chicken breasts, cut in half

Preheat oven to 325°F. Chop pickled ginger in food processor fitted with steel blade, add soy sauce and garlic. Arrange chicken breasts on a non-stick cookie sheet or shallow non-stick casserole. Brush chicken with ginger mixture. Bake for 35 minutes or until done.

4 servings   *1 serving: ½ breast*

Nutritive values per serving:

CHO (g)	PRO (g)	FAT (g)	CAL —	Fiber (g)	Sodium (mg)	Chol (mg)
2	29	4	169	1.4	222	99

Food Exchanges per serving: 3 Lean Meat Exchanges.
Low-sodium diets: This recipe is suitable for occasional use.

Jellied Chicken Mold

1½ tablespoons granulated gelatin
½ cup cold water
2¼ cups hot chicken broth
1 tablespoon fresh lemon juice
1½ cups finely chopped cooked chicken
¼ cup finely chopped celery
2 tablespoons finely chopped black olives
2 tablespoons finely chopped green onion
2 tablespoons diced pimientos
10 teaspoons regular mayonnaise
Lettuce (optional)

Soak gelatin in cold water. Add very hot chicken broth and lemon juice; stir to dissolve. Cool and then chill in the refrigerator until mixture is the consistency of unbeaten egg whites. Carefully fold in all remaining ingredients except mayonnaise and lettuce. Turn into a 4-cup ring mold, a 7½″ × 3¾″ × 2″ loaf pan, or five 6-ounce individual molds. Cover with plastic wrap. Chill about 3 hours before unmolding. If molded in a loaf pan, unmold, cut into five slices about 1½ inches thick, and place 2 teaspoons regular mayonnaise on top of each serving. If molded in a 4-cup ring mold, unmold onto crisp lettuce and place a small bowl with mayonnaise in the center of the ring.

5 servings   *1 serving: ⅔ cup plus 2 teaspoons*
(yield: 3⅓ cups)   *regular mayonnaise*

Nutritive values per serving:

CHO (g)	PRO (g)	FAT (g)	CAL —	Fiber (g)	Sodium (mg)	Chol (mg)
2	17	10	170	0.2	462	41

*Food Exchanges per serving:** 3 Lean Meat Exchanges.

Low-sodium diets: Use unsalted broth and low-sodium
                    mayonnaise.

*The nutritive values of the mayonnaise are calculated into the recipe. The calories and fat indicated above include fat and calories from the mayonnaise. The protein value of chicken is high, but the fat value of chicken is even lower than that in a Lean Meat Exchange. So the regular mayonnaise is a free bonus. Do not count additional Fat Exchanges for it.

Stewed Chicken

Sometimes we want cooked chicken to use in salads, in sandwich fillings, for cold sliced chicken, and in casserole dishes. It's a good idea to buy stewing chickens when they are available because they are the most flavorful kind for cooking in water. They are usually larger than roasters or fryers. Whatever kind you get, have it cut up into pieces, including the neck but excluding the giblets.

When stewing chickens are not available, select the largest whole or cut-up chicken you can find. Place chicken in a large deep kettle. For every pound of chicken pieces, add ½–1 cup water and ½ teaspoon salt. For added flavor also add to water ½ cup sliced carrot, ½ sliced onion, 1–2 stalks celery cut up with leaves, and 1 dried red pepper pod, 1–2 inches long (no larger). Bring to a rapid boil and remove any froth from surface. Cover the pot, reduce heat, and let simmer gently until the thickest parts of the chicken are fork-tender, which will be 2½–4 hours. The cooking time depends upon the age and the size of the chicken. Remove kettle from heat. With tongs, lift out chicken pieces carefully and place in a large shallow pan to cool quickly. Strain liquid, discard vegetables, and pour liquid into jars; cool, cover, and chill. When cold, the fat may be removed easily from the surface.

Cool the chicken as quickly as possible. Separate the good white and dark meat from the skin, bones, and gristle; discard these inedible parts. Wrap cooked chicken meat in plastic wrap or bags and store in refrigerator. Do not slice or dice the chicken until ready to use in a recipe or ready to serve.

The strained cooking liquid, when chilled, may form a gel, which will make a delicious jellied chicken consommé. Or it may be used as a base (diluted with some water) to make chicken soup, a sauce, or a gravy or used in recipes calling for chicken broth.

6–8 servings   *1 serving: 3½ ounces boneless chicken*

			Nutritive values per serving:			
CHO (g)	PRO (g)	FAT (g)	CAL —	Fiber (g)	Sodium (mg)	Chol (mg)
0	30	12	237	0	150	83

Food Exchanges per serving: 4 Lean Meat Exchanges.

Low-sodium diets: Omit salt.

Rock Cornish Hens with Grapes

1½ tablespoons margarine
1 teaspoon salt
¼ teaspoon freshly ground pepper
2 1¼-pound Rock Cornish hens, thawed
½ cup chicken broth
½ cup dry white wine
¼ cup unsweetened grape juice
½ cup seedless grapes, halved

Preheat oven to 350°F. Melt margarine in a saucepan; add salt and pepper. Split hens and place in a shallow baking pan, skin side up. Baste with margarine mixture. Roast hens, uncovered, for 1¼–1½ hours or until tender and browned; baste them several times with drippings. When hens are done, remove them from pan. Pour pan drippings into a small saucepan and add chicken broth, wine, and grape juice. Simmer 15 minutes or until volume is reduced to ¾ cup. Add grapes and cook 2 minutes over moderate heat.

4 servings (yield: 2 hens plus   *1 serving: ½ hen plus*
1 cup sauce)   *¼ cup sauce*

			Nutritive values per serving:			
CHO (g)	PRO (g)	FAT (g)	CAL —	Fiber (g)	Sodium (mg)	Chol (mg)
6	16	12	213	0.2	683	48

Food Exchanges per serving: 2½ Medium-Fat Meat Exchanges plus ½ Fruit Exchange.

Low-sodium diets: Omit salt. Substitute unsalted chicken broth.

TURKEY

Roast Turkey

Today's meat markets generally have a choice of frozen, stuffed, and unstuffed turkeys. The packages give clear, easy-to-follow directions for thawing, roasting temperatures, and cooking times depending upon the size of the bird. You may use prestuffed turkeys, but we remind you that our Bread Stuffing (*see* Index) is much lower in calorie and fat values than commercial stuffings. It is delicious for the entire family. The full recipe is ample for a 5- to 6-pound bird, so double the recipe for a 10- to 12-pound bird or triple it for a very large turkey. The amount of stuffing needed can be based on ½ cup prepared stuffing for each pound of turkey.

There is no "must" rule about stuffing any poultry. If you want to cook turkey or chicken unstuffed, go ahead! With a damp cloth, simply wipe out the body cavity and season it lightly as desired. Fold the piece of neck skin up and over the top end of the back and fasten it with a skewer. Either tie the legs together over the body opening or tuck them into that band of skin under the tail. When preparing turkey for roasting, remove and discard any separable fat from around and under skin near the body cavity, just as you do when preparing a chicken.

When your bird is ready for roasting, place it on a rack in a shallow roasting pan. Spread a few tablespoons of softened margarine around the sides and top of bird. Cover the roasting pan with a tent of heavy-duty foil and place in oven preheated to 325°F.

About 45 minutes before cooking time is completed, remove the tent of foil and baste bird.

The following roasting times are based on a preheated oven and on the bird being at room temperature.

Whole Turkey (Stuffed)

For unstuffed birds, reduce cooking time by about ½ hour.

Pounds	Approximate Cooking Times
6–8	3–3½ hours
8–12	3½–4½ hours
12–16	4½–5½ hours
16–20	5½–6½ hours
20–24	6½–7 hours

Turkey (Halves or quarters)

Pounds	Approximate Cooking Times
3–8	2–3 hours
8–12	3–4 hours

If the poultry is to be cooked from the frozen state, then extra time must be allowed to make sure the meat is completely cooked to be safe to eat as well as tasty. Unless the package directions state otherwise, commercially frozen stuffed poultry should not be thawed before cooking.

It is wise to plan the cooking time so that the bird will be done about 15–30 minutes before serving. Roast turkey can be carved much more easily after it has been at room temperature for this period.

Never store cooked turkey with stuffing inside it. If there is leftover turkey and stuffing, remove the stuffing and store it separately. Wipe out the inside of the cooked turkey before refrigerating. This will guard against food poisoning.

1 serving: 3½ ounces boneless roast turkey

			Nutritive values per serving:			
CHO (g)	PRO (g)	FAT (g)	CAL —	Fiber (g)	Sodium (mg)	Chol (mg)
0	29	5	170	0	70	76

Food Exchanges per serving: 4 Lean Meat Exchanges.

Low-sodium diets: This recipe is excellent. Avoid salt in the stuffing if you stuff the bird.

| NEW | Turkey Garden Scaloppine

6 tablespoons beef bouillon
½ cup chopped onion
½ cup chopped celery
½ cup chopped green pepper
1 cup chopped tomato, including liquid
3 tablespoons minced fresh parsley
½ teaspoon crumbled dried oregano
¼ teaspoon freshly ground pepper
1 pound sliced turkey breast (8 thin scallops)

Heat bouillon in a large nonstick frying pan. Add onion and celery and cook quickly over moderately high heat until soft. Add green pepper, tomato, parsley, oregano, and ground pepper. Continue cooking until tender, stirring with a wooden spoon. Remove vegetables, leaving some liquid in bottom of frying pan. Quickly fry turkey scallops in pan juices, about 1 minute on each side or until cooked. Arrange turkey slices on individual dishes and spoon 3 tablespoons of vegetables over them. Serve immediately.

4 servings   *1 serving: 2 turkey scallops plus*
                                3 tablespoons vegetables

Nutritive values per serving:

CHO (g)	PRO (g)	FAT (g)	CAL —	Fiber (g)	Sodium (mg)	Chol (mg)
6	35	4	207	1.9	166	79

Food Exchanges per serving: 4 Lean Meat Exchanges plus
                            1 Vegetable Exchange.

Low-sodium diets: This recipe is suitable.

$\boxed{NEW}$ Turkey Louis

This delicious recipe was provided by The National Turkey Federation. Try it over spinach noodles.

2 tablespoons margarine
1 pound boneless turkey breast, cut into 1-inch
   cubes
¼ cup thinly sliced green onion
¼ teaspoon salt
¼ teaspoon freshly ground pepper
3 tablespoons all-purpose flour
1 cup chicken broth
½ cup dry sherry
¼ cup sliced stuffed green olives
1 cup sliced fresh mushrooms
½ teaspoon dried tarragon

Preheat oven to 350°F. Heat margarine in skillet over medium-high heat. Quickly brown turkey cubes on all sides. Place cubes in 1½-quart casserole. To reserved drippings in skillet, add onion, salt, pepper, and flour; cook and stir for about 1 minute. Remove pan from heat and slowly add chicken broth and sherry; stir until smooth. Return to heat and cook, stirring constantly, until mixture thickens. Add olives, mushrooms, and tarragon, mixing well. Pour over turkey cubes. Cover; bake 20–25 minutes or until turkey is done. Do not overcook.

4 servings (yield: 3 cups)   *1 serving: ¾ cup*

Nutritive values per serving:

CHO (g)	PRO (g)	FAT (g)	CAL —	Fiber (g)	Sodium (mg)	Chol (mg)
8	29	9	238	0.2	678	70

Food Exchanges per serving: 4 Lean Meat Exchanges plus 1 Vegetable Exchange.

Low-sodium diets: Omit salt. Substitute unsalted chicken broth, unsalted margarine.

$\boxed{NEW}$ No-Fat Oven-Fried Turkey

This recipe was adapted from one developed by the National Turkey Federation.

3 tablespoons reduced-sodium (light) soy sauce
1 tablespoon dry sherry
⅛ teaspoon ground ginger
½ teaspoon minced garlic
1 pound turkey steaks, cutlets, or slices, ¼–½ inch thick
1 egg, beaten
4–5 tablespoons dry bread crumbs

Preheat oven to 350°F. Combine soy sauce, sherry, ginger, and garlic. Marinate turkey in mixture for 10–15 minutes. Dip turkey into beaten egg, then coat one side only with bread crumbs. Arrange, breaded side up, on a lightly greased baking sheet. Bake 10–15 minutes or until done. Do not overcook.

4 servings   *1 serving: 3 ounces*

Nutritive values per serving:

CHO (g)	PRO (g)	FAT (g)	CAL —	Fiber (g)	Sodium (mg)	Chol (mg)
6	24	2	153	0	330	91

Food Exchanges per serving: 3 Lean Meat Exchanges.

Low-sodium diets: Choose turkey with no salt added in processing. Substitute white wine Worcestershire sauce for soy sauce.

Turkey Patties in Mushroom Wine Sauce

½ pound fresh mushrooms, sliced
½ cup chopped onion
2 teaspoons margarine
1 pound ground turkey
1 egg
½ teaspoon salt
1 teaspoon Italian herb blend
½ cup dry red wine
¼ teaspoon cracked pepper

Sauté half the mushrooms and the chopped onion in margarine in a large frying pan. Combine sautéed vegetables with turkey, egg, salt, and herbs. Shape turkey mixture into 4 patties. Broil 3–5 minutes on each side until cooked through. While patties are cooking, add remaining mushrooms, wine, and pepper to frying pan. Simmer gently and serve sauce over patties.

4 servings   *1 serving: 1 patty with sauce*

CHO (g)	PRO (g)	FAT (g)	CAL —	Fiber (g)	Sodium (mg)	Chol (mg)
3	23	13	230	0.5	359	89

Nutritive values per serving:

Food Exchanges per serving: 3½ Lean Meat Exchanges.

Low-sodium diets: Omit salt. Use unsalted margarine.

NEW Spinach-Stuffed Turkey Birds

1½ cups chopped cooked spinach
¼ teaspoon freshly ground pepper
¼ teaspoon crumbled dried basil
¼ teaspoon minced garlic
½ cup seasoned croutons
4 tablespoons grated Parmesan cheese, divided
1 pound sliced turkey breast (8 thin scallops)

Drain cooked spinach on paper towels to remove excess moisture. Toss spinach, pepper, basil, garlic, and croutons in a deep bowl and set aside. Prepare a large nonstick frying pan with vegetable pan-coating. Sprinkle pan with 2 tablespoons of the Parmesan cheese and heat until cheese is browned. Put 2 tablespoons of the spinach mixture in center of each turkey scallop and roll scallop to enclose stuffing. Place in heated pan, seam side down. Cook over moderate heat on all sides until turkey is cooked and browned. Place 2 birds on each plate and sprinkle with remaining Parmesan cheese. Serve immediately.

4 servings   *1 serving: 2 turkey birds*

Nutritive values per serving:

CHO (g)	PRO (g)	FAT (g)	CAL —	Fiber (g)	Sodium (mg)	Chol (mg)
4	38	3	200	0.7	238	99

Food Exchanges per serving: 5 Lean Meat Exchanges plus
1 Vegetable Exchange.

Low-sodium diets: This recipe is suitable.

NEW Mideast Turkey Balls with Yogurt Dill Sauce

1 pound ground turkey
1 cup plain low-fat yogurt, divided
½ cup chopped onion
1 tablespoon fresh lemon juice
¼ cup chopped fresh parsley
½ teaspoon minced fresh garlic
½ teaspoon salt
¼ teaspoon ground cinnamon
⅛ teaspoon ground cloves
¼ teaspoon chili powder
½ teaspoon dried dill weed
¼ teaspoon cracked pepper

Preheat oven to 400°F. Combine turkey, 3 tablespoons of the yogurt, onion, lemon juice, parsley, garlic, salt, cinnamon, cloves, and chili powder. Shape into 20 balls, each about 1½ inches in diameter. Place on shallow pan and bake 25 minutes, turning balls once midway through cooking time. While turkey balls are cooking, mix remaining yogurt, dill weed, and pepper as the sauce.

5 servings   1 serving: 4 meatballs plus 2 tablespoons sauce

Nutritive values per serving:

CHO (g)	PRO (g)	FAT (g)	CAL —	Fiber (g)	Sodium (mg)	Chol (mg)
5	19	9	192	0.4	288	19

Food Exchanges per serving: 2 Lean Meat Exchanges plus ½ Low-Fat Milk Exchange.

Low-sodium diets: Omit salt.

DUCK

Roast Duckling

1 4½- to 5-pound duckling, fresh, or frozen and
   thawed
1 lemon, quartered lengthwise
1 medium apple, quartered
1 medium onion, quartered
2 cups water
1 cup Sweet and Sour Sauce (*see* Index)
1 tablespoon grated orange rind
1 thin slice orange, cut into quarters for garnish

Preheat oven to 400°F. Wash duckling and remove and discard
any separable fat around and under skin. Remove any pin-
feathers. Rub duckling all over, inside and out, with quartered
lemon, squeezing juice at the same time. Place apple and onion
pieces inside body cavity. (These are to be discarded before
eating and are used only for flavoring.) With a two-tined
kitchen fork, pierce skin of duckling all over in 10–15 places to
allow fat to drain out. Place duck on rack in a shallow roasting
pan. Pour water into bottom of pan at one corner of pan. Roast
duckling, uncovered, for 1½ hours. Again, prick skin with fork
in many places. Reduce oven heat to 350°F and roast another
45 minutes until duckling is cooked and skin is crisp. Meanwhile, prepare Sweet and Sour Sauce. Add grated orange rind
to the sauce. Serve the sauce with the duckling. Garnish the
duckling with orange slices.

4 servings   *1 serving: 3½ ounces boneless*
                                 duck meat plus ¼ cup sauce

Nutritive values per serving:

CHO (g)	PRO (g)	FAT (g)	CAL —	Fiber (g)	Sodium (mg)	Chol (mg)
8	25	24	343	0.3	376	89

Food Exchanges per serving: 3 High-Fat Meat Exchanges plus
                              ½ Fruit Exchange.

Low-sodium diets: Omit Sweet and Sour Sauce and substitute
                    Cooked Cranberry Sauce (*see* Index).

21
Seafood

COOKING FISH

There are a few things to remember about the cooking of fish:

- Because fish has very little connective tissue, it does not take long to cook.
- Overcooking fish always toughens it, so follow directions closely and watch the cooking time.
- The best tests for "cooked right" fish are (1) the flesh flakes easily when pierced with a fork; (2) the flesh loses its translucent look and becomes opaque.
- Serve fish as soon after cooking as possible. It always tastes best when piping hot!

Baking is an especially suitable method for cooking fish. It can be used for cleaned whole fish, fish fillets, or fish steaks. The recipe for World's Fastest Fish in this chapter is a fine example of baking fillets. There are also several other recipes for baking fish.

The Foil-Baked Fish Fillets recipe is really a combination of *oven-cooking* and *steaming*. The fish makes its own sauce, comes out tender and full of flavor, and the pan is so clean!

Poaching fish is a method of cooking fish gently in liquid, usually in either a seasoned water or milk. It is very simple, and again it results in a tasty fish. Try our recipe for Poached Fish.

Fish may also be prepared by *steaming* over boiling water. You may use a strainer with little "legs" that will sit above

boiling water or buy a regulation steamer for fish. Some cooks like to use their vegetable steamer for shrimp, scallops, fish steaks, or thick fillets cut into 2-inch cubes. Fish may even be tied in a cheesecloth bag for ease of handling. When steaming fish, don't let the water touch the fish, but do remember to cover the pot tightly. Generally, fish should be steamed for 10 minutes per inch of thickness of fish—twice as long if fish is frozen.

Broiling is also an acceptable method of cooking some fish, such as small whole fish or fish sticks.

We have not included any recipes for *deep-fat frying* of fish. Diabetics are usually advised not to deep-fry foods unless caloric needs are particularly high. The methods we have used in this book result in such good-tasting fish dishes that we hope you will try them all.

From a nutrition standpoint fish is a winner. Most varieties are very low in fat and high in protein, and all are counted as Lean Meat Exchanges. Because most types of fish have so little fat, you can safely eat some additional fat at the same meal without using up Fat Exchanges. In addition, the fat of fish is unsaturated and contains protective omega-3 fatty acids. Fish is highly encouraged by the American Heart Association and others concerned about your serum cholesterol.

World's Fastest Fish

½ teaspoon vegetable oil (to prepare pan)
1 pound low-fat fish fillet (walleye pike, sole,
    flounder, whitefish)
1 cup milk
1 teaspoon salt
24 soda crackers, crushed fine
1 tablespoon vegetable oil
Lemon wedges

Preheat oven to 500°F. Lightly oil baking pan with ½ teaspoon
vegetable oil and set aside. Cut fish fillets into four serving
pieces. Mix milk and salt together. Turn cracker crumbs into a
large pie plate. Dip each piece of fish into milk, then crumbs,
then milk, then crumbs again to coat thoroughly. Place fish
pieces in the oiled baking pan. Liberally sprinkle 1 tablespoon
of oil all over tops of fish pieces. Bake 10–12 minutes or until
fish flakes lightly with a fork. Serve with wedges of lemon.

4 servings   *1 serving: 3½ ounces cooked fish*

Nutritive values per serving:

CHO (g)	PRO (g)	FAT (g)	CAL —	Fiber (g)	Sodium (mg)	Chol (mg)
14	23	7	220	0.3	414	62

Food Exchanges per serving: 3 Lean Meat Exchanges plus
                    1 Starch Exchange.

Low-sodium diets: Omit salt. Use unsalted crackers. Choose a
                    freshwater fish.

*Only ¼ cup of the milk plus salt for dipping is used up;
therefore, only that amount is calculated.

Poached Fish

Use this method to poach any fish fillets or salmon steaks.

1½ pounds fresh or frozen haddock fillets, thawed
2 cups water
3 tablespoons white vinegar
¼ cup finely chopped onion
3 whole peppercorns
2 sprigs fresh parsley or dill
1 bay leaf, crushed
¼ teaspoon salt

Cut fish into six serving portions and place them in a large frying pan. Combine all other ingredients and add to pan. Bring to a boil; cover pan and reduce heat to low. Simmer 6–8 minutes or until fish flakes easily with a fork. Lift fish out of liquid carefully with a pancake turner. Serve with lemon wedges or with Sunshine Sauce, Cucumber Sauce, or Dill Sauce (*see* Index).

6 servings   *1 serving: 3½ ounces cooked fish*

Nutritive values per serving:

CHO (g)	PRO (g)	FAT (g)	CAL —	Fiber (g)	Sodium (mg)	Chol (mg)
1	17	6	124	0.1	142	72

Food Exchanges per serving: 2½ Lean Meat Exchanges. Because poached fish has even less fat than allowed in the Lean Meat Exchanges, feel free to use 1 teaspoon of a sauce or lemon butter over each serving without counting the Fat Exchange for the butter.

Low-sodium diets: Omit salt. Choose a freshwater fish.

Foil-Baked Fish Fillets

1 pound fresh or thawed frozen fish fillets, thawed
1½ teaspoons vegetable oil (to oil foil)
1½ teaspoons fresh lemon juice
1 tablespoon finely chopped onion
1 tablespoon finely chopped celery with leaves
⅛ teaspoon salt
Dash of freshly ground pepper
1 tablespoon vegetable oil

Preheat oven to 400°F. Cut fresh or thawed fillets into three individual serving pieces. Tear or cut three separate pieces of heavy-duty foil about 12–14 inches square. Brush with 1½ teaspoons vegetable oil to coat centers of each piece of foil. Place fish on top of oiled areas, then sprinkle fish with lemon juice. On top of fish spread a layer of each: onion, celery, salt, and pepper. Sprinkle 1 tablespoon vegetable oil over all. Lift foil up from opposite sides of fish to come together across top; fold over twice; then pinch together to seal tightly. Seal ends in same way. Place foil packages in a shallow pan. Bake 25 minutes. To serve, lift each package onto a dinner plate, unwrap, and transfer cooked fish and sauce with a wide pancake turner.

3 servings   *1 serving: 1 foil package of fish
(about 4 ounces cooked)*

Nutritive values per serving:

CHO (g)	PRO (g)	FAT (g)	CAL —	Fiber (g)	Sodium (mg)	Chol (mg)
1	23	14	222	0.1	161	74

Food Exchanges per serving: 3 Medium-Fat Meat Exchanges.
Low-sodium diets: Omit salt. Choose a freshwater fish.

Cod Southwestern Style

FISH
2 pounds fresh or frozen cod or other fish fillets,
    thawed
¼ teaspoon salt
⅛ teaspoon freshly ground pepper
⅔ cup white wine
⅔ cup chicken broth

SAUCE
4 tablespoons margarine
½ cup chopped onion
1⅓ cup diced green pepper
3 large tomatoes, peeled and diced
2 tablespoons fresh lemon juice
1 teaspoon chili powder
½ teaspoon salt
⅛ teaspoon freshly ground pepper
¼ teaspoon garlic powder *or* 1 clove garlic, crushed
¼ teaspoon ground thyme
¼ teaspoon dried oregano
6 slices (about ½ ounce each) mozzarella cheese

Preheat oven to 350°F. Divide cod into six equal portions. Place cod in a large frying pan, season with salt and pepper, pour wine and chicken broth over fish, and cover. Bring to a boil, reduce heat to low, and poach fish for 10 minutes.

Meanwhile, prepare the sauce. Melt margarine; sauté onion, add green pepper, and cook gently for 3 minutes. Add the remaining sauce ingredients except the cheese slices; simmer for 10 minutes. Place fish on ovenproof serving platter. Cover fish entirely with sauce. Place a thin slice of cheese over each portion of fish. Place in oven for a few minutes, just long enough to melt cheese.

6 servings   1 serving: 4 ounces cooked fish plus ⅓ cup sauce

		Nutritive values per serving:				
CHO (g)	PRO (g)	FAT (g)	CAL —	Fiber (g)	Sodium (mg)	Chol (mg)
10	28	20	329	2.5	797	62

Food Exchanges per serving: 4 Medium-Fat Meat Exchanges plus 2 Vegetable Exchanges.

Low-sodium diets: Omit salt. Use unsalted chicken broth and low-sodium cheese. Substitute unsalted margarine.

Herb Seasoning for Fish

1 tablespoon finely chopped onion
1½ teaspoons dried parsley flakes *or* 1 tablespoon
    snipped fresh parsley
1 tablespoon Worcestershire sauce
½ teaspoon salt
¼ teaspoon crushed dried rosemary
Dash of freshly ground pepper
4 teaspoons melted margarine

Combine all ingredients. Spread over fillets. Use regular method for baking or broiling fish.

4 servings (yield: ¼ cup)   *1 serving: 1 tablespoon*

		Nutritive values per serving:				
CHO (g)	PRO (g)	FAT (g)	CAL —	Fiber (g)	Sodium (mg)	Chol (mg)
1	0	4	38	0.1	326	0

Food Exchanges per serving: 1 Fat Exchange.

Low-sodium diets: Omit salt. Substitute white wine for Worcestershire sauce, use unsalted margarine.

Red Snapper Creole

2 pounds fresh or frozen red snapper fillets,
    thawed
2 tablespoons margarine, melted
½ cup finely chopped celery
½ cup finely diced carrot
¼ cup chopped black olives
½ cup finely chopped green pepper
1 cup chopped onion
1 16-ounce can tomatoes, cut up
½ cup tomato sauce
2 tablespoons margarine

Preheat oven to 350°F. Cut fish into six serving pieces. Pour 2
tablespoons melted margarine into a large baking pan and set
aside. Combine celery, carrot, olives, green pepper, onion, tomatoes, and tomato sauce. Spread half of this mixture in bottom of pan. Place fish pieces on top; cover with remaining
mixture. Dot with 2 tablespoons margarine. Bake 30–35 minutes or until fish flakes with a fork.

6 servings   *1 serving: 3½ ounces cooked fish*
                                              plus ½ cup sauce

Nutritive values per serving:

CHO (g)	PRO (g)	FAT (g)	CAL —	Fiber (g)	Sodium (mg)	Chol (mg)
9	32	11	258	1.8	486	98

Food Exchanges per serving: 4 Lean Meat Exchanges plus
                                          2 Vegetable Exchanges.

Low-sodium diets: Use unsalted margarine, unsalted canned
                              tomatoes, and unsalted tomato sauce. Omit
                              the olives if sodium restriction is 1 gram per
                              day or less.

NEW Grilled Mackerel with Chopped Tomatoes

A delicious barbecue entree that can also be prepared indoors under a broiler. Mackerel is a fish particularly high in omega-3 fatty acids.

6 5-ounce mackerel fillets
3 teaspoons fresh lemon juice
1/4 teaspoon freshly ground pepper
1/2 teaspoon crumbled dried oregano
2 cups chopped fresh tomato
1/2 cup chopped fresh parsley

Arrange mackerel pieces in a shallow baking pan. Combine lemon juice, pepper, and oregano; sprinkle over fish. Prepare a wire grilling basket with vegetable pan-coating and secure fish in basket. Grill fish over medium-hot coals about 3–4 minutes on each side, depending on the thickness of the fish. Fish is done when it flakes easily when tested with a fork. Place mackerel on individual serving dishes. Combine tomato and parsley and spread decoratively around and over the mackerel. Serve fish hot.

6 servings   *1 serving: 1 mackerel fillet with tomato topping*

			Nutritive values per serving:			
CHO (g)	PRO (g)	FAT (g)	CAL —	Fiber (g)	Sodium (mg)	Chol (mg)
4	32	11	246	1.6	122	57

Food Exchanges per serving: 4 Lean Meat Exchanges.
Low-sodium diets: This recipe is excellent.

Caspian Cod Fillets

2 pounds fresh or frozen cod fillets, thawed (not
    salted)
3 tablespoons vegetable oil
½ cup chopped onion
¼ cup minced fresh parsley
½ teaspoon Worcestershire sauce
¼ teaspoon salt
⅛ teaspoon crushed dried rosemary
⅛ teaspoon garlic powder *or* 1 clove garlic, crushed
Dash of freshly ground pepper
Lemon wedges for garnish

Preheat oven to 350°F. Prepare large baking pan with vegetable pan-coating. Cut fish into six equal serving pieces. Place in prepared pan. Combine remaining ingredients except lemon wedges; mix well. Spread on top of fish. Bake 30–40 minutes or until fish flakes easily with a fork. Serve with lemon wedges.

6 servings   *1 serving: 4 ounces cooked fish*

Nutritive values per serving:

CHO (g)	PRO (g)	FAT (g)	CAL —	Fiber (g)	Sodium (mg)	Chol (mg)
2	23	15	243	0.4	339	53

Food Exchanges per serving: 3 Medium-Fat Meat Exchanges.

Low-sodium diets: Omit salt.

NEW Grilled Catfish with Creole Sauce

The fish can be prepared on a sheet of aluminum foil or on a nonstick cookie sheet in the broiler if an outdoor grill is not available.

6 5-ounce catfish (or whitefish) fillets
1 teaspoon minced garlic
1 teaspoon paprika
½ teaspoon crumbled dried tarragon
1½ cups Creole Gumbo Sauce (*see* Index)

Sprinkle catfish fillets with garlic, paprika, and tarragon. Prepare a wire grilling basket with vegetable pan-coating and secure fish in basket. Grill fish over medium-hot coals for 3–4 minutes on each side, depending on the thickness of the fish and the distance from the coals. Fish is done when it flakes easily when tested with a fork. Arrange a piece of fish on each plate and serve with Creole Gumbo Sauce.

6 servings   *1 serving: 1 fish fillet and ¼ cup sauce*

Nutritive values per serving:

CHO (g)	PRO (g)	FAT (g)	CAL —	Fiber (g)	Sodium (mg)	Chol (mg)
11	35	20	360	1.6	977	65

Food Exchanges per serving: 4 Medium-Fat Meat Exchanges plus 1 Vegetable Exchange.

Low-sodium diets: Prepare grilled fish as directed and top with chopped fresh tomatoes.

Hearty Halibut

2 pounds fresh or frozen halibut steaks, thawed
¾ cup thinly sliced onion
1 4-ounce can sliced mushrooms, drained *or* 1 cup
    fresh mushrooms, sliced
¾ cup chopped fresh or drained canned tomato
¼ cup chopped green pepper
¼ cup minced fresh parsley
3 tablespoons finely chopped pimiento
½ cup dry white wine
2 tablespoons white vinegar
1 teaspoon salt
⅛ teaspoon freshly ground pepper
2 tablespoons margarine
Lemon wedges for garnish

Preheat oven to 350°F. Prepare large baking pan with vegetable pan-coating. Cut fish into six serving pieces. Arrange onion in bottom of baking pan. Place fish on top of onion. Combine remaining ingredients except margarine and lemon wedges. Spread on top of fish. Dot with margarine. Bake 25–30 minutes or until fish flakes easily with a fork. Serve with lemon wedges.

6 servings   *1 serving: 4 ounces cooked fish*

Nutritive values per serving:

CHO (g)	PRO (g)	FAT (g)	CAL —	Fiber (g)	Sodium (mg)	Chol (mg)
6	32	6	228	1.3	466	76

Food Exchanges per serving: 4 Lean Meat Exchanges plus 1 Vegetable Exchange. One Fat Exchange may be used elsewhere in the same meal because this recipe is very low in fat.

Low-sodium diets: This recipe is not suitable unless you substitute a freshwater fish for the halibut. Also omit the salt. Use fresh mushrooms and unsalted margarine.

Salmon Loaf

*Canned mackerel may be used in place of salmon in this recipe
to make a very good budget fish loaf.*

  1 16-ounce can salmon (*see* note below)
  1 tablespoon vinegar or fresh lemon juice
  Cold water
  2 medium eggs, beaten
  ½ teaspoon salt
  ⅛ teaspoon freshly ground pepper
  1 slice fresh bread, crumbled fine
  ¼ cup finely chopped celery with leaves
  2 tablespoons finely chopped green onion
  1 tablespoon finely chopped green pepper

Preheat oven to 350°F. Prepare a 7½" × 2¼" loaf pan with
vegetable pan-coating. Drain salmon, saving liquid. Discard
skin but save bones. Flake salmon lightly but well with a fork
(yield will be 3 cups). Crush bones (a free calcium bonus) and
mix with salmon. Add vinegar to salmon liquid and add
enough cold water to make ½ cup total liquid; add to salmon.
Add all remaining ingredients and mix thoroughly. Pack into
the prepared loaf pan. Bake 1 hour. Leave loaf in pan for 5
minutes before unmolding onto a serving plate. To serve, cut
across width into four thick or eight thin slices.

  Note: Canned pink and chum salmon are less expensive and
as nutritious as sockeye, coho, and red salmon.

4 servings   *1 serving: ¼ loaf*

Nutritive values per serving:

CHO (g)	PRO (g)	FAT (g)	CAL —	Fiber (g)	Sodium (mg)	Chol (mg)
4	26	10	221	0.4	907	182

Food Exchanges per serving: 3 Lean Meat Exchanges plus
                                                    1 Vegetable Exchange.

Low-sodium diets: This recipe is not suitable.

NEW Teriyaki Scallop and Salmon Rolls

¾ pound fresh salmon, cut into very thin strips
¾ pound large sea scallops

SAUCE
3 tablespoons reduced-sodium (light) soy sauce
2 tablespoons white wine
1 tablespoon light brown sugar
½ teaspoon grated fresh gingerroot

Arrange salmon slices and scallops in a shallow glass bowl.
Combine sauce ingredients and marinate fish for 30 minutes.
Drain seafood and reserve marinade. Wrap sea scallops in salmon strips and secure, if necessary, with a short bamboo
skewer that has been soaked in water.

To oven-broil: Place a sheet of aluminum foil over broiler
rack; arrange seafood on foil and broil about 4 inches from
heat until lightly done, about 4 minutes. Baste with marinade
during cooking. Serve immediately.

To charcoal broil: Arrange skewers on oiled grill in single
layer and grill for about 3 minutes on each side or until
cooked.

6 servings   1 serving: 3 rolls of salmon-wrapped scallops

Nutritive values per serving:

CHO (g)	PRO (g)	FAT (g)	CAL —	Fiber (g)	Sodium (mg)	Chol (mg)
2	28	5	173	0	216	57

Food Exchanges per serving: 4 Lean Meat Exchanges.
Low-sodium diet: This recipe is suitable.

NEW Grilled Salmon Steaks with Rosemary

Salmon is a popular fish, rich in healthy omega-3 fatty acids.

1 tablespoon crumbled dried sage
¼ teaspoon white pepper
3 tablespoons crumbled dried rosemary, divided
2 tablespoon fresh lemon juice
2 tablespoons olive oil
6 5-ounce salmon steaks
1 lemon, cut into 6 wedges

Mix together sage, pepper, and half the rosemary. Add the lemon juice and olive oil. Brush both sides of each salmon steak with the mixture. Prepare a wire grilling basket with vegetable pan-coating and arrange salmon steaks securely in the basket. Sprinkle remaining rosemary over hot coals for extra flavor. Grill steaks about 6 minutes on each side, depending on the thickness of the fish and the distance from the coals. Fish is cooked when it flakes easily when tested with a fork. The salmon steaks can also be prepared indoors in the broiler on a sheet of aluminum foil. Be sure not to overcook the fish. Serve with lemon wedges.

6 servings   *1 serving: 1 fish steak*

Nutritive values per serving:

CHO (g)	PRO (g)	FAT (g)	CAL —	Fiber (g)	Sodium (mg)	Chol (mg)
4	39	15	311	0.2	167	67

Food Exchanges per serving: 5 Lean Meat Exchanges.

Low-sodium diets: This recipe is excellent.

NEW Grilled Salmon with Cilantro Spinach Sauce

This recipe is shown on the cover.

SAUCE
½ cup fresh cilantro, washed and trimmed
2 cups fresh spinach, washed and trimmed
½ cup light mayonnaise
½ cup sour half-and-half
½ teaspoon Dijon mustard
½ teaspoon salt
¼ teaspoon freshly ground pepper

FISH
6 7-ounce salmon fillets
1 tablespoon margarine, melted
Additional cilantro for garnish

Prepare sauce: Pat greens dry with paper towel. Puree cilantro, spinach, and mayonnaise in a food processor fitted with steel blade. Add remaining sauce ingredients and continue processing only until all ingredients are combined. Sauce may be prepared in advance and refrigerated until serving time.

Brush salmon fillets with melted margarine and place on prepared grill over ashen coals or on a broiler rack about 3–4 inches from heat source. Cook salmon for 3 minutes, depending on the thickness of the fillets and the distance from the heat source. Turn fillets with a spatula and continue cooking for 2–3 minutes or until fish begins to flake when tested with a fork. Fish is best when slightly undercooked. Drizzle sauce decoratively around and/or over salmon fillets. Garnish with fresh cilantro and serve immediately.

6 servings   1 serving: 1 salmon fillet and ¼ cup sauce

Nutritive values per serving:

CHO (g)	PRO (g)	FAT (g)	CAL —	Fiber (g)	Sodium (mg)	Chol (mg)
1	34	18	308	0.7	418	71

Food Exchanges per serving: 5 Lean Meat Exchanges plus 1 Fat Exchange.

Low-sodium diets: Omit salt. Use unsalted margarine.

~~NEW~~ Sesame Shrimp

1 tablespoon margarine
1 tablespoon sesame oil
½ cup diced green pepper
1 pound raw shrimp, peeled and deveined
⅓ cup diagonally sliced green onion
2 tablespoons minced fresh gingerroot
1½ tablespoons sesame seeds
1 tablespoon reduced-sodium (light) soy sauce

Heat margarine and sesame oil together in large frying pan or wok. Mix all other ingredients together in a bowl; stir to blend. Add shrimp mixture to hot oil and stir-fry about 4–5 minutes, until shrimp are opaque and vegetables are crisp but tender. Taste and add more soy sauce if desired.

4 servings (yield: 2⅔ cups)   *1 serving: ⅔ cup*

Nutritive values per serving:

CHO (g)	PRO (g)	FAT (g)	CAL —	Fiber (g)	Sodium (mg)	Chol (mg)
4	23	9	194	0.5	345	170

Food Exchanges per serving: 3 Lean Meat Exchanges plus 1 Vegetable Exchange.

Low-sodium diets: This recipe is suitable for occasional use unless sodium restriction is severe.

Cantonese Shrimp and Green Beans

This one tastes so delicious that Kay's nondiabetic taste-testers asked for more.

3 tablespoons vegetable oil
¼ cup diagonally sliced green onion
1 clove garlic, crushed, *or* ⅛ teaspoon garlic powder
1½ pounds thawed large, raw frozen shrimp,
    deveined, *or* 2 pounds fresh raw shrimp, peeled
    and deveined
1 teaspoon salt
½ teaspoon ground ginger *or* ½ teaspoon minced
    fresh gingerroot
Dash of freshly ground pepper
1 9-ounce package frozen cut green beans
1¼ cups chicken broth
1 tablespoon cornstarch
1 tablespoon cold water

Heat oil in a deep skillet. Cook onion, garlic, and shrimp in hot oil over medium heat for 3 minutes, stirring frequently. Stir in salt, ginger, pepper, green beans, and chicken broth; stir to mix well, then cover. Let simmer for 5–8 minutes, until beans are crisp-tender. Stir cornstarch into cold water. Add cornstarch mixture to shrimp. Cook, stirring constantly, until thick and clear. Serve over cooked rice if desired.

6 servings (yield: 4 cups)　　　　　　　　　*1 serving: ⅔ cup*

Nutritive values per serving:

CHO (g)	PRO (g)	FAT (g)	CAL —	Fiber (g)	Sodium (mg)	Chol (mg)
5	23	8	190	0.8	652	180

Food Exchanges per serving: 3 Lean Meat Exchanges plus 1 Vegetable Exchange. If served on ⅓ cup hot cooked rice, add 1 Starch Exchange.

Low-sodium diets: This recipe is not suitable.

Shrimp Creole

3 cups Creole Gumbo Sauce (*see* Index)
1 pound ready-to-cook fresh or frozen shrimp,
    peeled and deveined

Put sauce in saucepan. Add shrimp; bring to a boil, stirring with a wooden spoon frequently to separate shrimp. When boiling point is reached, turn heat to medium low, cover, and let simmer gently for 10 minutes; stir occasionally. Serve over cooked rice if desired.

6 servings (yield: 4½ cups)   *1 serving: ¾ cup*

Nutritive values per serving:

CHO (g)	PRO (g)	FAT (g)	CAL —	Fiber (g)	Sodium (mg)	Chol (mg)
9	16	5	147	1.6	960	119

Food Exchanges per serving: 2 Lean Meat Exchanges plus 1 Vegetable Exchange. If you serve this on rice, add 1 Starch Exchange, which is 80 calories, and CHO 15, PRO 3, for each ⅓ cup hot cooked rice.

Low-sodium diets: This recipe is not suitable.

NEW Crabmeat Mushroom Crepes

This recipe can be made with canned tuna or salmon instead of crabmeat.

½ cup sliced fresh mushrooms
⅓ cup chopped green onion
½ teaspoon dried thyme
1 teaspoon margarine, melted
1½ teaspoons all-purpose flour
⅓ cup skim milk
1 cup frozen, canned, or fresh lump crabmeat,
    drained and flaked
1 tablespoon chopped fresh parsley
1½ teaspoons fresh lemon juice
1 teaspoon Dijon mustard
⅛ teaspoon salt
Pinch cayenne pepper
8 Basic Crepes (*see* Index)

Sauté mushrooms, green onion, and thyme in margarine in a skillet until vegetables are tender. Reduce heat to low and add flour. Cook 1 minute, stirring constantly. Gradually add milk, cooking over medium heat, stirring constantly, until thickened and bubbly. Remove from heat; stir in crabmeat, parsley, lemon juice, mustard, salt, and cayenne.

Preheat oven to 350°F. Spoon 2 tablespoons crabmeat mixture down center of each crepe; roll up crepes and arrange in a baking pan prepared with vegetable pan-coating. Cover and bake for 25 minutes or until thoroughly heated. Broil crepes four to six inches from heat 1 minute or until golden brown.

4 servings   *1 serving: 2 filled crepes*

Nutritive values per serving:

CHO (g)	PRO (g)	FAT (g)	CAL —	Fiber (g)	Sodium (mg)	Chol (mg)
23	12	9	224	1.0	426	172

Food Exchanges per serving: 1½ Starch Exchanges plus
1 High-Fat Meat Exchange.

Low-sodium diets: Omit salt. Use frozen, not canned crabmeat.
(Frozen is packed without salt.) Or prepare
Tuna Mushroom Crepes using unsalted tuna.

NEW Mussels Dijonnaise

2 pounds mussels, scrubbed and beards discarded
½ cup chopped fresh parsley
4 bay leaves
1 cup dry white wine
1 cup Mustard Dressing (*see* Index)
Fresh parsley sprigs for garnish

Cover mussels with water and soak for 45 minutes; drain. In a
large 6-quart pot place chopped parsley, bay leaves, and wine.
Heat to a boil and add mussels. Cover pan and cook mussels
over high heat for 3–4 minutes or until mussels have opened.
Shake pan or stir during the cooking time. Drain and discard
any unopened mussels. Arrange mussels in a large bowl or in
four deep soup bowls. Pour Mustard Dressing over the mussels
and garnish with parsley sprigs.

4 servings   *1 serving: ½ pound mussels*

Nutritive values per serving:

CHO (g)	PRO (g)	FAT (g)	CAL —	Fiber (g)	Sodium (mg)	Chol (mg)
5	9	3	86	0.3	158	100

Food Exchanges per serving: 1 Lean Meat Exchange plus
1 Vegetable Exchange.

Low-sodium diets: This recipe is excellent.

NEW   Spiced Grilled Scallops on Leeks

1 pound leeks (about 2 leeks)
1 tablespoon margarine
1 tablespoon olive oil (for leeks)
¼ teaspoon salt
¼ teaspoon freshly ground pepper
1 pound large sea scallops
1 teaspoon olive oil (to baste scallops)
1 teaspoon "blacken spice," or Cajun spice

Wash leeks well and discard root ends. Dry with paper toweling. Cut leeks into ⅛- to ¼-inch slices, including green tops. Heat margarine and 1 tablespoon olive oil in a nonstick skillet. Sauté leeks over medium heat until tender, stirring often. Season with salt and pepper. Set aside. Brush scallops with 1 teaspoon olive oil and sprinkle with blacken spice. Arrange scallops on a broiler rack suitable for indoor cooking, on a sheet of aluminum foil, in an oiled rack for outdoor grilling, or on skewers. Broil scallops until they are just opaque, turning once. Serve scallops on a bed of sautéed leeks.

4 servings   *1 serving: 3 ounces cooked scallops*
                                       and ⅓ cup leeks

Nutritive values per serving:

CHO (g)	PRO (g)	FAT (g)	CAL —	Fiber (g)	Sodium (mg)	Chol (mg)
11	27	9	230	1.2	468	60

Food Exchanges per serving: 3 Lean Meat Exchanges plus
2 Vegetable Exchanges.

Low-sodium diets: Omit salt. Acceptable for occasional use if
sodium restriction is not severe. Sea scallops
are high in sodium.

NEW Clambake

This recipe can be made outdoors on a charcoal grill or on the kitchen stove. This is great served with Buttermilk Corn Bread (see Index) and a green salad.

3 pounds clams, small cherrystones, littlenecks, or
    soft steamer clams (about 6–8 per person)
Seaweed (traditional but optional)
6 small ears corn in husks
6 tablespoons margarine, melted

Cover clams with water and let stand for 30 minutes; drain to remove sand. Place 1 inch of water and a layer of wet seaweed (if available at fish market) in the bottom of a large heavy kettle. Bring water to simmer. Top seaweed with corn, still in husks, and the clams. Arrange a layer of seaweed on top. Cover kettle and steam over high heat for about 10 minutes or until clams have opened and are cooked. Discard any clams that do not open. Discard seaweed unless using it to decorate the platter. Arrange clams and corn on a large platter or in individual bowls. Strain pan juices and serve with clams. Dip into reserved strained pan juices and melted margarine.

6 servings   *1 serving: ½ pound clams, 1 ear corn,*
                           1 tablespoon margarine for dipping

			Nutritive values per serving			
CHO (g)	PRO (g)	FAT (g)	CAL —	Fiber (g)	Sodium (mg)	Chol (mg)
29	11	7	213	2.7	75	28

Food Exchanges per serving: 2 Starch Exchanges plus 1 Lean Meat Exchange plus 1 Fat Exchange.

Low-sodium diets: This recipe is excellent, but don't use seaweed.

22
Eggs, Cheese, and Yogurt

Scrambled Egg Whites

Cholesterol-free scrambled eggs!

 2 tablespoons skim milk
 2 egg whites
 Pinch salt
 Few grains pepper
 Few specks crushed dried marjoram
 Few specks crushed dried thyme or basil
 1–2 drops yellow food color
 ½ teaspoon minced fresh parsley
 ½ teaspoon minced onion
 ½ teaspoon margarine

Combine all ingredients except margarine and mix well. Beat gently with a fork until foamy and very well blended. Melt margarine in a small frying pan to coat bottom. Add beaten egg whites. Scramble as usual over low heat.

1 serving

			Nutritive values per serving:			
CHO (g)	PRO (g)	FAT (g)	CAL —	Fiber (g)	Sodium (mg)	Chol (mg)
2	7	2	58	0	129	1

Food Exchange per serving: 1 Lean Meat Exchange.

Low-sodium diets: Omit salt. Use salt substitute if your doctor allows.

Eggs Benedict

The timing in making this takes a bit of practice to get the eggs poached, the muffins toasted, and the bacon and sauce all hot at the same time. Get all ingredients measured and pans ready before you start. You will need a large frying pan for the bacon, a toaster or broiler for the muffins, and a suitable pan of simmering water for poaching the eggs. Ready?

¾ cup Mock Hollandaise Sauce (*see* Index)
3 English muffins, split
6 large eggs
6 1-ounce slices Canadian bacon
Chopped fresh parsley for garnish

Prepare the Mock Hollandaise Sauce, set aside, and cover to keep hot. Now, all at the same time, toast the split muffins, poach the eggs in simmering water, and grill bacon in a separate pan with no added fat. Place toasted muffin halves split side up on a plate; top each with 1 slice bacon, then a poached egg, and, finally, 2 tablespoons Mock Hollandaise Sauce. Garnish with parsley. For each serving, serve 2 muffin halves.

3 servings   *1 serving: 2 muffin halves plus 2 eggs plus 2 bacon slices plus 4 tablespoons sauce*

			Nutritive values per serving:			
CHO (g)	PRO (g)	FAT (g)	CAL —	Fiber (g)	Sodium (mg)	Chol (mg)
33	32	19	437	0	1421	669

Food Exchanges per serving: 4 Medium-Fat Meat Exchanges plus 2 Starch Exchanges.

Low-sodium diets: This recipe is not suitable.

Puffy Omelet

Kay's friend, the late Kathryn Bele Niles, was a cookbook au-thor and the all-time expert on cooking eggs and poultry. Kay said Mrs. Niles always recommended a 10-inch pan for a four-egg omelet "to give it room to puff up and not over." The following was adapted from one of Mrs. Niles's basic recipes. Have eggs at room temperature before beating.

4 large eggs, separated
½ teaspoon salt
3 tablespoons cold water
⅛ teaspoon finely ground pepper
Dash paprika
1 tablespoon margarine

Preheat oven to 325°F. Place egg whites in a 1-quart mixing bowl. Add salt and cold water. Beat until high peaks form but whites are still bright and shiny. Add pepper and paprika to egg yolks; beat until thick, lemon-colored, and well mixed. Fold carefully but thoroughly into egg whites. Heat margarine in a 10-inch skillet over moderate heat until hot enough to sizzle a few drops of water. Pour in egg mixture and reduce heat to low. With flat side of spatula, gently even out top surface of egg mixture. Cook slowly about 5 minutes, until evenly puffed and lightly browned on bottom. To peek at bottom, carefully lift omelet at edge with tip of spatula. Place in oven and bake about 12–14 minutes or until a knife tip inserted in center comes out clean. Serve immediately on warmed plates. To di-vide, use two forks and tear gently into pie-shaped pieces. In-vert omelet on plates so browned bottom is on top. If desired, fold over before serving.

2 servings   *1 serving: ½ omelet*

Nutritive values per serving:

CHO (g)	PRO (g)	FAT (g)	CAL —	Fiber (g)	Sodium (mg)	Chol (mg)
1	12	17	209	0	693	548

Food Exchanges per serving: 2 High-Fat Meat Exchanges.

Low-sodium diets: Omit salt. Use unsalted margarine.

Classic French Omelet

This omelet is best made in a small nonstick frying pan or an 8-inch omelet pan. It may be served plain or filled with cheese or a vegetable mixture. Especially tasty omelets include those stuffed with Ratatouille or Sautéed Sweet Peppers (see Index).

2 large eggs
2 tablespoons water
¼ teaspoon salt
Dash freshly ground pepper
2 teaspoons margarine

Mix eggs, water, salt, and pepper with a fork. Heat margarine in a skillet until hot enough to sizzle a drop of water. Reduce heat to medium. Pour in egg mixture; allow edges to set and lift mixture at edges with pancake turner to allow egg liquid to flow under the center. Slide pan back and forth over heat to keep omelet in motion so that it does not stick. When bottom is set and top is still moist, fill if desired or fold omelet in half and slide out onto a heated plate to serve.

1 serving   *1 serving: 1 omelet*

Nutritive values per serving:

CHO (g)	PRO (g)	FAT (g)	CAL —	Fiber (g)	Sodium (mg)	Chol (mg)
1	12	19	226	0	715	548

Food Exchanges per serving: 2 Medium-Fat Meat Exchanges
plus 2 Fat Exchanges.

Low-sodium diets: Omit salt. Use unsalted margarine.

Note: The same technique can be used to make an omelet with half the cholesterol and less fat. Substitute 1 egg and 1 egg white for the 2 whole eggs.

Baked Eggs-in-Baskets

4 small hamburger buns, unsliced
1 cup (4 ounces) grated American cheese
4 teaspoons catsup
4 medium eggs
Pinch salt
Dash freshly ground pepper
2 tablespoons finely chopped green onion
2 tablespoons light cream

Preheat oven to 375°F. Cut thin slice off of each bun. With a
fork, lift out most of the white bread and crumbs from centers
of buns and discard, leaving "baskets" ½ inch thick. Place the
baskets in a shallow baking pan. Spoon 2 tablespoons grated
cheese into each shell; top each with 1 teaspoon catsup. One at
a time, break eggs into a saucer, then slide an egg carefully
into each basket. Sprinkle each lightly with salt and pepper
and the remaining grated cheese; top each with onion and
cream. Bake 20–25 minutes or until eggs are firm.

4 servings   *1 serving: 1 egg in bun*

Nutritive values per serving:

CHO (g)	PRO (g)	FAT (g)	CAL —	Fiber (g)	Sodium (mg)	Chol (mg)
13	14	17	264	0.1	656	306

Food Exchanges per serving: 2 High-Fat Meat Exchanges plus
1 Starch Exchange.

Low-sodium diets: Omit salt. Use low-sodium cheese.

Jeanette's Dutch Babies

This recipe is from our friend Jeanette Hoyt, R.D., who super-vised the calculation of all recipes in this book. Serve this as a dessert or as a main dish for a brunch or luncheon meal. If used as a main course, double the portion.

2 medium eggs
⅓ cup all-purpose flour
⅓ cup skim milk
¼ teaspoon salt
¼ teaspoon grated lemon rind
1½ teaspoons sugar
1 tablespoon very soft margarine
1 tablespoon fresh lemon juice
1 lemon, sliced thin

Preheat oven to 400°F. Prepare an 8- or 9-inch-round cake pan with vegetable pan-coating. Beat eggs until light yellow, then mix in flour, milk, salt, lemon rind, sugar, and margarine; beat until smooth. Pour into prepared pan. Bake 20 minutes, then reduce heat to 350°F and continue baking for another 10 minutes. To serve, cut into 4 wedges, sprinkle with fresh lemon juice, and garnish with lemon slices.

4 servings (yield: 9-inch pancake)   *1 serving: ¼ pancake*

Nutritive values per serving:

CHO (g)	PRO (g)	FAT (g)	CAL —	Fiber (g)	Sodium (mg)	Chol (mg)
10	5	6	113	0.2	201	137

Food Exchanges per serving: 1 Medium-Fat Meat Exchange and ½ Fruit Exchange.

Low-sodium diets: Omit salt. Use unsalted margarine.

Apple Pancake

A great brunch or luncheon entree.

CINNAMON TOPPING
1 teaspoon ground cinnamon
Sugar substitute equivalent to ¼ cup sugar
    (granulated or in packets)

PANCAKE
1 large cooking apple
½ cup skim milk
½ cup all-purpose flour
3 medium eggs, beaten
1 teaspoon sugar (needed for browning)
Dash salt
2 tablespoons margarine
2 tablespoons fresh lemon juice

Preheat oven to 400°F. For cinnamon topping, combine cinnamon and sugar substitute and mix well; set aside. Cut apple into very thin slices, removing core. Combine the skim milk, flour, eggs, sugar, and salt and mix until smooth; do not beat. Melt 1 tablespoon of the margarine in a 10-inch frying pan and "roll" it around so sides and bottom are covered. Add sliced apples and sauté slightly. Pour batter evenly on top. Bake in oven about 10 minutes or until pancake is puffy and nearly cooked. Sprinkle top with cinnamon mixture, dot with remaining 1 tablespoon margarine, and return to oven to brown pancake. Before serving, sprinkle with lemon juice. Cut into quarters to serve.

4 servings   *1 serving: ¼ pancake*

Nutritive values per serving:

CHO (g)	PRO (g)	FAT (g)	CAL —	Fiber (g)	Sodium (mg)	Chol (mg)
29	7	10	234	2.3	135	206

Food Exchanges per serving: 1 Starch Exchange plus 1 Fruit Exchange plus 1 High-Fat Meat Exchange.

Low-sodium diets: Omit salt. Use unsalted margarine.

Orange French Toast

Serve this warm with a sweet spread (see Index) or with fresh fruit (remember to add the nutritive values and exchanges).

    2 medium eggs, beaten very lightly
    ⅓ cup unsweetened orange juice *or* the juice of 1
        medium orange
    ½ teaspoon pure vanilla extract
    1 teaspoon grated orange rind
    4 slices bread (day-old bread is better than fresh)
    2 teaspoons margarine

Mix together the eggs, orange juice, vanilla, and orange rind; pour into a pie plate. Dip each slice of bread into mixture until all liquid is absorbed into bread. Heat margarine in a large frying pan over medium heat and lightly brown bread on both sides.

2 servings   *1 serving: 2 slices toast*

Nutritive values per serving:

CHO (g)	PRO (g)	FAT (g)	CAL —	Fiber (g)	Sodium (mg)	Chol (mg)
29	10	11	265	1.7	372	274

Food Exchanges per serving: 2 Starch Exchanges plus 1 High-Fat Meat Exchange.

Low-sodium diets: Use unsalted margarine.

Baked Welsh Rarebit

4 slices white bread
8 1-ounce slices American cheese
2 large eggs, beaten
2 tablespoons prepared mustard
1 cup skim milk
1 teaspoon salt
1 teaspoon Worcestershire sauce
Paprika or minced fresh parsley for garnish

Preheat oven to 350°F. Place bread slices in a large shallow casserole or oblong baking pan; do not overlap slices. Place 2 slices cheese on each slice of bread. Combine remaining ingredients except garnish; mix well. Pour on top of cheese and bread. Bake 25 minutes. Garnish with paprika or minced parsley.

4 servings   *1 serving: 1 slice bread plus cheese sauce*

			Nutritive values per serving:			
CHO (g)	PRO (g)	FAT (g)	CAL —	Fiber (g)	Sodium (mg)	Chol (mg)
17	20	22	351	0.7	1616	193

Food Exchanges per serving: 2½ High-Fat Meat Exchanges plus 1 Starch Exchange.

Low-sodium diets: This recipe is not suitable.

Cheese and Onion Pie

A hearty, full-flavored treat for lunch or brunch!

CRUST
1¼ cups soda cracker crumbs (20 crackers crushed)
¼ cup melted margarine

FILLING
2 tablespoons margarine
2½ cups thinly sliced onion
3 medium eggs, beaten
½ cup instant nonfat dry milk powder
⅔ cup water
6 ounces Swiss cheese, shredded
¼ teaspoon salt
Dash freshly ground pepper
Dash ground nutmeg

Make the crust: Prepare a 9-inch pie plate with vegetable pan-coating. Combine crumbs and margarine thoroughly; press evenly with the back of a spoon into the bottom and sides of prepared pie plate. Set aside.

Prepare the filling: Preheat oven to 325°F. Melt margarine in a frying pan. Add onion and sauté over low heat, stirring until clear and tender but not brown. Turn onion into cracker crust and spread evenly. Combine all remaining filling ingredients and mix well. Heat over low heat, stirring only until cheese melts. Pour carefully on top of onion. Bake about 45 minutes or until custard is set. Knife tip inserted in center should come out clean.

6 servings (yield: 9-inch pie)   *1 serving: ⅙ pie*

Nutritive values per serving:

CHO (g)	PRO (g)	FAT (g)	CAL —	Fiber (g)	Sodium (mg)	Chol (mg)
15	15	23	329	0.9	483	167

Food Exchanges per serving: 2 High-Fat Meat Exchanges plus 1½ Fat Exchanges plus 1 Starch Exchange.

Low-sodium diets: This recipe is not suitable.

Never-Fail Blintzes

FILLING
1 pound dry cottage cheese (or farmer's cheese)
1 medium egg, beaten
1 tablespoon margarine
Sugar substitute equivalent to 1 tablespoon sugar
Dash salt

BATTER
2 eggs, beaten until light and foamy
½ teaspoon salt
1 teaspoon sugar (needed for browning)
1¼ cups water
½ teaspoon grated orange rind
2 tablespoons margarine, melted
¼ teaspoon baking powder
1 cup sifted all-purpose flour

Make the filling: Press cheese through a ricer or fine strainer; mix well with remaining filling ingredients; set aside.

Prepare the blintzes: Preheat oven to 400°F. Prepare a 7-inch frying pan and a shallow baking pan with vegetable pan-coating. To make the batter, combine eggs, salt, sugar, water, orange rind, 1 tablespoon melted margarine, baking powder, and flour; beat until smooth. Pour 2½ tablespoonfuls at a time into a heated, prepared frying pan. Tip pan so batter spreads thinly over entire pan. Pour off excess. Cook over low to medium heat until top is dry and starts to blister. Turn out onto board. Put 1 tablespoon of filling on the blintz, fold in the sides, and roll until filling is enclosed. Place them in the prepared baking pan. When all blintzes are in the pan, brush tops with remaining 1 tablespoon melted margarine. Bake for 30 minutes, until lightly browned.

15 blintzes   *1 serving: 3 small filled blintzes*

Nutritive values per serving:

CHO (g)	PRO (g)	FAT (g)	CAL —	Fiber (g)	Sodium (mg)	Chol (mg)
21	22	11	274	0.6	346	171

Food Exchanges per serving: 3 Lean Meat Exchanges plus 1 Starch Exchange.

Low-sodium diets: Omit salt. Use unsalted margarine.

Blueberry Yogurt

½ cup fresh blueberries
Sugar substitute equivalent to 1 tablespoon sugar
¼ teaspoon vanilla extract
1 cup plain low-fat yogurt

Wash blueberries; mash them with sweetener. Stir vanilla into yogurt; fold in blueberries. Chill in a small covered container for several hours or overnight.

2 servings (yield: 1⅓ cups)   *1 serving: ⅔ cup*

Nutritive values per serving:

CHO (g)	PRO (g)	FAT (g)	CAL —	Fiber (g)	Sodium (mg)	Chol (mg)
14	6	2	97	1.0	82	7

Food Exchanges per serving: ½ Low-Fat Milk Exchange plus ½ Fruit Exchange.

Low-sodium diets: This recipe is excellent.

[NEW] **Banana Yogurt**

1 medium-size ripe fresh banana, sliced
1 teaspoon fresh lemon juice
1 cup plain low-fat yogurt

Mash sliced banana with lemon juice. Stir in yogurt; blend well. Chill in a covered container several hours or overnight.

2 servings (yield: 1½ cups)   *1 serving: ¾ cup*

Nutritive values per serving:						
CHO (g)	PRO (g)	FAT (g)	CAL —	Fiber (g)	Sodium (mg)	Chol (mg)
22	7	2	127	1.4	80	7

Food Exchanges per serving: 1 Low-Fat Milk Exchange plus ½ Fruit Exchange.

Low-sodium diets: This recipe is excellent.

Nectarine or Peach Yogurt

⅔ cup diced pared fresh ripe nectarines or peaches
½ teaspoon fresh lemon juice
Sugar substitute equivalent to 1 tablespoon sugar
1 cup plain low-fat yogurt

Slightly mash diced fruit with lemon juice and sweetener. Stir in yogurt; blend well. Chill in a covered container several hours or overnight.

2 servings (yield: 1⅓ cups)   *1 serving: ⅔ cup*

Nutritive values per serving:

CHO (g)	PRO (g)	FAT (g)	CAL —	Fiber (g)	Sodium (mg)	Chol (mg)
15	6	2	100	1.3	80	7

Food Exchanges per serving: ½ Fruit Exchange plus ½ Low-Fat Milk Exchange.

Low-sodium diets: This recipe is excellent.

Raspberry Yogurt

½ cup fresh raspberries
Sugar substitute equivalent to 1 tablespoon sugar
1 cup plain low-fat yogurt

Wash raspberries; mash them with the sweetener. Stir in yogurt and mix well. Chill in a covered container several hours or overnight.

2 servings (yield: 1⅓ cups)   *1 serving: ⅔ cup*

Nutritive values per serving:

CHO (g)	PRO (g)	FAT (g)	CAL —	Fiber (g)	Sodium (mg)	Chol (mg)
13	6	2	91	1.4	80	7

Food Exchanges per serving: ½ Fruit Exchange plus ½ Low-Fat Milk Exchange.

Low-sodium diets: This recipe is excellent.

Strawberry Yogurt

¾ cup whole ripe strawberries
1 teaspoon fresh lemon juice
Sugar substitute equivalent to 1 tablespoon sugar
1 cup plain low-fat yogurt

Wash and hull strawberries; cut them into small pieces. Add lemon juice and sweetener; mix well. Combine with yogurt; mix thoroughly. Chill in a small covered container for several hours or overnight.

2 servings (yield: 1⅓ cups)   *1 serving: ⅔ cup*

Nutritive values per serving:

CHO (g)	PRO (g)	FAT (g)	CAL —	Fiber (g)	Sodium (mg)	Chol (mg)
13	6	2	94	1.2	80	7

Food Exchanges per serving: ½ Low-Fat Milk Exchange plus ½ Fruit Exchange.

Low-sodium diets: This recipe is excellent.

23
Potatoes, Rice, Pasta, and Grains

POTATOES

Baked "French Fries"

2 large potatoes
1 tablespoon vegetable oil
½ teaspoon salt
⅛ teaspoon paprika

Preheat oven to 450°F. Peel potatoes and cut into slices 4 inches long and ¼ inch wide; place in a bowl of iced water to crisp. Just before cooking, turn onto paper towels and pat dry. Spread pieces in one layer on a shallow baking pan. Sprinkle with the vegetable oil. Shake pan to spread oil evenly over potatoes. Bake 30–40 minutes, turning frequently, until golden brown. Empty potatoes onto paper towels. Sprinkle with salt and paprika.

5 servings (yield: 50–60 pieces)   *1 serving: 10–12 pieces*

Nutritive values per serving:

CHO (g)	PRO (g)	FAT (g)	CAL —	Fiber (g)	Sodium (mg)	Chol (mg)
15	2	3	93	1.8	198	0

Food Exchanges per serving: 1 Starch Exchange plus ½ Fat Exchange.

Low-sodium diets: Omit salt. Use a seasoned salt substitute, if allowed by your doctor.

Roasted Potatoes

This is also lovely made with small new red potatoes. If you use these, do not peel the potatoes. The skins are tender and delicious.

1 pound (about 2 medium) potatoes
Boiling water
1 teaspoon salt (for the cooking water)
2 tablespoons margarine, melted
½ teaspoon salt
⅛ teaspoon freshly ground pepper
1 tablespoon finely minced fresh parsley *or* fresh
    dill

Prepare a pie plate with vegetable pan-coating. Wash potatoes; boil them in their skins in enough salted boiling water to cover for 20–25 minutes or until tender when pierced with a fork. Preheat oven to 400°F. Drain potatoes and peel them immediately. Cut each potato into four pieces and place potatoes on prepared pie plate; baste each potato with melted margarine and sprinkle with salt, pepper, and parsley. Roast in oven 15 minutes, until potatoes are nicely browned.

4 servings   *1 serving: 2 pieces of potato*

Nutritive values per serving:

CHO (g)	PRO (g)	FAT (g)	CAL —	Fiber (g)	Sodium (mg)	Chol (mg)
16	2	6	124	1.8	318	0

Food Exchanges per serving: 1 Starch Exchange plus 1 Fat Exchange.

Low-sodium diets: Omit salt. Use unsalted margarine.

Giant Potato Pancake

Use Idaho potatoes in this recipe because they are more solid and grate better than most other varieties. The turning is tricky!

1½ pounds Idaho potatoes
¼ cup finely chopped onion
1 teaspoon salt
¼ teaspoon freshly ground pepper
1 tablespoon margarine

Pare potatoes with a vegetable peeler. Grate potatoes on medium grater into a large bowl. Add onion, salt, and pepper and mix lightly but well with a blending fork. Melt margarine in a 10-inch frying pan and rotate to coat bottom and sides of pan. Turn potatoes into pan; pat down and spread evenly. Cover pan tightly; turn heat low and let cook about 15 minutes or until underside is browned. Take pan off heat temporarily. Put a 12-inch plate (or very large pie plate) upside down on top of potatoes and, with one hand on handle of frying pan and the other hand guiding the plate, turn frying pan upside down, then lift off of the pancake. This puts the pancake on the plate. Next, immediately slide pancake back into the frying pan, browned side up. Return to low heat. Do not cover. Let cook for another 15 minutes or until bottom is browned. To serve, cut evenly into 6 pie-shaped wedges.

6 servings   *1 serving: ⅙ pancake*

Nutritive values per serving:

CHO (g)	PRO (g)	FAT (g)	CAL —	Fiber (g)	Sodium (mg)	Chol (mg)
18	2	2	97	1.9	351	0

Food Exchanges per serving: 1 Starch Exchange plus ½ Fat Exchange.

Low-sodium diets: Omit salt. Use unsalted margarine.

Scalloped Potatoes

1 pound potatoes (about 3 medium potatoes)
2 tablespoons all-purpose flour
½ teaspoon salt
⅛ teaspoon freshly ground pepper
2 tablespoons margarine
3 tablespoons finely chopped onion
Hot water

Preheat oven to 400°F. Prepare a 1½-quart casserole with vegetable pan-coating. Pare potatoes; slice potatoes crosswise in ⅛-inch slices; if potatoes are large, cut slices in half. Mix together flour, salt, and pepper. Place half of potatoes in prepared casserole. Dot with half the margarine, sprinkle half the seasoned flour on top, then half the onion. Repeat with remaining potatoes, margarine, seasoned flour, and onion. Pour enough hot water in, at one corner only, so that the water barely comes to the top of the potatoes. Cover and bake 50 minutes; then uncover and bake for another 25–30 minutes or until potatoes are browned and tender.

5 servings (yield: 2½ cups)   *1 serving: ½ cup*

Nutritive values per serving:						
CHO (g)	PRO (g)	FAT (g)	CAL —	Fiber (g)	Sodium (mg)	Chol (mg)
17	2	5	117	2.0	251	0

Food Exchanges per serving: 1 Starch Exchange plus 1 Fat Exchange.

Low-sodium diets: Omit salt. Use unsalted margarine.

Pratie Cakes

Certain Irish folk refer to potato cakes as "praties." They are great! Mix and shape ahead, then chill before cooking.

    2 cups cold mashed potatoes (fresh or prepared
        from flakes)
    ½ cup unsifted all-purpose flour (reserve
        1 tablespoon for flouring board)
    ¼ teaspoon salt
    2 tablespoons finely chopped onion
    2 tablespoons margarine

Turn mashed potatoes into a large bowl. Add flour, salt, and onion. Mix thoroughly with hands and fingers until completely mixed and smooth. Pat on a lightly floured board until ½ inch thick. Cut with a 3-inch floured cookie cutter. Place on a cookie sheet, cover lightly with waxed paper, and chill in refrigerator until just before cooking. To cook, use 1 tablespoon margarine at a time. Melt margarine in a large frying pan or stovetop griddle. Fry cakes over moderately hot heat, turning to brown on both sides. Serve immediately.

7 servings (yield: 7 cakes)   *1 serving: a 3-inch cake*

Nutritive values per serving:

CHO (g)	PRO (g)	FAT (g)	CAL —	Fiber (g)	Sodium (mg)	Chol (mg)
15	2	5	110	0.3	248	1

Food Exchanges per serving: 1 Starch Exchange plus 1 Fat Exchange.

Low-sodium diets: Omit salt from original mashed potato mixture and from recipe.

German Potato Salad

4 medium-sized potatoes (about 1½ pounds)
½ teaspoon salt (for cooking potatoes)
4 medium slices bacon
¾ cup chopped onion
¾ cup chopped celery
¾ cup water
¼ cup cider vinegar
1 tablespoon all-purpose flour
1½ tablespoons sugar
½ teaspoon salt
¼ teaspoon freshly ground pepper
1 tablespoon minced fresh parsley

Pare and cook potatoes in boiling water to cover until tender, about 25 minutes. Meanwhile, fry bacon in a large frying pan over low heat until crisp. Lift bacon out of fat and place on paper towel. To bacon fat in the frying pan add onion and celery; cook and stir over medium heat until onions are slightly browned. Add remaining ingredients except parsley, potatoes, and bacon to the frying pan and cook, stirring, about 10 minutes, until sauce is thick and smooth. Drain potatoes and slice them into thin rounds. Add potatoes to frying pan and toss with hot sauce. Chop bacon strips and toss bacon bits and chopped parsley into potatoes. Serve this potato salad warm.

8 servings (yield: about 4 cups)   *1 serving: ½ cup*

Nutritive values per serving:

CHO (g)	PRO (g)	FAT (g)	CAL —	Fiber (g)	Sodium (mg)	Chol (mg)
17	3	8	146	2.2	334	9

Food Exchanges per serving: 2 Fat Exchanges plus
1 Starch Exchange.

Low-sodium diets: Omit salt.

Zesty Potato Salad

If red potatoes are used, leave skins on for extra color and fiber.

2½ cups diced cooked potato
½ cup finely chopped onion
¼ cup chopped fresh parsley
¼ cup finely chopped celery
½ cup plain low-fat yogurt
1 tablespoon prepared mustard
¾ teaspoon herb or Italian seasoning
1 hard-cooked egg, sliced
¼ teaspoon paprika

Combine the potato, onion, parsley, and celery; then mix. In a small bowl combine the yogurt, mustard, and seasoning; add to vegetables and mix carefully. Cover and chill several hours to allow flavors to blend. To serve, garnish with slices of egg and paprika.

6 servings (yield: almost 4 cups)   *1 serving: ⅔ cup*

			Nutritive values per serving:			
CHO (g)	PRO (g)	FAT (g)	CAL —	Fiber (g)	Sodium (mg)	Chol (mg)
12	3	1	77	2.1	64	47

Food Exchange per serving: 1 Starch Exchange.

Low-sodium diets: This recipe is excellent.

Mashed Sweet Potatoes

Because sweet potatoes are high in carbohydrates, only ¼ cup of mashed, cooked sweet potatoes yields 19 grams CHO, which may be counted as 1 Starch Exchange. If you eat ½ cup, count it as 2 Starch Exchanges and 1 Fat Exchange.

> 1½ pounds sweet potatoes
> Boiling water
> 1½ tablespoons margarine, cut into pieces
> ¼ teaspoon pumpkin pie spice mixture

Scrub potatoes thoroughly; cut off and discard small ends and inedible knobs. If potatoes are large, cut into halves or thirds. Place in a deep cooking pot, then cover with boiling water. Cover pot, bring to a boil, and cook over moderate heat until potatoes are soft (about 25 minutes). Drain at once. Hold each potato with a fork and peel quickly. Place potatoes in a bowl, mash, and beat with margarine and pumpkin pie spice.

5 servings (yield: 2 cups)   *1 serving: for the diabetic serve ¼ cup*

Nutritive values per serving:						
CHO (g)	PRO (g)	FAT (g)	CAL —	Fiber (g)	Sodium (mg)	Chol (mg)
19	1	2	98	1.4	33	0

Food Exchanges per serving: 1 Starch Exchange plus ½ Fat Exchange.

Low-sodium diets: This recipe is excellent.

RICE

In all of the rice recipes, brown rice may be substituted for white rice. This will increase the fiber content of the recipes. Brown rice usually takes about 40 minutes to cook, so adjust cooking times. Canned or homemade broth can be substituted for the bouillon cubes and water. Use whatever is handy.

NEW Brown Rice Pilaf

3 tablespoons margarine
1 cup crumbled uncooked thin noodles
1 cup raw brown rice
3 cups chicken broth

Heat margarine in a large nonstick skillet. Sauté noodles until coated, stirring often. Add the rice and stir to combine. Add broth; cover, and continue cooking until broth is absorbed and the rice is tender, about 40 minutes. Let stand, covered, for 5 minutes before serving.

8 servings (yield: 4 cups)   *1 serving: ½ cup*

Nutritive values per serving:

CHO (g)	PRO (g)	FAT (g)	CAL —	Fiber (g)	Sodium (mg)	Chol (mg)
26	5	5	175	0.7	343	0

Food Exchanges per serving: 1½ Starch Exchanges plus 1 Fat Exchange.

Low-sodium diets: Use unsalted chicken broth. Use unsalted margarine.

Rizzi Bizzi

This is one of Mary's "specials"—try it with Chicken Paprika (see Index).

1½ cups water
1 chicken bouillon cube
½ teaspoon salt
1 tablespoon margarine
¾ cup raw rice
1 10-ounce package frozen peas
¼ cup finely chopped green onion

Bring water, chicken bouillon cube, salt, and margarine to a boil. Add rice slowly, stirring with a fork, and cook according to package directions. Cook peas according to package directions until crisp-tender. When rice is cooked, add peas and green onion; mix well.

6 servings (yield: 4 cups)   *1 serving: ⅔ cup*

		Nutritive values per serving:				
CHO (g)	PRO (g)	FAT (g)	CAL —	Fiber (g)	Sodium (mg)	Chol (mg)
26	4	2	141	2.2	371	0

Food Exchanges per serving: 2 Starch Exchanges.

Low-sodium diets: Omit salt. Use low-sodium chicken bouillon cube and unsalted margarine.

Curried Rice

2½ cups cold water
3 chicken bouillon cubes
1 cup raw rice
1½ teaspoons margarine
1 teaspoon curry powder

Combine all ingredients in a heavy saucepan. Bring to a boil, stirring with a fork until bouillon cubes are dissolved. Cover tightly, reduce heat to simmer, and cook 15–20 minutes. Turn

heat off, remove lid, and let stand 2–3 minutes; stirring occasionally with a fork until rice is fluffy and dry.

6 servings (yield: 3 cups)   *1 serving: ½ cup*

		Nutritive values per serving:				
CHO (g)	PRO (g)	FAT (g)	CAL —	Fiber (g)	Sodium (mg)	Chol (mg)
17	2	1	83	0.2	296	0

Food Exchange per serving: 1 Starch Exchange.

Low-sodium diets: Use low-sodium chicken bouillon cubes and unsalted margarine.

Rice Palau

⅛ teaspoon saffron
2 tablespoons water
1 cup raw rice
½ teaspoon cumin seed
2 cups water
½ teaspoon salt
1 tablespoon minced fresh parsley

Soak saffron in 2 tablespoons water (to get color). Combine the rice, saffron water, cumin seed, 2 cups water, and salt in a 1½-quart cooking pot. Bring to a boil, cover, and cook over low heat about 20 minutes or until water is just absorbed. If necessary, toss lightly with a fork. Mix parsley with rice before serving.

9 servings (yield: 3 cups)   *1 serving: ⅓ cup (Many will want double portions.)*

		Nutritive values per serving:				
CHO (g)	PRO (g)	FAT (g)	CAL —	Fiber (g)	Sodium (mg)	Chol (mg)
17	1	0	75	0.2	110	0

Food Exchange per serving: 1 Starch Exchange.

Low-sodium diets: Omit salt.

Beef-Flavored Pilaf

2 teaspoons vegetable oil
½ cup raw rice
¼ cup finely chopped onion
1 cup beef broth
¼ cup water
2 tablespoons snipped fresh parsley

Combine oil, rice, and onion in a 1½-quart saucepan. Stir over medium heat with a wooden spoon until rice is lightly browned. Add broth and water; bring to boil. Cover and simmer 20 minutes or until rice is tender and liquid is absorbed. Stir occasionally with a fork and use a lifting motion to prevent rice grains from lumping. Just before serving, use a fork to gently mix in the parsley.

4 servings (yield: 2 cups)   *1 serving: ½ cup*

Nutritive values per serving:

CHO (g)	PRO (g)	FAT (g)	CAL —	Fiber (g)	Sodium (mg)	Chol (mg)
13	2	2	76	0.3	132	0

Food Exchange per serving: 1 Starch Exchange.

Low-sodium diets: Substitute 1 low-sodium beef bouillon cube dissolved in 1¼ cups water for the broth and water in the recipe.

Rice with Mushrooms

2 cups water
2 chicken bouillon cubes
½ teaspoon salt
1 cup raw rice
1 4-ounce can mushroom stems and pieces
2 tablespoons margarine
⅛ teaspoon freshly ground pepper
Few sprigs parsley for garnish

Bring water, bouillon cubes, and salt to a boil. Add rice slowly, stirring with a fork, and cook according to cooking time indicated on rice package. (Different types of rice vary in cooking times.) Drain mushrooms and pour liquid from can into water with the rice. All liquid should be absorbed when the rice is cooked. Heat margarine in a small saucepan; sauté drained mushrooms in margarine until they are slightly browned. When rice is cooked, toss mushrooms and pepper into rice and stir with a fork to mix. Serve in a bowl topped with parsley sprigs.

5 servings (yield: 3⅓ cups)   *1 serving: ⅔ cup*

Nutritive values per serving:

CHO (g)	PRO (g)	FAT (g)	CAL —	Fiber (g)	Sodium (mg)	Chol (mg)
17	2	3	102	0.5	331	0

Food Exchanges per serving: 1 Starch Exchange plus ½ Fat Exchange.

Low-sodium diets: Omit salt. Use low-sodium bouillon cubes, unsalted margarine, and fresh mushrooms.

PASTA

Pasta Primavera

A typical Italian preparation of pasta without a hint of tomato sauce. It is scrumptious hot but may also be served at room temperature as a pasta salad for a buffet or picnic.

> ½ pound thin spaghetti, cooked according to
>   package directions
> ½ pound broccoli (*see* note below)
> 2 tablespoons olive oil
> 2 cloves garlic, crushed
> ½ pound young zucchini (*see* note below) sliced
>   thin
> ½ pound fresh mushrooms, sliced
> 1½ teaspoons dried basil
> ½ teaspoon salt
> ½ teaspoon coarsely ground pepper
> 2 tablespoons water
> 2 tablespoons grated Parmesan cheese

While spaghetti is cooking, wash broccoli and cook it in a small amount of boiling water until crisp-tender. Meanwhile, heat 1 tablespoon of the olive oil in a large frying pan and sauté garlic 3 minutes; add zucchini and cook until slightly browned. Add mushrooms; cook until mushrooms are tender. Drain broccoli; slice into bite-sized pieces and add to zucchini and mushrooms. Stir in seasonings. When spaghetti is *al dente*, stop cooking by pouring cold water into pot; drain spaghetti. Return it to the pot, stir in 2 tablespoons water, remaining 1 tablespoon olive oil, Parmesan cheese, and vegetable mixture. Cover and reheat over low heat.

Note: You may substitute eggplant, red or green peppers, green beans, onions, or other vegetables in season.

6 servings (yield: 6¼ cups)   *1 serving: 1 cup*

			Nutritive values per serving:			
CHO (g)	PRO (g)	FAT (g)	CAL —	Fiber (g)	Sodium (mg)	Chol (mg)
34	8	6	217	3.3	215	2

Food Exchanges per serving: 2 Starch Exchanges plus 1 Vegetable Exchange plus 1 Fat Exchange.

Low-sodium diets: Omit salt.

Mary's Macaroni Salad

3 cups firmly cooked and drained hot macaroni
⅓ cup Low-Calorie Cooked Dressing (*see* Index)
⅓ cup thinly sliced celery
2 tablespoons finely minced fresh parsley
1 tablespoon chopped green onion with tops
2 hard-cooked eggs, sliced
½ teaspoon salt
¼ teaspoon coarsely ground pepper

Mix all ingredients together in a large bowl while macaroni is hot. Cover and chill in the refrigerator several hours before serving.

7 servings (yield: 3½ cups)   *1 serving: ½ cup*

			Nutritive values per serving:			
CHO (g)	PRO (g)	FAT (g)	CAL —	Fiber (g)	Sodium (mg)	Chol (mg)
15	4	3	101	0.6	238	87

Food Exchanges per serving: 1 Starch Exchange plus ½ Fat Exchange.

Low-sodium diets: Omit salt from cooking water for macaroni and in this recipe. Omit salt from Low-Calorie Cooked Dressing recipe.

NEW Fettuccine with Garlic, Tomatoes, and Basil

12 fresh tomatoes, seeded and diced
2 tablespoons olive oil
2 teaspoons minced fresh garlic
½ teaspoon cracked pepper
¼ teaspoon salt
6 ounces dry fettuccine
¼ cup chopped fresh basil
5 whole fresh basil leaves for garnish

In saucepan combine tomatoes, olive oil, garlic, pepper, and salt; simmer for 15 minutes. While sauce is simmering, cook fettuccine according to package directions. Drain pasta and toss with sauce and chopped fresh basil. Garnish each serving with a fresh basil leaf.

5 servings (yield: 5 cups)   *1 serving: 1 cup*

			Nutritive values per serving:			
CHO (g)	PRO (g)	FAT (g)	CAL —	Fiber (g)	Sodium (mg)	Chol (mg)
32	6	7	215	3.7	113	13

Food Exchanges per serving: 2 Starch Exchanges plus 1 Fat Exchange.

Low-sodium diets: Omit salt from recipe and in cooking pasta.

GRAINS

NEW Bulgur Wheat with Raisins and Cinnamon

1 tablespoon margarine
½ cup chopped onion
½ cup chopped celery
1 cup bulgur wheat
2 cups chicken broth
½ teaspoon minced garlic
¼ teaspoon ground white pepper
½ teaspoon crumbled dried tarragon
½ cup raisins
½ teaspoon ground cinnamon
½ teaspoon salt

In a nonstick 2-quart pot melt margarine; sauté onion and celery until tender, stirring often. Stir in bulgur and continue cooking until bulgur is coated and turns a golden brown. Blend in broth, garlic, pepper, and tarragon. Add raisins, cinnamon, and salt, and mix well. Cover and continue cooking 15–17 minutes or until all liquid has been absorbed. Serve hot as cereal or as a grain side dish.

6 servings (yield: 3 cups)   *1 serving: ½ cup*

Nutritive values per serving:

CHO (g)	PRO (g)	FAT (g)	CAL —	Fiber (g)	Sodium (mg)	Chol (mg)
35	5	3	179	1.4	455	0

Food Exchanges per serving: 2 Starch Exchanges.

Low-sodium diets: Omit salt. Substitute unsalted broth.

⟦ NEW ⟧ Garlic Grits

Baking the garlic gives the grits a mild and nutty flavor. Serve this dish with an entree that has gravy or sauce.

4 cloves garlic, unpeeled
3 cups water
½ teaspoon salt
¼ teaspoon freshly ground white pepper
¾ cup quick-cooking white hominy grits

Place garlic on baking sheet and bake at 375°F for 10 minutes. Remove and discard outer skin. Chop garlic; reserve. Bring water to a rolling boil; add salt and pepper. Stir grits into boiling water in a slow, steady stream. Cook, stirring constantly, for 3 minutes. Turn off heat; let stand, covered, for 5 minutes. Stir chopped garlic into grits.

6 servings (yield: 3 cups)   *1 serving: ½ cup*

Nutritive values per serving:						
CHO (g)	PRO (g)	FAT (g)	CAL —	Fiber (g)	Sodium (mg)	Chol (mg)
16	2	0	76	0.1	196	0

Food Exchange per serving: 1 Starch Exchange.
Low-sodium diets: Omit salt.

NEW Pioneer Buckwheat Cereal

2½ cups water
¼ teaspoon salt
½ cup roasted buckwheat kernels
1 tablespoon margarine
2 cups skim milk
¼ cup raisins

Bring water and salt to a rapid boil in medium-size saucepan. Stir in buckwheat and margarine. Cook, uncovered, stirring occasionally, for 10 minutes. Serve with skim milk and sprinkle with raisins. Serve hot.

4 servings (yield: 3 cups)   *1 serving: ¾ cup cereal plus*
                                       ½ cup skim milk

Nutritive values per serving:

CHO (g)	PRO (g)	FAT (g)	CAL —	Fiber (g)	Sodium (mg)	Chol (mg)
24	5	3	146	0.9	246	0

Food Exchanges per serving: 1 Starch Exchange plus ½ Low-Fat Milk Exchange.

Low-sodium diets: Omit salt. Use unsalted margarine.

24
Vegetables

Vegetables that are cooked just right are a wonderful addition to meals. They are colorful, flavorful, and crunchy—and excellent sources of many vitamins and minerals. Vegetables fresh and in season are usually the tastiest as well as the most economical choice. So don't think of vegetables as just another food or something you *have* to include. Choose them and cook them to enjoy them!

American cooks are notorious for ruining vegetables by overcooking them. No food can become so unappetizing and tasteless as badly cooked vegetables.

There is an art to cooking vegetables, and it is very simple:

- Any vegetable should be cooked only long enough to make it tender. Overcooking makes vegetables soft and mushy and destroys the nutritive values.
- Cook strong-flavored vegetables in a large quantity of boiling water, uncovered, only long enough to make them tender. Place a slice of stale bread on top to absorb cooking odors. The bread is discarded, so it is not included in the calculations for nutritive values and Food Exchanges.
- Cook mild-flavored vegetables (when cooked in water) in only a small amount of rapidly boiling water in a covered pan with a tight-fitting lid.

To prepare greens, such as spinach, beet tops, collards, or kale, for cooking, wash them under lots of running water. Spinach needs no additional water except that which clings to

the leaves. Other greens will need the addition of a few table-spoons of water. Greens like privacy; be sure to cover the pot tightly and cook quickly.

There are four especially fine methods of vegetable cookery that we recommend for any home kitchen. Each is used in one or more vegetable recipes in this book.

Baking or *oven-cooking* may be used for fresh, frozen, or canned vegetables or for dried vegetables prepared for cook-ing. Choose the right temperature, the right casserole size, and the right timing.

The *boiling* method has been covered briefly in the reference to strong-flavored and mild-flavored vegetables. We advise no more than $\frac{1}{2}$ to 1 inch water in the pan. Some vegetables, such as new potatoes and sweet potatoes, take very well indeed to being boiled in their jackets. Peel the sweet potatoes imme-diately, but leave the tender skins on the new potatoes.

Steaming is an excellent cooking method that helps preserve the flavor and food values of vegetables. A regulation vegeta-ble steamer basket that may be used in most pots is a handy piece of equipment. Make sure the bottom of the steamer does not touch the water and keep the saucepan tightly covered. That way the steam will cook the vegetable in its own liquids. Steamed vegetables are so tasty that they need little additional seasoning.

Sautéing may also be called *stir-frying* when applied to cer-tain types of foods or recipes. A small amount of fat, some-times with a small amount of liquid, is used in a large frying pan or wok. Vegetables alone, or meat and vegetables together, may be cooked over rather high heat and stirred with a wooden spoon during this quick cooking method. Vegetables should be hot but crisp and crunchy.

Try our vegetable recipes! Good eating!

Asparagus au Gratin

1 pound (16–24 spears) asparagus
Boiling water
½ teaspoon vegetable oil (to oil pan)
3 tablespoons grated Parmesan cheese
3 tablespoons water
2 tablespoons chopped green onion
1 tablespoon margarine, melted
3 tablespoons fine dry bread crumbs
Dash freshly ground pepper

Preheat oven to 350°F. Snap stems of asparagus at breaking point to remove woody ends; discard ends. Wash spears well to remove all soil under leaf tips. Arrange in a large shallow frying pan and cover with boiling water. Cover pan, bring to a boil, and let cook briskly, about 8–10 minutes. Drain carefully. Arrange half the spears in a single layer in a lightly oiled shallow casserole or baking pan. Sprinkle with half the cheese; add the 3 tablespoons water. Cover with remaining asparagus; sprinkle with remaining cheese. Mix together all the other ingredients with a fork, then spread on top of asparagus. Bake, covered, for 15 minutes.

4 servings   *1 serving: 4–6 spears*

Nutritive values per serving:

CHO (g)	PRO (g)	FAT (g)	CAL —	Fiber (g)	Sodium (mg)	Chol (mg)
9	6	5	97	1.4	160	4

Food Exchanges per serving: 2 Vegetable Exchanges plus 1 Fat Exchange.

Low-sodium diets: Substitute unsalted margarine.

NEW Jade Green Gingered Broccoli

Beautiful, tasty, nutritious—this broccoli recipe is a winner!

6 cups sliced trimmed broccoli pieces
⅓ cup chicken broth
2 cloves garlic, minced fine
1 teaspoon grated peeled fresh gingerroot
3 tablespoons reduced-sodium (light) soy sauce
1 tablespoon brown sugar
1 teaspoon sesame oil
1 tablespoon cornstarch
2 tablespoons cold water

Place broccoli in large pan of boiling water. Return to boil and cook for 2 minutes; drain and set aside. Heat chicken broth in a wok or large skillet over medium heat. Add garlic and ginger; stir for 1 minute. Add soy sauce, brown sugar, and sesame oil. Combine cornstarch and cold water; add to skillet. Cook and stir until sauce thickens. Stir in broccoli.

6 servings (yield: 4½ cups loosely packed)   1 serving: ¾ cup

Nutritive values per serving:						
CHO (g)	PRO (g)	FAT (g)	CAL	Fiber (g)	Sodium (mg)	Chol (mg)
8	4	1	48	1.1	359	0

Food Exchanges per serving: 2 Vegetable Exchanges.

Low-sodium diets: This recipe is not suitable.

Broccoli "Hollandaise"

1½ pounds broccoli
¼ teaspoon salt
¾ cup Mock Hollandaise Sauce (*see* Index)

Wash broccoli and trim off tough stems. Cut each stalk of broccoli into several pieces from top to bottom for more uniform cooking. Put broccoli into a vegetable steamer basket over boiling water. Sprinkle with salt; cover pan tightly. Simmer 12–15 minutes or until broccoli is crisp-tender. Meanwhile, prepare Mock Hollandaise Sauce. Drain broccoli, put on platter, and top with sauce before serving.

8 servings (yield: 6 cups, loosely packed)   1 serving: ¾ cup

			Nutritive values per serving:			
CHO (g)	PRO (g)	FAT (g)	CAL —	Fiber (g)	Sodium (mg)	Chol (mg)
5	3	1	34	2.5	61	18

Food Exchange per serving: 1 Vegetable Exchange.

Low-sodium diets: Omit salt from this recipe and from Mock Hollandaise Sauce.

Broccoli with Lemon

Broccoli is rich in many nutrients—terrific in vitamin A, vitamin C, many minerals, and fiber. And, as a cruciferous vegetable, it may help to prevent cancer.

1½ pounds broccoli
¼ teaspoon salt
2 tablespoons margarine
2 tablespoons fresh lemon juice
½ lemon, cut into thin wedges, for garnish

Wash broccoli and trim off tough stems. Cut each stalk of broccoli into several pieces from top to bottom for more uniform cooking. Put broccoli into a vegetable steamer basket over boiling water. Sprinkle with salt; cover pan tightly.

Simmer 12–15 minutes or until broccoli is crisp-tender. Meanwhile, melt margarine; add lemon juice. Arrange broccoli in a serving dish; drizzle margarine-lemon mixture over broccoli and garnish with lemon wedges.

8 servings (yield: 6 cups, loosely packed)   *1 serving: ¾ cup*

Nutritive values per serving:

CHO (g)	PRO (g)	FAT (g)	CAL —	Fiber (g)	Sodium (mg)	Chol (mg)
5	2	2	36	2.5	70	0

Food Exchanges per serving: 1 Vegetable Exchange plus ½ Fat Exchange.

Low-sodium diets: Omit salt. Use unsalted margarine.

Brussels Sprouts with Cheese Crumbs

    1 10-ounce package frozen or 1 pound fresh
        brussels sprouts
    1 cup boiling water
    ¼ teaspoon salt
    1 teaspoon fresh lemon juice
    2 tablespoons cheese cracker crumbs (10 small
        crackers, crushed)

Cook sprouts in boiling salted water in an uncovered pan. Simmer over medium heat 10–12 minutes or until tender when pierced with a fork; drain sprouts. Sprinkle with lemon juice and crumbs; mix to blend.

5 servings (yield: 2½ cups, loosely packed)   *1 serving: ½ cup*

Nutritive values per serving:

CHO (g)	PRO (g)	FAT (g)	CAL —	Fiber (g)	Sodium (mg)	Chol (mg)
8	2	2	54	1.8	182	0

Food Exchanges per serving: 1 Vegetable Exchange plus ½ Fat Exchange.

Low-sodium diets: Omit salt.

Orange Spiced Carrots

1 pound young tender carrots, without tops
½ cup water
½ cup orange juice
1 tablespoon margarine
½ teaspoon pure vanilla extract
¼ teaspoon ground nutmeg
1½ teaspoons grated fresh orange rind

Wash carrots and pare them with a vegetable peeler; remove ends. Cut carrots crosswise into ¼-inch rounds. Put water, orange juice, and margarine into a saucepan and add carrots. Cover tightly and simmer over low heat 25 minutes or until carrots are crisp-tender. Check to make sure that carrots don't burn because most of the liquid will be absorbed; add a few tablespoons of water if necessary. Sprinkle carrots with vanilla, nutmeg, and orange rind; mix well.

4 servings (yield: 2 cups)   *1 serving: ½ cup*

Nutritive values per serving:

CHO (g)	PRO (g)	FAT (g)	CAL —	Fiber (g)	Sodium (mg)	Chol (mg)
14	1	3	84	3.1	69	0

Food Exchanges per serving: 1 Vegetable Exchange plus ½ Fruit Exchange plus ½ Fat Exchange.

Low-sodium diets: This recipe is excellent.

Dilled Carrots

1 pound young tender carrots, without tops
1½ tablespoons margarine
¼ teaspoon dried dill weed
¼ teaspoon salt
Dash freshly ground pepper
1 tablespoon water

Preheat oven to 375°F. Pare carrots with vegetable peeler or scrub them very well with a vegetable brush. Cut carrots into strips, like french fries. Place carrots in the middle of a piece of heavy-duty foil; dot with margarine and sprinkle with seasonings and water. Wrap carrots securely in foil and crimp edges. Bake 45 minutes or until carrots are tender.

5 servings (yield: 2½ cups)   1 serving: ½ cup (about 7 strips)

				Nutritive values per serving:		
CHO (g)	PRO (g)	FAT (g)	CAL —	Fiber (g)	Sodium (mg)	Chol (mg)
9	1	4	70	2.6	169	0

Food Exchanges per serving: 1 Vegetable Exchange plus 1 Fat Exchange.

Low-sodium diets: Omit salt. Use unsalted margarine.

Sweet and Sour Red Cabbage

1 pound red cabbage, shredded
½ cup cider vinegar
½ cup water
2 tablespoons margarine
½ teaspoon salt
Sugar substitute equivalent to 2 tablespoons sugar

Put cabbage, vinegar, water, margarine, and salt in a deep cooking pot. Cover and cook about 15 minutes or until crisp-tender, lifting and turning with a large kitchen fork two or three times. Remove from heat. Add sweetener to cabbage gradually, lifting and mixing well with a fork. Drain off any liquid.

8 servings (yield: 6 cups)   *1 serving: ¾ cup*

Nutritive values per serving:

CHO (g)	PRO (g)	FAT (g)	CAL —	Fiber (g)	Sodium (mg)	Chol (mg)
5	1	3	42	1.5	100	0

Food Exchanges per serving: 1 Vegetable Exchange plus ½ Fat Exchange.

Low-sodium diets: Omit salt. Use unsalted margarine.

Braised Celery and Mushrooms

2 cups diagonally sliced celery
1 4-ounce can mushroom pieces, drained
¼ cup chopped onion
1 chicken bouillon cube
1 cup boiling water
½ teaspoon Worcestershire sauce

Place celery in a large frying pan. Scatter mushroom pieces and onion on top. Dissolve bouillon cube in boiling water, add Worcestershire sauce, and stir. Pour on top of vegetables. Bring to a boil, cover, reduce heat, and simmer 10 minutes or until celery is crisp-tender.

4 servings (yield: 2 cups)   *1 serving: ½ cup*

Nutritive values per serving:

CHO (g)	PRO (g)	FAT (g)	CAL —	Fiber (g)	Sodium (mg)	Chol (mg)
5	1	0	22	1.3	275	0

Food Exchange per serving: 1 Vegetable Exchange.

Low-sodium diets: This recipe is not suitable.

Cauliflower Crown

1 small (1½-pound head) cauliflower
1 quart boiling water
1 teaspoon fresh lemon juice
1 teaspoon salt
1 slice bread
¼ cup plain low-fat yogurt
1 tablespoon margarine
¼ teaspoon paprika

Trim tough stem and old leaves off whole head of cauliflower,
leaving tender leaves and stems. Even off the bottom. Place in
a deep pot with boiling water, lemon juice, and salt. Place
bread slice on top to absorb odor. Preheat oven to 350°F.

Let cauliflower cook briskly for about 20 minutes or until
cauliflower stem is fork-tender. Discard bread slice. Drain cauliflower carefully but thoroughly. Place cauliflower stem side
down on a foil-lined baking sheet. Put yogurt just in the center
of the top of the cauliflower to form a "crown." Divide the
margarine into small bits and dot margarine around yogurt.
Sprinkle evenly with paprika. Bake for 10 minutes.

6 servings   *1 serving: ⅙ head (about ¾ cup)*

Nutritive values per serving:

CHO (g)	PRO (g)	FAT (g)	CAL —	Fiber (g)	Sodium (mg)	Chol (mg)
7	2	2	52	2.3	85	0

Food Exchanges per serving: 1 Vegetable Exchange plus ½ Fat
Exchange.

Low-sodium diets: Omit salt. Use unsalted margarine.

Cauliflower in Cheese Sauce

1 very small (1-pound) head cauliflower
1 slice bread
1 teaspoon salt
1 tablespoon fresh lemon juice
½ cup skim milk
½ cup (2 ounces) shredded cheddar cheese
1 tablespoon margarine
1 tablespoon all-purpose flour
1 tablespoon chopped fresh parsley
Dash cayenne pepper

Preheat oven to 325°F. Prepare a 1½-quart ovenproof casserole with vegetable pan-coating. Wash cauliflower, remove leaves and core, and divide into flowerets. Put in a pot with boiling water to cover; add bread, salt, and lemon juice. Cook cauliflower over medium heat about 15–20 minutes, until it is fork-tender. Meanwhile, in the top of a double boiler, heat the milk, add the cheese, and stir to blend; add remaining ingredients and cook until cheese mixture is thick and smooth. Drain the cauliflower and discard bread; place cauliflower in the prepared casserole. Pour cheese sauce evenly over top. Bake, uncovered, 15 minutes.

6 servings (yield: approximately 3¾ cups)   *1 serving: ⅔ cup*

Nutritive values per serving:

CHO (g)	PRO (g)	FAT (g)	CAL —	Fiber (g)	Sodium (mg)	Chol (mg)
7	5	5	91	1.6	240	10

Food Exchanges per serving: 1 Vegetable Exchange plus 1 Fat Exchange.

Low-sodium diets: Omit salt. Use low-sodium cheese and unsalted margarine.

Corn Creole

1 tablespoon margarine
½ cup finely chopped onion
½ cup finely chopped green pepper
1 16-ounce can whole kernel corn, drained
½ cup canned tomatoes, cut up, with liquid
½ teaspoon chili powder (more or less to taste)
½ teaspoon salt
¼ teaspoon freshly ground pepper

Melt margarine in a 1½-quart pot; add onion and green pepper and stir over medium heat 5 minutes. Add remaining ingredients; mix well and stir over medium heat for 5 more minutes.

4 servings (yield: 2 cups)   *1 serving: ½ cup*

Nutritive values per serving:

CHO (g)	PRO (g)	FAT (g)	CAL —	Fiber (g)	Sodium (mg)	Chol (mg)
25	4	4	134	2.3	645	0

Food Exchanges per serving: 1 Starch Exchange plus
                    1 Vegetable Exchange plus
                    1 Fat Exchange.

Low-sodium diets: Omit salt. Use unsalted margarine, unsalted canned corn, and unsalted canned tomatoes.

NEW Corn and Bean Medley

3 tablespoons liquid drained from canned corn
¼ cup chopped onion
1 cup canned whole-kernel corn, drained
¾ cup canned red kidney beans, drained
¾ teaspoon chili powder
¼ teaspoon red pepper flakes (or to taste)

Heat liquid from canned corn in a nonstick saucepan. Sauté onion in liquid until tender, about 2 minutes, adding more

liquid if necessary. Add remaining ingredients and heat, stirring often. Adjust seasonings and serve hot.

4 servings (yield: 2 cups)   *1 serving: ½ cup*

Nutritive values per serving:

CHO (g)	PRO (g)	FAT (g)	CAL —	Fiber (g)	Sodium (mg)	Chol (mg)
17	4	0	81	3.4	160	0

Food Exchange per serving: 1 Starch Exchange.

Low-sodium diets: This recipe is suitable. Substitute unsalted
canned vegetables if available.

Green Beans Almandine

1 9-ounce package French-cut green beans
½ teaspoon salt
⅓ cup boiling water
1½ tablespoons margarine
1 tablespoon slivered almonds

Cook green beans in salted boiling water in a small covered
saucepan, separating beans with a fork, for 8 minutes, until
crisp-tender. Meanwhile, heat margarine in a small pan; sauté
almonds in margarine until they are golden and margarine is
slightly browned. Drain beans and toss with almond mixture.

4 servings (yield: 2 cups)   *1 serving: ½ cup*

Nutritive values per serving:

CHO (g)	PRO (g)	FAT (g)	CAL —	Fiber (g)	Sodium (mg)	Chol (mg)
4	1	5	66	1.2	180	0

Food Exchanges per serving: 1 Vegetable Exchange plus 1 Fat
Exchange.

Low-sodium diets: Omit salt. Use unsalted margarine.

Green Beans Italiano

1 tablespoon margarine
1 medium cooking onion
2 cloves garlic, crushed
1 8-ounce can tomatoes
1 16-ounce can cut green beans
¼ cup chopped green pepper
¼ teaspoon salt
½ teaspoon crushed dried oregano
1 tablespoon wine vinegar

Melt margarine in a heavy deep saucepan. Peel onion and slice crosswise into thin rings; sauté onion and garlic in melted margarine. Stir over medium heat with a wooden spoon until onion is tender but not browned. Cut tomatoes into bite-sized pieces. Add to onions with tomato liquid, green beans and their liquid, and all remaining ingredients. Mix well. Bring to a boil and simmer gently about 10 minutes to blend flavors.

5 servings (yield: 4 cups)   *1 serving: ¾ cup*

Nutritive values per serving:						
CHO (g)	PRO (g)	FAT (g)	CAL —	Fiber (g)	Sodium (mg)	Chol (mg)
11	2	3	71	2.4	202	0

Food Exchanges per serving: 2 Vegetable Exchanges plus ½ Fat Exchange.

Low-sodium diets: Omit salt. Use unsalted margarine, unsalted canned tomatoes, and unsalted canned green beans.

Mary's Easy Mushrooms

1 pound fresh mushrooms
1 tablespoon margarine, broken into bits
¼ teaspoon salt
Dash freshly ground pepper

Preheat oven to 350°F. Wash mushrooms thoroughly and re-move tough tips from bottom of stems. Cut a large piece of aluminum foil; place mushrooms in the middle of the foil, dot with margarine, and sprinkle with salt and pepper. Fold foil around mushrooms; seal package tightly by crimping edges. Bake for 20–30 minutes in oven or on a barbecue grill. Open package very carefully to avoid spilling the delicious juices from the mushrooms. These mushrooms with their juices are great with steak or roast beef.

7 servings (yield: 3½ cups)   *1 serving: ½ cup*

Nutritive values per serving:						
CHO (g)	PRO (g)	FAT (g)	CAL —	Fiber (g)	Sodium (mg)	Chol (mg)
3	1	2	31	1.2	91	0

Food Exchange per serving: 1 Vegetable Exchange.

Low-sodium diets: Omit salt. Use unsalted margarine.

Yummy Onions

4 cups onion wedges
1 cup water
1 chicken bouillon cube
¼ cup finely diced green pepper
1 tablespoon vegetable oil
½ teaspoon salt
½ teaspoon Italian seasoning
¼ teaspoon garlic powder
Dash ground cloves

Combine all ingredients in a saucepan. Cover tightly and simmer over medium heat 25 minutes.

5 servings (yield: 2½ cups)   *1 serving: ½ cup*

Nutritive values per serving:

CHO (g)	PRO (g)	FAT (g)	CAL —	Fiber (g)	Sodium (mg)	Chol (mg)
3	1	3	36	0.3	371	0

Food Exchange per serving: 1 Vegetable Exchange.

Low-sodium diets: Omit salt. Use low-sodium chicken bouillon cube.

Spinach with Nutmeg

2 10-ounce packages frozen chopped spinach
½ teaspoon salt
1 cup boiling water
½ cup Lemon Mayonnaise (*see* Index)
¼ teaspoon coarsely ground pepper
¼ teaspoon ground nutmeg

Cook spinach in salted boiling water in a saucepan. Separate spinach with a fork; cook over moderate heat, covered, 8–10 minutes or until tender. Drain in a strainer, pressing out ex-

cess liquid with the back of a wooden spoon. Return spinach to pan; stir in Lemon Mayonnaise, pepper, and nutmeg. Reheat gently 2 minutes.

5 servings (yield: 2½ cups)   *1 serving: ½ cup*

Nutritive values per serving:

CHO (g)	PRO (g)	FAT (g)	CAL —	Fiber (g)	Sodium (mg)	Chol (mg)
8	4	1	49	2.5	400	37

Food Exchanges per serving: 2 Vegetable Exchanges.

Low-sodium diets: Omit salt from recipe and in preparing Lemon Mayonnaise.

Baked Spinach Casserole

2 10-ounce packages frozen chopped spinach
2 eggs, beaten
1 tablespoon all-purpose flour
½ teaspoon salt
⅛ teaspoon freshly ground pepper
⅛ teaspoon fresh lemon juice
½ teaspoon vegetable oil (to oil casserole)

Preheat oven to 350°F. Cook spinach as directed on package, but simmer only 3 minutes; drain. To beaten eggs add flour, seasonings, and lemon juice; beat with a hand beater. Add cooked spinach and mix well. Turn into lightly oiled 1-quart casserole. Bake, uncovered, for 20–25 minutes.

5 servings (yield: 2½ cups)   *1 serving: ½ cup*

Nutritive values per serving:

CHO (g)	PRO (g)	FAT (g)	CAL —	Fiber (g)	Sodium (mg)	Chol (mg)
8	6	3	74	2.5	321	110

Food Exchanges per serving: 1 Vegetable Exchange plus ½ Medium-Fat Meat Exchange.

Low-sodium diets: Omit salt.

Sautéed Sweet Peppers

This very colorful vegetable may be served alone, but it's beautiful over a beef patty or over a plain omelet.

2 medium (9 ounces) green peppers
2 medium (9 ounces) red peppers
2 tablespoons margarine
2 tablespoons water
½ teaspoon salt
½ teaspoon dried basil *or* 1 tablespoon chopped
    fresh basil
⅛ teaspoon coarsely ground pepper

Wash peppers; remove stems, seeds, and cores. Cut peppers into 1-inch squares. Heat margarine in a large frying pan over medium heat; add peppers and cook 3–4 minutes, stirring often. Add water and continue stirring and cooking another 4–5 minutes, until peppers are crisp-tender. Add seasonings and serve.

6 servings (yield: 3 cups)   *1 serving: ½ cup*

Nutritive values per serving:

CHO (g)	PRO (g)	FAT (g)	CAL —	Fiber (g)	Sodium (mg)	Chol (mg)
4	1	4	51	0.9	209	0

Food Exchanges per serving: 1 Vegetable Exchange plus ½ Fat Exchange.

Low-sodium diets: Omit salt. Use unsalted margarine.

Mashed Winter Squash

Use butternut, Hubbard, or acorn squash as you prefer.

1¾ pounds winter squash
½ teaspoon vegetable oil
1½ tablespoons margarine, cut into pieces
Ground cinnamon for garnish (optional)

Preheat oven to 350°F. Cut each squash into lengthwise quarters; scoop out seeds and discard. Score yellow meaty part of each quarter with a knife. Brush bottom of a shallow baking pan with the vegetable oil. Place squash pieces in pan with skin sides up. Bake 45 minutes or until very tender. Carefully remove skin from squash and put squash pulp into a bowl; beat until fluffy; add margarine and beat it in well. If desired, garnish with sprinkle of cinnamon.

4 servings (yield: 2 cups)   *1 serving: ½ cup*

Nutritive values per serving:

CHO (g)	PRO (g)	FAT (g)	CAL —	Fiber (g)	Sodium (mg)	Chol (mg)
22	2	2	101	3.1	23	0

Food Exchanges per serving: 1 Starch Exchange plus ½ Fat Exchange.

Low-sodium diets: This recipe is excellent.

Pineapple Squash

2 medium acorn squash (2 pounds), 4½ inches in
   diameter
1 8-ounce can unsweetened crushed pineapple with
   juice
2 teaspoons margarine
½ teaspoon ground cinnamon
Hot water

Preheat oven to 375°F. Cut each squash in half; scoop out and
discard seeds and pulp. Trim tip off bottom if necessary so
that each squash cup stands up straight. Fill each squash cup
with ¼ cup crushed pineapple, ½ teaspoon margarine, and a
sprinkle of cinnamon. Put squash into a flat baking dish and
pour hot water around bottoms of squash to a depth of ½ inch.
Cover pan tightly with foil. Bake 1 hour or until squash is
tender and can be easily pierced with a fork.

4 servings   *1 serving: ½ stuffed squash*

Nutritive values per serving:

CHO (g)	PRO (g)	FAT (g)	CAL —	Fiber (g)	Sodium (mg)	Chol (mg)
34	2	2	148	4.1	31	0

Food Exchanges per serving: 1 Starch Exchange plus 1 Fruit
                              Exchange.

Low-sodium diets: This recipe is excellent.

Mashed Turnips

1 pound turnips, without tops
2 cups boiling water
1½ tablespoons margarine
½ teaspoon salt
⅛ teaspoon freshly ground pepper
Paprika or chopped fresh parsley for garnish
     (optional)

Remove tops and root ends and pare turnips; cut turnips into small cubes. Measure boiling water into a small heavy saucepan. Add cubed turnips; cover pan, bring to a boil, reduce heat to low, and cook for about 20 minutes or until tender. Drain any remaining water (most of it should be cooked away). Mash turnips thoroughly with a hand masher or an electric beater; add margarine, salt, and pepper. Beat until blended and fluffy. If garnish is desired, sprinkle paprika or finely cut parsley on top.

4 servings (yield: 2 cups)   *1 serving: ½ cup*

CHO (g)	PRO (g)	FAT (g)	CAL —	Fiber (g)	Sodium (mg)	Chol (mg)
6	1	4	59	1.5	351	0

Nutritive values per serving:

Food Exchanges per serving: 1 Vegetable Exchange plus 1 Fat Exchange.

Low-sodium diets: Omit salt. Use unsalted margarine.

Baked Tomatoes

4 small tomatoes (about 1 pound)
1 slice bread, crumbled fine (¾ cup soft crumbs)
½ teaspoon herb or Italian seasoning
½ teaspoon salt
⅛ teaspoon coarsely ground pepper
1 tablespoon finely chopped green onion
1 teaspoon margarine, melted

Preheat oven to 350°F. Wash tomatoes and cut a thin slice off tops; scoop out pulp into a bowl, leaving shells. Mix pulp, ½ cup of the bread crumbs, the seasonings, and the green onion. Place tomato shells in an 8-inch square pan or a pie pan. Divide pulp mixture evenly among the tomatoes, placing in hollows carefully. Mix melted margarine with remaining ¼ cup bread crumbs and sprinkle on top of tomatoes. Bake about 25 minutes, until tomatoes are tender.

4 servings · *1 serving: 1 tomato*

Nutritive values per serving:

CHO (g)	PRO (g)	FAT (g)	CAL —	Fiber (g)	Sodium (mg)	Chol (mg)
8	2	1	49	2.1	297	0

Food Exchange per serving: 1 Vegetable Exchange *or*
½ Starch Exchange.

Low-sodium diets: Omit salt.

Zucchini and Tomatoes au Gratin

1 10-ounce can tomatoes with liquid
1 tablespoon vegetable oil
¾ cup thinly sliced onion rings
1½ pounds zucchini, sliced thin
½ cup tomato juice
¼ teaspoon salt
⅛ teaspoon freshly ground pepper
½ cup grated Parmesan cheese

Preheat oven to 350°F. Cut tomatoes into bite-sized pieces. Use ½ teaspoon of oil to prepare casserole. Heat remaining oil in a large frying pan. Add onion rings and cook over medium heat, stirring until limp. Add zucchini slices, cover, and cook over low heat 5 minutes. Add tomatoes, juice from can, tomato juice, salt, and pepper; mix carefully. Turn into a lightly oiled 1½- to 2-quart casserole. Sprinkle with grated cheese. Bake about 20 minutes, until top is golden brown.

10 servings (yield: 5 cups)　　　　　　　*1 serving: ½ cup*

			Nutritive values per serving:			
CHO (g)	PRO (g)	FAT (g)	CAL —	Fiber (g)	Sodium (mg)	Chol (mg)
5	3	3	56	1.6	234	4

Food Exchanges per serving: 1 Vegetable Exchange plus ½ Fat Exchange.

Low-sodium diets: Omit salt. Use unsalted canned tomatoes and unsalted tomato juice.

Zucchini Sauté

2–3 medium zucchini (1 pound)
1 tablespoon vegetable oil
½ cup thinly sliced red onion
¼ teaspoon dried oregano or basil
¼ teaspoon salt
Dash freshly ground pepper

Clean and slice zucchini into thin strips or bite-sized pieces. Heat oil in a large frying pan. Add onion and stir-fry quickly until onion is translucent, not browned. Add zucchini, cover pan, and cook 3–4 minutes, until zucchini is wilted. Sprinkle with all seasonings and mix well.

4 servings (yield: 2⅔ cups)   *1 serving: ⅔ cup*

CHO (g)	PRO (g)	FAT (g)	CAL —	Fiber (g)	Sodium (mg)	Chol (mg)
5	2	4	54	2.1	125	0

Nutritive values per serving:

Food Exchanges per serving: 1 Vegetable Exchange plus ½ Fat Exchange.

Low-sodium diets: Omit salt.

Ratatouille

This versatile vegetable mixture is great served either hot or cold. Mary likes to serve it warm on toast points as an appetizer or chilled on Boston lettuce with additional capers on top. She always makes enough so that she can serve it hot once and cold once.

¼ cup olive oil
4 tablespoons margarine
3 cloves garlic, crushed
3 medium onions, chopped (2 cups)

1 medium (1-pound) eggplant, peeled and cubed
2 medium green peppers (8–9 ounces), cored and
  sliced
2 medium zucchini (about 12 ounces), sliced
3 tablespoons all-purpose flour
1 16-ounce can tomatoes, cut up, with liquid
¾ cup water
1 6-ounce can tomato paste
1 teaspoon salt
½ teaspoon coarsely ground pepper
¼ cup fresh chopped parsley
2 teaspoons drained capers

Heat the oil and margarine in a large pot. Add garlic and onions and cook until onions are translucent. Add eggplant, green pepper, and zucchini and cook, stirring often, until vegetables wilt. Sprinkle flour over vegetable mixture; stir in tomatoes with liquid, water, and tomato paste. Cover and cook over low heat 20 minutes, stirring often to prevent sticking to the bottom of pot. Add remaining ingredients and cook, uncovered, 10 more minutes; stir often.

16 servings (yield: 8 cups)   *1 serving: ½ cup*

Nutritive values per serving:

CHO (g)	PRO (g)	FAT (g)	CAL —	Fiber (g)	Sodium (mg)	Chol (mg)
9	2	7	97	1.7	297	0

Food Exchanges per serving: 2 Vegetable Exchanges plus 1 Fat Exchange.

Low-sodium diets: Omit salt and capers. Substitute unsalted margarine, 4 small fresh tomatoes for the canned tomatoes, and unsalted tomato paste.

NEW Sautéed Vegetable Filling for Buckwheat Crepes

This sautéed vegetable mixture can also be served as a vegetable.

- 1 tablespoon margarine
- 1 cup thinly sliced red onion
- 1 cup zucchini or other summer squash strips
- 1 cup red or green pepper strips
- ½ teaspoon dried basil
- ½ teaspoon dried oregano
- ½ teaspoon dried tarragon
- 2 tablespoons beef broth

Melt margarine in a large nonstick frying pan over medium heat. Sauté onion, stirring often, until tender. Mix in remaining ingredients except beef broth and cook until vegetables are crisp but tender, stirring often. Add beef broth during cooking. Cool vegetable filling before placing in crepes.

Yield: 2 cups   *1 serving: ¼ cup as filling*
                                   or ½ cup as vegetable

Nutritive values per serving (¼ cup as filling):

CHO (g)	PRO (g)	FAT (g)	CAL —	Fiber (g)	Sodium (mg)	Chol (mg)
3	0	2	27	0.8	30	0

Food Exchange per serving: 1 Vegetable Exchange.

Nutritive values per serving (½ cup as vegetable):

CHO (g)	PRO (g)	FAT (g)	CAL —	Fiber (g)	Sodium (mg)	Chol (mg)
6	1	3	55	1.6	61	0

Food Exchanges per serving: 1 Vegetable Exchange plus ½ Fat Exchange.

Low-sodium diets: This recipe is excellent.

25
Desserts

PIES AND COBBLERS

Graham Cracker Pie Shell

Do not use packaged graham cracker crumbs for this recipe because their carbohydrate content is higher than that of graham wafers. Fill this crust with your favorite flavor of sugar-free pudding.

>   7 large plain graham wafers (each 2½ by 5 inches)
>   3 tablespoons margarine, melted

Break graham wafers into small pieces, place in a plastic bag, fasten opening with a bag tie, and press with a rolling pin or a large jar to make crumbs. Continue until all crumbs are fine (total of 1¼ cups). Empty into a bowl. Melt the margarine, add to crumbs, and mix well with a fork. Set aside 2 tablespoons to use later as the garnish on the pie filling. Using the back of a spoon, press remainder of crumb mixture evenly on bottom and sides of a 9-inch pie plate. Chill in refrigerator for 3 hours or longer before filling.

8 servings (yield: 9-inch pie shell)   *1 serving: ⅛ pie shell*

Nutritive values per serving:

CHO (g)	PRO (g)	FAT (g)	CAL —	Fiber (g)	Sodium (mg)	Chol (mg)
9	1	5	86	0.1	108	0

Food Exchanges per serving (crust only): 1 Fat Exchange plus
                                          ½ Starch Exchange.

Low-sodium diets: Use unsalted margarine.

Vanilla Wafer Crumb Crust

Use this unbaked shell for Chocolate Whipped Cream Pie, Jo's Cranberry Pie (see Index), or for other fillings.

> 2 tablespoons margarine, melted
> 30 vanilla wafers (1¾ inches in diameter)
> ¼ teaspoon pure vanilla extract

Prepare a 9-inch pie plate by rubbing inside, bottom, and sides with 1 teaspoon of the margarine; set aside. Crush vanilla wafers to make very fine crumbs (1¼ cups). Place crumbs in a large bowl; combine vanilla and melted margarine and drizzle all over crumbs. Mix thoroughly with a blending fork to make sure all is well blended. Remove about 2 tablespoons of crumb mixture and set aside to use if desired as a garnish on top of pie. With back of a large spoon, press remaining crumbs evenly all over bottom and sides of prepared pie pan. Chill in refrigerator 2 hours or longer before filling.

8 servings (yield: 9-inch pie shell)   *1 serving: ⅛ pie shell*

Nutritive values per serving:						
CHO (g)	PRO (g)	FAT (g)	CAL —	Fiber (g)	Sodium (mg)	Chol (mg)
11	1	5	95	0	71	9

Food Exchanges per serving (crust only): 1 Starch Exchange
plus ½ Fat Exchange.

Low-sodium diets: Use unsalted margarine.

Lemon Cheese Pie

Some of Kay's nondiabetic friends asked for double-sized servings of this one!

> 1½ tablespoons granulated gelatin
> ½ cup cold water

1 cup skim milk
3 medium eggs, beaten
¼ teaspoon salt
1 tablespoon grated lemon rind
⅓ cup fresh lemon juice
½ teaspoon pure lemon extract
Sugar substitute equivalent to ½ cup sugar
1 pound (2 cups) small-curd cream-style cottage
   cheese
1 Graham Cracker Pie Shell (*see* Index)
3–4 fresh strawberries or thin lemon slices for
   garnish

Soak gelatin in cold water. Scald milk in top of a double boiler. Pour slowly on top of gently beaten eggs and salt, stirring constantly. Return to top of the double boiler; cook over slowly simmering water, stirring constantly, until mixture coats spoon. Remove from heat. Turn into a bowl; add gelatin, lemon rind, lemon juice, lemon extract, and sweetener; mix well until gelatin is dissolved. Chill until mixture is the consistency of unbeaten egg whites; stir gently several times while chilling. Add cottage cheese. Beat with an electric mixer at high speed for 8–10 minutes. If filling thins, chill for 5–10 minutes. Turn into prepared 9-inch Graham Cracker Pie Shell. Sprinkle reserved 2 tablespoons cracker crumbs on top; garnish with sliced strawberries or lemons. Chill 3 hours or longer.

8 servings (yield: 9-inch pie)   *1 serving: ⅛ pie*

Nutritive values per serving:						
CHO (g)	PRO (g)	FAT (g)	CAL —	Fiber (g)	Sodium (mg)	Chol (mg)
10	12	9	171	0.3	396	111

Food Exchanges per serving: 1 Starch Exchange plus 1 High-Fat Meat Exchange.

Low-sodium diets: Omit salt. Use unsalted cottage cheese if available. Use unsalted margarine in the crust recipe.

Holiday Pumpkin Chiffon Pie

1 tablespoon granulated gelatin
½ cup cold water
3 eggs, separated
½ cup whole milk
1¼ cups solid-pack canned pumpkin
½ teaspoon salt
¼ teaspoon ground nutmeg
¾ teaspoon ground cinnamon
½ teaspoon ground ginger
½ teaspoon ground allspice
Sugar substitute equivalent to ½ cup sugar
2 tablespoons sugar
2 teaspoons brandy
1 Graham Cracker Pie Shell (*see* Index)

Dissolve gelatin in cold water; set aside. Beat egg yolks lightly and stir in milk, pumpkin, salt, and spices; blend well. Cook in the top of a double boiler, stirring constantly until thick and smooth, about 8 minutes. Remove from heat, add gelatin and sweetener, and stir until completely dissolved. Cool, then chill in refrigerator until mixture thickens to consistency of un-beaten egg white. Remove from refrigerator. Beat egg whites until soft peaks form. Add sugar and brandy gradually to egg whites, beating constantly until stiff, glossy, and shiny. Fold carefully but thoroughly into pumpkin mixture. Turn care-fully into the prepared pie shell; scatter reserved 2 tablespoons graham cracker crumbs on top as garnish. Chill about 8 hours. Slice into 8 equal portions.

8 servings (yield: 9-inch pie)   *1 serving: ⅛ pie*

		Nutritive values per serving:				
CHO (g)	PRO (g)	FAT (g)	CAL —	Fiber (g)	Sodium (mg)	Chol (mg)
13	4	7	138	0.9	237	105

Food Exchanges per serving: 1 Starch Exchange plus 1 Fat
Exchange.

Low-sodium diets: Omit salt. Use unsalted margarine in crust
recipe. When available, use unsalted canned
pumpkin for filling.

NEW Chocolate Whipped Cream Pie

*This is Rachel Hess's favorite recipe in the whole book. She
recently made it for a party for her teenage friends.*

1 Vanilla Wafer Crumb Crust (*see* Index)
1 1.5-ounce package sugar-free chocolate instant
    pudding mix
2 cups skim milk
1½ cups frozen whipped topping

Prepare Vanilla Wafer Crumb Crust (reserve 2 tablespoons
crumb mixture), pack into a 9-inch pie shell, and chill in refrigerator at least 2 hours before making filling. Prepare pudding
according to package directions using the 2 cups skim milk.
Allow it to cool for one-half hour. Spoon pudding carefully into
chilled pie shell and chill until pudding is firm. Spread
whipped topping gently across top of pie with a small spatula.
Scatter the reserved crumb mixture on top as a garnish.

6 servings (yield: 9-inch pie)   *1 serving: ⅙ pie*

Nutritive values per serving:

CHO (g)	PRO (g)	FAT (g)	CAL —	Fiber (g)	Sodium (mg)	Chol (mg)
24	5	8	190	0	211	14

Food Exchanges per serving: 1½ Fat Exchanges plus
1 Starch Exchange plus
½ Skim Milk Exchange.

Low-sodium diets: This recipe is suitable unless sodium is
severely restricted. Use unsalted margarine in
crust recipe.

Banana Cream Pie

1 Vanilla Wafer Crumb Crust (*see* Index)
1½ teaspoons granulated gelatin
¼ cup cold water
1½ cups hot skim milk
¼ cup flour
¼ teaspoon salt
½ cup cold skim milk
2 eggs, beaten
Sugar substitute equivalent to 3 tablespoons sugar
1½ teaspoons pure vanilla extract
1 pound firm-ripe bananas

Prepare pie crust and chill 2 hours or longer before filling.
Soak gelatin in cold water and set aside. Heat 1½ cups milk in
the top of a double boiler over simmering water. In a small
bowl combine flour, salt, and ½ cup cold milk; mix until
smooth and without lumps. Slowly pour ½ cup of the hot milk
into the bowl with the flour mixture; stir to mix well. Then
slowly pour contents of the bowl back into the pot of hot milk.
Cook and stir over simmering water until thick and smooth.
Pour mixture slowly on top of beaten eggs, stirring constantly.
Return to top of double boiler. Cook and stir over simmering
water about 4 minutes; remove from heat. Add gelatin, sweetener, and vanilla; mix well to dissolve gelatin. Cool and chill
until mixture begins to gel. Peel bananas, slice thin, and measure 1½ cups. Arrange 1 cup sliced bananas in bottom of pie
shell, then very carefully spoon and pour filling evenly on top.
Arrange remaining ½ cup sliced bananas on top and garnish
with the vanilla crumbs saved when making pie shell. Cover
whole pie carefully with plastic wrap. Chill 2–3 hours, until set
and firm. To serve, cut into eight equal pieces.

8 servings (yield: 9-inch pie)   *1 serving: ⅛ pie*

Nutritive values per serving:						
CHO (g)	PRO (g)	FAT (g)	CAL —	Fiber (g)	Sodium (mg)	Chol (mg)
24	5	7	174	0.8	174	79

Food Exchanges per serving: 1 Fruit Exchange plus 1 Low-Fat Milk Exchange.

Low-sodium diets: Omit salt. Use unsalted margarine in crust recipe.

NEW Strawberry Tart

This beautiful dessert is shown on the book cover.

- 1 Graham Cracker Pie Shell (*see* Index)
- 2 cups low-fat (2%) milk
- 1 1.1-ounce package sugar-free vanilla instant pudding mix
- 1 teaspoon freshly grated orange rind
- 2 cups cleaned and hulled strawberries or other berries

Use an 8- or 9-inch tart pan with removable bottom. Firmly pat graham cracker pie shell into tart pan. Set aside. Blend milk with instant pudding mix in deep bowl using a whisk or an electric mixer. Continue mixing at low speed for 1 minute or until pudding is dissolved. Add grated orange rind. Let stand for 5 minutes and pour into pie shell. Let stand for 15 minutes or until set. Arrange strawberries or other berries decoratively over pudding shortly before serving.

8 servings (yield: 8- or 9-inch pie)   *1 serving: ⅛ pie*

			Nutritive values per serving:			
CHO (g)	PRO (g)	FAT (g)	CAL —	Fiber (g)	Sodium (mg)	Chol (mg)
18	3	5	134	1.2	320	1

Food Exchanges per serving: 1 Starch Exchange plus 1 Fat Exchange.

Low-sodium diets: This recipe is suitable for occasional use. Use unsalted margarine in pie shell.

Jo's Cranberry Pie

This is a really great pie and is unique and low in calories. Josephine Anderson's original recipe is the Thanksgiving favorite at Mary's home and is not for diabetics. But Kay has made a very good "diabetic copy."

> 1 Vanilla Wafer Crumb Crust (*see* Index)
> 1 tablespoon granulated gelatin
> 2 cups cold water
> 3 cups raw fresh or frozen cranberries
> ¼ teaspoon grated orange rind
> ¼ teaspoon pure orange extract
> Sugar substitute equivalent to 10 tablespoons sugar
>   (15 packets)
> 1½ cups frozen whipped topping

Make crumb crust according to recipe and chill in refrigerator at least 2 hours before filling. Soak gelatin in ½ cup cold water; set aside. Pick over fresh or frozen cranberries, wash, and measure; put in a deep, heavy saucepan with 1½ cups water and orange rind. Cook over moderate heat until all cranberries pop, stirring occasionally. Remove from heat. Stir in gelatin, orange extract and sweetener; mix until gelatin is dissolved. Let cool for about 30 minutes, stirring occasionally. Taste to see if enough sweetener has been added because cranberries vary greatly in tartness. Spoon carefully and slowly into pie crust and smooth evenly with the back of a spoon. Chill in refrigerator. When cool, spread whipped topping on pie, smoothing and swirling evenly. Chill in refrigerator for 3–4 hours before serving.

8 servings (yield: 9-inch pie)   *1 serving: ⅛ pie*

Nutritive values per serving:

CHO (g)	PRO (g)	FAT (g)	CAL —	Fiber (g)	Sodium (mg)	Chol (mg)
16	2	9	149	0.4	84	10

Food Exchanges per serving: 2 Fat Exchanges plus 1 Starch Exchange.

Low-sodium diets: This recipe is excellent.

NEW French Apple Clafouti

4 cups sliced peeled Granny Smith or Rome apples
   (4 medium-large)
1½ cups whole milk
4 eggs
½ cup all-purpose flour, sifted
¼ cup sugar
1½ teaspoons pure vanilla extract
½ teaspoon ground cinnamon

Preheat oven to 350°F. Use a 10-inch nonstick deep pie plate or spray the pan with vegetable pan-coating. Arrange apple slices evenly in pan. Use a blender or food processor to combine milk and eggs. Add remaining ingredients and blend for 5 seconds. Scrape down sides of blender with a spatula and blend until ingredients are mixed together, about 30 seconds. A bowl and whisk can be used to prepare batter by hand. Spread the batter over the apples. Bake for 1 hour or until custard forms and the cake tests done by inserting a toothpick that comes out clean. Serve warm or at room temperature.

8 servings (yield: 10-inch clafouti)   1 serving: 2½-inch wedge

			Nutritive values per serving:			
CHO (g)	PRO (g)	FAT (g)	CAL —	Fiber (g)	Sodium (mg)	Chol (mg)
22	5	5	148	3.5	57	143

Food Exchanges per serving: 1 Fruit Exchange plus ½ Whole Milk Exchange.

Low-sodium diets: This recipe is excellent.

$\boxed{NEW}$ **Pear Crumble**

¼ cup margarine, cut into ½-inch pieces
⅓ cup uncooked quick-cooking oats
¼ cup all-purpose flour
Sugar substitute equivalent to 2 tablespoons sugar
2 cups chopped cored firm-ripe pears (½-inch
    pieces)
2 teaspoons fresh lemon juice
½ teaspoon ground cinnamon
¼ teaspoon ground nutmeg
½ teaspoon grated lemon rind

Preheat oven to 400°F. Prepare an 8-inch pie plate with vegetable pan-coating. Toss margarine, oats, flour, and sweetener together in a medium mixing bowl; reserve. Place pears in a mixing bowl and toss with lemon juice, cinnamon, nutmeg, and lemon rind. Arrange pears in the prepared pan. Sprinkle oat mixture over fruit. Bake for 15 minutes. Serve warm or cool.

6 servings (yield: 8-inch pie)   *1 serving: ⅙ of pie*

| | | | *Nutritive values per serving:* | | | |
CHO (g)	PRO (g)	FAT (g)	CAL —	Fiber (g)	Sodium (mg)	Chol (mg)
16	1	8	137	1.8	89	0

Food Exchanges per serving: 1½ Fat Exchanges plus 1 Starch Exchange.

Low-sodium diets: This recipe is excellent.

Apple Cobbler

1¾ pounds (about 4) medium-sized cooking apples
   (Jonathans or Wealthies)
1½ tablespoons fresh lemon juice
½ teaspoon grated lemon rind
1 tablespoon cornstarch
1 teaspoon apple pie spice
¼ teaspoon salt, divided
Sugar substitute equivalent to 4 tablespoons sugar
½ cup flour
3 tablespoons margarine

Preheat oven to 425°F. Prepare inside of a 9-inch pie plate with vegetable pan-coating. Pare apples, remove cores, and cut apples into ⅛-inch slices; measure 4 cups. Combine apple slices, lemon juice, and rind. Combine cornstarch, spice, ⅛ teaspoon salt, and sweetener; mix thoroughly. Add to apples and stir lightly with a fork to coat all slices. Spread apples evenly in prepared pie plate; set aside. Mix together flour and remaining ⅛ teaspoon salt. Cut in margarine with pastry blender or fork until crumbly; scatter all over top of apples. Bake about 35 minutes or until top is golden brown. Serve warm.

8 servings (yield: 9-inch pie)   *1 serving: ⅛ pie*

Nutritive values per serving:

CHO (g)	PRO (g)	FAT (g)	CAL —	Fiber (g)	Sodium (mg)	Chol (mg)
19	1	5	117	1.8	111	0

Food Exchanges per serving: 1 Fruit Exchange plus 1 Fat Exchange.

Low-sodium diets: Omit salt. Use unsalted margarine.

CAKES

Cheesecake

6 plain graham wafers (2½ by 2½ inches each)
1½ tablespoons margarine, melted
1 tablespoon granulated gelatin
½ cup cold water
⅓ cup boiling water
½ teaspoon grated lemon rind
½ cup fresh lemon juice
Sugar substitute equivalent to ¼ cup sugar
2 tablespoons water
2 cups (16 ounces) cream-style cottage cheese (4% fat)
½ teaspoon lemon extract
4 large strawberries

Prepare an 8″ × 8″ × 2″ cake pan with vegetable pan-coating; set aside. Make fine crumbs with graham crackers (½ cup) and mix thoroughly with melted margarine; set aside. Soak gelatin in cold water. Combine boiling water and lemon rind; add to gelatin; add lemon juice and sweetener, stirring until completely dissolved. Chill until it is the consistency of unbeaten egg whites. Put 2 tablespoons water, cottage cheese, and lemon extract into a blender or food processor and cover; turn to high speed for 10–15 seconds. Add partially set gelatin mixture; turn to high speed 15 seconds or until well blended. Pour into

prepared pan. Sprinkle graham cracker crumbs evenly over top. Wash, hull, and dry strawberries. Slice in halves lengthwise. Arrange on top of cake so that, when cut into eight servings (4 by 2 inches), each will have a strawberry garnish in center. Chill several hours, until set.

8 servings   *1 serving: 1 piece, 4 by 2 inches*

Nutritive values per serving:

CHO (g)	PRO (g)	FAT (g)	CAL —	Fiber (g)	Sodium (mg)	Chol (mg)
8	8	5	106	0.3	263	8

Food Exchanges per serving: 1 Medium-Fat Meat Exchange plus ½ Fruit Exchange.

Low-sodium diets: This recipe is suitable for occasional use if sodium restriction is not severe.

Refrigerator No-Cheese Cake

4 large (2½- by 2½-inches) graham crackers
1 teaspoon margarine
1 tablespoon granulated gelatin
½ cup cold water
2 cups plain low-fat yogurt
Sugar substitute equivalent to 1 tablespoon sugar
½ cup iced water
1½ teaspoons grated lemon rind
1 egg white
½ cup instant nonfat dry milk powder
2 tablespoons fresh lemon juice
1½ teaspoons pure vanilla extract
Sugar substitute equivalent to 1 tablespoon sugar
3 maraschino cherries, halved, *or* 6 small
     strawberries for garnish

Put crackers in a plastic bag and tie top; crush with a rolling
pin or jar to make fine crumbs. Melt margarine in the bottom
of an 8- or 9-inch round cake pan. Spread margarine evenly
over bottom of pan. Sprinkle crumbs evenly on bottom only;
press gently. Chill in refrigerator. Soak gelatin in cold water.
Heat over boiling water to dissolve the gelatin. Combine
yogurt and first measure of sweetener; beat at moderate speed
with rotary beaters, adding dissolved gelatin gradually. Chill
until it is the consistency of unbeaten egg whites. Meanwhile,
place iced water, lemon rind, egg white, and dry milk powder
in a large bowl. Beat with rotary beaters until soft peaks form.

Add lemon juice, vanilla, and second measure of sweetener. Beat at high speed until stiff. Fold into partially set yogurt; blend very well. Spoon mixture on top of crumbs in pan. Chill 4 hours or longer until set. To unmold, loosen around edge of mold with thin spatula right down to the bottom of pan. Place larger plate upside down on top of mold. Turn plate and pan over; cover top of pan for a few seconds with a hot cloth that has been run under hot water and then wrung out. Remove cloth and lift pan from mold. When ready to serve, garnish with cherries or strawberries and cut into six equal slices.

6 servings   *1 serving: ⅙ cake*

Nutritive values per serving:

CHO (g)	PRO (g)	FAT (g)	CAL —	Fiber (g)	Sodium (mg)	Chol (mg)
13	8	2	104	0.3	124	6

Food Exchange per serving: 1 Low-Fat Milk Exchange.

Low-sodium diets: This recipe is suitable.

NEW Louis's Boston Cream Cake

This cake is dedicated to Dr. Louis Kraus, who has just moved to Boston to begin his residency. Louis is Barbara Grunes's son, and Barbara is our superstar recipe developer.

    5 eggs
    ½ cup sugar
    3 packets Sweet'n Low or other heat-stable sugar
        substitute
    1 teaspoon pure vanilla extract
    ¾ cup flour
    2 tablespoons cornstarch
    1 teaspoon baking powder
    2 cups skim milk
    1 1.1-ounce package sugar-free vanilla instant
        pudding mix
    ½ teaspoon ground cinnamon
    1 teaspoon cocoa powder

Preheat oven to 400°F. Grease and line two 8-inch round cake pans with parchment paper or waxed paper. Beat eggs with electric mixer until light and fluffy. Sprinkle sugar, Sweet'n Low, and vanilla over eggs; continue beating for 2 minutes. Sift flour, cornstarch, and baking powder together; sprinkle half the mixture over batter. Fold in with rubber spatula. Repeat with remaining flour mixture. Use a rubber spatula to spread batter evenly in pans. Bake on center rack of oven for 15–20 minutes or until cake is golden and springs back when lightly touched. Invert cake onto wire rack and cool for 5 minutes; remove pan. Set aside to cool.

Blend milk with instant pudding mix in mixing bowl using electric mixer. Continue mixing at low speed for 1 minute or until pudding mix is dissolved. Set pudding aside for 10 minutes or until set.

To assemble: Arrange a single cake layer on serving dish. Spread two-thirds of firm pudding evenly over bottom cake layer. Place remaining cake layer evenly on top. Stir cinnamon and cocoa into remaining pudding. Spread over top of cake as chocolate frosting. Refrigerate until ready to serve. Cut with serrated knife.

8 servings (yield: 8-inch cake)   *1 serving: ⅛ cake*

Nutritive values per serving:						
CHO (g)	PRO (g)	FAT (g)	CAL —	Fiber (g)	Sodium (mg)	Chol (mg)
28	7	4	176	0.3	165	172

Food Exchanges per serving: 2 Starch Exchanges plus 1 Fat Exchange.

Low-sodium diets: This recipe is suitable.

NEW Chocolate-Filled Cake Roll

CAKE

5 eggs
½ cup sugar
3 packets Sweet'n Low or other heat-stable sugar
    substitute
1 teaspoon pure vanilla extract
¾ cup all-purpose flour
2 tablespoons cornstarch
1 teaspoon baking powder

FILLING

2 cups skim milk
1 1.5 ounce package sugar-free chocolate instant
    pudding mix

TOPPING

2 teaspoons sugar-free cocoa mix

Preheat oven to 400°F. Grease and line the bottom of a 10″ ×
15″ jelly roll pan with waxed paper. Beat eggs in large bowl
with electric mixer until fluffy. Sprinkle sugar, Sweet'n Low and
vanilla over eggs; continue beating for 2 minutes. Sift flour,
cornstarch, and baking powder together. Sprinkle half the
mixture over batter; fold in with spatula. Repeat with remaining flour mixture. Spread batter evenly in pan. Bake on center
rack in oven for 10–12 minutes or until cake is golden and
springs back when lightly touched. Arrange a towel on work
surface and cover with aluminum foil. Loosen edges of cake;
unmold on foil. Roll cake jelly roll style, with towel as a guide.
Leave cake rolled until it cools into jelly roll shape.

Meanwhile, to make filling, blend milk with pudding mix according to package directions. Refrigerate pudding until it thickens.

Unroll cake, spread evenly with pudding, and reroll. Sprinkle sugar-free cocoa over the top to decorate. Cut into 1-inch slices and serve.

15 servings   *1 serving: 1-inch-wide slice*

Nutritive values per serving:

CHO (g)	PRO (g)	FAT (g)	CAL —	Fiber (g)	Sodium (mg)	Chol (mg)
21	5	2	122	0.2	197	92

Food Exchanges per serving: 1 Fruit Exchange plus ½ Skim Milk Exchange plus ½ Fat Exchange.

Low-sodium diets: Omit cocoa topping. This recipe is suitable for occasional use if sodium restriction is not severe.

NEW Plum Jelly Roll

This jelly roll can also be made with other sweet spreads (see Index), especially the ones with the stronger flavors such as apricot or Concord grape.

    5 eggs
    ½ cup sugar
    3 packets Sweet'n Low or other heat-stable sugar
        substitute
    1 teaspoon pure vanilla extract
    ¾ cup all-purpose flour
    2 tablespoons cornstarch
    1 teaspoon baking powder
    1¼ cups Red Plum Spread (*see* Index)

Preheat oven to 400°F. Grease and line the bottom of a 10″ × 15″ jelly roll pan with waxed paper. Beat eggs in large bowl with electric mixer until fluffy. Sprinkle sugar, Sweet'n Low and vanilla over eggs; continue beating for 2 minutes. Sift flour, cornstarch, and baking powder together. Sprinkle half the mixture over batter; fold in with spatula. Repeat with remaining flour mixture. Spread batter evenly in pan. Bake on center rack in oven for 10–12 minutes or until cake is golden and springs back when lightly touched. Arrange a towel on work surface and cover with aluminum foil. Loosen edges of cake; unmold on foil. Roll cake jelly roll style, with towel as a guide. Leave cake rolled until it cools into jelly roll shape. Unroll formed roll and spread with the sweet spread. Reroll. Cut into 1-inch slices and serve.

15 servings   *1 serving: 1-inch-wide slice*

			Nutritive values per serving:			
CHO (g)	PRO (g)	FAT (g)	CAL —	Fiber (g)	Sodium (mg)	Chol (mg)
15	3	2	88	0.5	46	91

Food Exchange per serving: 1 Starch Exchange.

Low-sodium diets: This recipe is excellent.

COOKIES AND BARS

NEW   Brownie Squares

⅓ cup margarine
1 1-ounce square unsweetened chocolate
½ cup sugar
1 large egg
1 teaspoon pure vanilla extract
½ cup Oat Bran cereal
⅓ cup all-purpose flour
½ cup chopped walnuts, divided

Heat oven to 350°F. Prepare an 8-inch square pan with vegetable pan-coating. In medium saucepan, melt margarine and chocolate over medium heat; cool. Add sugar, egg, and vanilla; mix well. Add Oat Bran cereal, flour, and ¼ cup nuts; mix just until well blended. Spread into prepared pan; sprinkle with remaining nuts. Bake about 18 minutes or until firm to the touch. Cool; cut into squares.

8 servings   *1 serving: 2 2-inch-square brownies*
(yield: 16 brownies)

Nutritive values per servings:

CHO (g)	PRO (g)	FAT (g)	CAL —	Fiber (g)	Sodium (mg)	Chol (mg)
20	4	14	208	1.0	100	34

Food Exchanges per serving: 2 Fat Exchanges plus 1½ Starch Exchanges.

Low-sodium diets: This recipe is suitable.

$\boxed{NEW}$ Almond Slices

3 large eggs
⅓ cup sugar
3 tablespoons vegetable shortening at room
    temperature
¾ teaspoon pure almond extract
¾ teaspoon pure vanilla extract
1½ cups all-purpose flour
1 teaspoon baking powder
½ cup golden raisins

Preheat oven to 350°F. Prepare bottom of 9″ × 13″ pan with vegetable pan-coating. With an electric mixer beat eggs and sugar until light. Add the shortening, almond extract, vanilla extract, flour, and baking powder; mix well. Blend in raisins. Divide batter and arrange into two 2-inch tube-shape loaves in the prepared pan. Bake for 25 minutes. Remove pan from oven and cut cookies into slices, ⅓ inch thick. Turn cookies on their sides and continue cooking for 5 minutes more or until firm to touch. Cool cookies and store in a tightly covered container. a tightly covered container.

22 servings (yield: 44 almond slices)   *1 serving: 2 cookies*

Nutritive values per serving:

CHO (g)	PRO (g)	FAT (g)	CAL —	Fiber (g)	Sodium (mg)	Chol (mg)
15	3	1	78	0.5	25	37

Food Exchange per serving: 1 Starch Exchange.
Low-sodium diets: This recipe is excellent.

Applesauce Bar Cookies

1¾ cups sifted cake flour
½ teaspoon baking soda
1 teaspoon ground cinnamon
½ teaspoon ground allspice
⅛ teaspoon ground cloves
½ teaspoon salt
¼ cup margarine
¾ cup sugar
1 medium egg
½ cup unsweetened applesauce
½ cup seedless raisins

Preheat oven to 375°F. Prepare bottom of an 11" × 7" pan with vegetable pan-coating. Sift together flour, baking soda, spices, and salt. Cream margarine until soft and fluffy; beat in sugar gradually. Add egg and beat until light and fluffy. Add sifted dry ingredients and applesauce, alternately, stirring in just enough to blend well. Add raisins; stir until all ingredients are thoroughly mixed. Turn into the prepared pan. Bake about 30 minutes. Let cool on a baking rack for 10 minutes, then cut into 24 squares, each 1¾ by 1¾ inches.

24 servings   *1 serving: a 1¾- by 1¾-inch square*

Nutritive values per serving:

CHO (g)	PRO (g)	FAT (g)	CAL —	Fiber (g)	Sodium (mg)	Chol (mg)
15	1	2	80	0.5	83	11

Food Exchange per serving: 1 Starch Exchange.

Low-sodium diets: Omit salt. Use unsalted margarine.

French Sponge Cookies

For best whipping volume, remove eggs from the refrigerator 30 minutes or more before using.

½ cup sifted cake flour
¾ teaspoon baking powder
¼ teaspoon salt
3 medium eggs, separated
½ teaspoon pure almond extract
¼ teaspoon pure vanilla extract
6 tablespoons sugar

Preheat oven to 350°F. Sift together flour, baking powder, and salt. Beat egg yolks in a small bowl, rapidly, until very thick and lemon-colored, adding almond and vanilla extracts during the beating. With clean beaters, beat the egg whites until stiff and shiny; begin to add sugar not more than 1 tablespoonful at a time, and beat constantly. Continue to beat rapidly until whites are very stiff and glossy. Gently and slowly fold in the beaten egg yolks. In same manner, fold in the dry ingredients until well mixed. Using a small spatula and a measuring tablespoon, measure and drop onto ungreased baking sheets 1 level tablespoon batter for each cookie, spacing them 2 inches apart. Bake 10 minutes, until light golden in color. Remove from oven and at once. Slide spatula under each cookie and transfer to wire cake rack to cool cookies. Let stand, uncovered, to dry and crisp. Store in a tightly covered container.

10 servings (yield: 40 cookies)   *1 serving: 4 cookies*

Nutritive values per serving:

CHO (g)	PRO (g)	FAT (g)	CAL —	Fiber (g)	Sodium (mg)	Chol (mg)
11	2	2	69	0.1	94	82

Food Exchange per serving: 1 Starch Exchange.
Low-sodium diets: Omit salt.

NEW Lemon Rings

1½ cups all-purpose flour
¼ cup sugar
Grated rind of 1 lemon
6 tablespoons margarine, cut into small pieces
1 large egg
1 egg white, beaten lightly

Preheat oven to 375°F. Prepare bottom of a cookie sheet with vegetable pan-coating. Using a food processor fitted with a steel blade, combine all ingredients except egg white. Flatten dough slightly; cover in plastic wrap. Chill for 30 minutes. Break off a tablespoonful of dough and roll out to form a 3-inch pencil-shaped rope. Attach edges to shape a ring. Place on prepared cookie sheet. Continue with remaining dough. Brush tops of cookies with lightly beaten egg white. Bake for 10–12 minutes or until lightly golden. Remove cookies from baking sheet and cool on a wire rack. Store in a covered container.

12 servings (yield: 24 cookies)   *1 serving: 2 cookies*

Nutritive values per serving:						
CHO (g)	PRO (g)	FAT (g)	CAL —	Fiber (g)	Sodium (mg)	Chol (mg)
16	2	6	130	0.4	77	22

Food Exchanges per serving: 1 Starch Exchange plus 1 Fat Exchange.

Low-sodium diets: This recipe is suitable.

NEW Refrigerator Raisin Cookies

½ cup margarine
¼ cup sugar
Sugar substitute equivalent to 2 tablespoons sugar
1 teaspoon pure vanilla extract
1 large egg
1½ cups all-purpose flour
½ cup uncooked quick-cooking oats
2 teaspoons baking powder
½ cup raisins
1 teaspoon all-purpose flour (to flour glass)

In a large bowl of electric mixer, cream together margarine, sugar, sugar substitute, vanilla, and egg until batter is light. Add 1½ cups flour, oats, baking powder, and raisins; blend well. Gather dough together, roll into a ball, and cover with plastic wrap. Chill dough for 2 hours or overnight. Preheat oven to 375°F. Roll dough into ¾-inch balls and place 1½ inches apart on a nonstick cookie sheet. Flatten cookies with bottom of a lightly floured glass. Bake cookies about 8–10 minutes or until they are firm and golden brown. Cool cookies before serving.

40 cookies   *1 serving: 2 cookies*

			Nutritive values per serving:			
CHO (g)	PRO (g)	FAT (g)	CAL —	Fiber (g)	Sodium (mg)	Chol (mg)
14	2	5	106	0.6	91	14

Food Exchanges per serving: 1 Starch Exchange plus 1 Fat Exchange.

Low-sodium diets: This recipe is suitable.

Peanut Butter Cookies

1½ cups sifted all-purpose flour
1½ teaspoons baking powder
½ teaspoon salt
¼ cup margarine
½ cup creamy peanut butter
½ teaspoon grated fresh orange rind
1½ teaspoons pure vanilla extract
1 egg, well beaten
⅓ cup orange juice
Sugar substitute equivalent to ½ cup sugar
¾ cup seedless raisins

Preheat oven to 400°F. Sift together flour, baking powder, and salt. Cream together margarine, peanut butter, orange rind, and vanilla. Add egg, orange juice, and sweetener; blend well. Add dry ingredients gradually; mix well after each addition. Add raisins; mix well. Measure 1 level tablespoonful of dough for each cookie. Roll between hands to form ball. Place 2 inches apart on an ungreased cookie sheet; flatten with fork. Bake about 15 minutes. Store cookies in a tightly covered tin. These cookies have better flavor and texture 24 hours after baking.

12 servings (yield: 24 cookies)   *1 serving: 2 cookies*

			Nutritive values per serving:			
CHO (g)	PRO (g)	FAT (g)	CAL —	Fiber (g)	Sodium (mg)	Chol (mg)
22	5	10	191	2.5	224	23

Food Exchanges per serving: 2 Fat Exchanges plus 1½ Starch Exchanges.

Low-sodium diets: Omit salt. Use unsalted margarine and unsalted peanut butter.

FRUIT

Grand Marnier Fruit Cup

1 small peach or nectarine
2 small purple plums
1 small red apple
24 green Thompson seedless grapes
2 teaspoons fresh lemon juice
Sugar substitute equivalent to 2 tablespoons sugar
1½ tablespoons Grand Marnier

Peel peach. Remove stones from peach or nectarine and plums and core from apple. Cut grapes in half; cut remaining fruit into small bite-sized pieces. Mix fruits well with remaining ingredients. Turn into a jar, cover, and chill for a few hours to blend flavors.

4 servings (yield: 2 cups)   *1 serving: ½ cup*

Nutritive values per serving:						
CHO (g)	PRO (g)	FAT (g)	CAL —	Fiber (g)	Sodium (mg)	Chol (mg)
14	1	0	59	2.0	1	0

Food Exchange per serving: 1 Fruit Exchange.

Low-sodium diets: This recipe is excellent.

Sherry Ambrosia

⅔ cup fresh orange sections
1 cup fresh grapefruit sections
2 medium red apples
2 tablespoons dry sherry
1 teaspoon fresh lemon juice
Sugar substitute equivalent to 2 teaspoons sugar
⅓ cup sliced banana
2 tablespoons shredded coconut
3 maraschino cherries, drained

Cut orange sections into halves, grapefruit sections into quarters, and cored (but not pared) apples into small bite-sized cubes. Mix these fruits with sherry, lemon juice, and sugar substitute. Turn into a jar, cover, and chill for 1 hour or longer. Just before serving, add banana; mix well. Spoon into 6 individual dessert dishes. With scissors, cut coconut into small pieces; scatter on top of fruits. Slice maraschino cherries; place a few slices on top of coconut.

6 servings (yield: 3 cups)   *1 serving: ½ cup*

Nutritive values per serving:

CHO (g)	PRO (g)	FAT (g)	CAL —	Fiber (g)	Sodium (mg)	Chol (mg)
11	1	1	53	1.8	1	0

Food Exchange per serving: 1 Fruit Exchange.

Low-sodium diets: This recipe is excellent.

Granny Smith Applesauce

We have had many compliments on this recipe. Be sure to try it. This recipe was kitchen-tested in June, early in the new apple season with Granny Smith apples, which were very firm, large, and yielded 3 cups of sauce for 4 apples. The sauce was a "solid" pack.

> 2 pounds firm Granny Smith apples
> 2 tablespoons fresh lemon juice
> 1 cup water
> ¼ teaspoon ground cinnamon
> Sugar substitute equivalent to 3 tablespoons sugar

Pare apples very thin, preferably with a vegetable parer. Remove cores; cut apples into 8–12 slices, then into bite-sized pieces. Measure 6 cups into a large heavy pot; add lemon juice and water; mix well. Bring to a boil; cover and cook gently until apples are very soft and tender. Remove from heat; add cinnamon and sweetener; mix thoroughly with a wooden spoon (a metal spoon may darken the sauce). Pack into jars, cover, and store in refrigerator. Serve warm or chilled.

9 servings (yield: 3 cups)   *1 serving: ⅓ cup*

Nutritive values per serving:						
CHO (g)	PRO (g)	FAT (g)	CAL —	Fiber (g)	Sodium (mg)	Chol (mg)
16	0	0	62	2.4	1	0

Food Exchange per serving: 1 Fruit Exchange.

Low-sodium diets: This recipe is excellent.

Pink Applesauce

1 pound red-skinned apples (Jonathan or McIntosh)
1½ cups water
1 tablespoon fresh lemon juice
⅛ teaspoon ground cinnamon
¹⁄₁₆ teaspoon ground mace
Sugar substitute equivalent to 2–3 tablespoons
    sugar

Wash apples and cut into quarters; leave skin on, but remove
and discard cores. Cut apples into small cubes; there will be
about 3 cups. Place apples in pot; add water and lemon juice.
Cover and bring to a boil. Cook gently over medium heat, stirring occasionally, until apples are soft, about 8–10 minutes.
Remove from heat; add cinnamon, mace, and sweetener; mix
well. Turn into a pint jar; cool, cover, and store in refrigerator.

4 servings (yield: 2 cups)   *1 serving: ½ cup*

Nutritive values per serving:

CHO (g)	PRO (g)	FAT (g)	CAL —	Fiber (g)	Sodium (mg)	Chol (mg)
14	0	0	53	1.9	0	0

Food Exchange per serving: 1 Fruit Exchange.

Low-sodium diets: This recipe is excellent.

Poached Pears Delight

*If you serve this dessert with Vanilla Crème Fraîche (see Index)
or with ladyfingers, count their values in addition.*

> 5 small, just underripe Anjou, Bartlett, or Bosc
>   pears (1 pound)
> 3½ cups water
> 2 tablespoons fresh lemon juice
> 2 teaspoons imitation rum flavor
> 1 teaspoon pure vanilla extract
> 1¼ teaspoons pure orange extract
> Sugar substitute equivalent to 2½ tablespoons sugar

Pare, halve lengthwise, and core the pears; the total weight of
the 10 halves will be approximately 11 ounces. Put prepared
pear halves, water, and lemon juice in a saucepan. Bring to a
boil, turn heat down, and let simmer gently 20–22 minutes or
until pears are tender but firm. Remove from heat. Lift pears
out carefully with a spoon and place in a pint jar or bowl. Add
all flavorings and sweetener to hot liquid; stir to blend well.
Pour on top of pears. Cover tightly. Chill and store in
refrigerator.

*5 servings (yield: 10 halves   1 serving: 2 pear halves plus
plus 1 cup liquid)   3–4 tablespoons liquid*

Nutritive values per serving:

CHO (g)	PRO (g)	FAT (g)	CAL —	Fiber (g)	Sodium (mg)	Chol (mg)
11	0	0	41	1.8	0	0

Food Exchange per serving: 1 Fruit Exchange when served
                                        plain.

Low-sodium diets: This recipe is excellent.

Stewed Rhubarb

Frozen unsweetened rhubarb is sold in 1-pound packages. The amount of fresh rhubarb to pick or buy, in order to end up with the same quantity—4 cups uncooked—depends upon how much top and bottom is left on before cleaning and cutting. Be sure all leaves are removed because they are poisonous.

   1 pound diced fresh or frozen rhubarb (4 cups)
   ¼ cup water
   Sugar substitute equivalent to 6 tablespoons sugar
       (*see* note below)

Place diced rhubarb and water in a deep saucepan. Cover and bring to a boil; turn heat down and simmer gently until rhubarb is very tender, about 10 minutes, stirring occasionally. Remove from heat, add sweetener, and mix well. Turn into a pint jar. Cover and store in refrigerator.

   Note: The amount of artificial sweetener required is largely dependent upon the acidity or "sour" taste of the rhubarb you use. Taste and adjust amount of sweetener accordingly.

4 servings (yield: 2 cups)   *1 serving: ½ cup*

| Nutritive values per serving: | | | | | | |
CHO (g)	PRO (g)	FAT (g)	CAL —	Fiber (g)	Sodium (mg)	Chol (mg)
8	1	0	31	1.9	2	0

Food Exchange per serving: ½ Fruit Exchange.

Low-sodium diets: This recipe is excellent.

Peter's Favorite Strawberries

Mary's husband, Peter, particularly likes this simple but elegant dessert. Mary serves it in champagne or brandy glasses. Never have vitamins and fiber looked and tasted so good!

    1 pint ripe, very red strawberries
    1 medium orange
    2 tablespoons orange juice
    2 tablespoons sweet vermouth
    Sugar substitute equivalent to 1 tablespoon sugar
        (optional)

Wash and hull strawberries; cut each in half. Slice ends off orange; quarter orange lengthwise and slice orange wedges crosswise with rinds left on, as thin as possible. Put strawberries and oranges in a bowl; mix well. Mix together the orange juice and sweet vermouth and drizzle over fruit mixture; stir to mix. Check to see if berries have enough natural sweetness for your taste; if not, add sweetener. Cover bowl and chill in refrigerator 2 hours before serving; stir gently several times to blend flavors.

4 servings (yield: 3 cups)   *1 serving: ¾ cup*

			Nutritive values per serving:			
CHO (g)	PRO (g)	FAT (g)	CAL —	Fiber (g)	Sodium (mg)	Chol (mg)
11	1	0	56	2.3	1	0

Food Exchange per serving: 1 Fruit Exchange.

Low-sodium diets: This recipe is excellent.

Strawberry Shortcake

3 cups fresh ripe strawberries
6 Baking Powder Biscuits (*see* Index)
¾ cup Vanilla Crème Fraîche (*see* Index) (*see* note
  below)

Hull and slice strawberries. Split each biscuit and arrange 2
halves on each plate. Spread ½ cup sliced strawberries over
each 2 halves and top each serving with 2 tablespoons Vanilla
Crème Fraîche. Enjoy! If you like the strawberries sweetened,
1 hour before serving slice berries into a bowl. Sprinkle with
sugar substitute equivalent to 1 tablespoon sugar; mix well.
Cover bowl and chill in refrigerator.

Note: If desired, you may substitute Phony Whipped Cream
(*see* Index) for the Vanilla Crème Fraîche and omit 1 Fat Exchange from the calculated value.

6 servings   *1 serving: 1 strawberry shortcake*

Nutritive values per serving:

CHO (g)	PRO (g)	FAT (g)	CAL —	Fiber (g)	Sodium (mg)	Chol (mg)
22	4	9	182	2.1	266	14

Food Exchanges per serving: 2 Fat Exchanges plus 1 Starch
                    Exchange plus ½ Fruit Exchange.

Low-sodium diets: Modify biscuit recipe as directed.

NEW | **Hot Summer Fruit Compote**

4 fresh peaches, peeled, pitted, and sliced
2 cups hulled fresh strawberries
30 fresh sweet cherries, pitted and halved
2 fresh pears, peeled, cored, and sliced thin
1 tablespoon brown sugar
½ teaspoon ground cinnamon
2 tablespoons orange juice
½ teaspoon brandy extract

Combine all ingredients in a large bowl; toss gently to coat. Spoon mixture into a 2-quart casserole. Bake at 350°F for 15 minutes. Serve immediately.

8 servings (yield: 4 cups)   *1 serving: ½ cup*

Nutritive values per serving:						
CHO (g)	PRO (g)	FAT (g)	CAL —	Fiber (g)	Sodium (mg)	Chol (mg)
22	1	1	87	3.7	2	0

Food Exchanges per serving: 1½ Fruit Exchanges.
Low-sodium diets: This recipe is excellent.

NEW | **Mango Sorbet**

The same technique can be used with peaches, berries, or other soft fruits. Use amounts equal to 1¼ cups pureed fruit.

2 large mangoes
¼ cup fresh orange juice
Sugar substitute equivalent to 1 tablespoon sugar

Peel and slice mangoes; puree in a food processor fitted with steel blade. Add orange juice and sweetener; mix well. Pour into a shallow pan; freeze mixture until solid. Remove sorbet from freezer; break into pieces with a fork. Return to food

processor and process 10 seconds until smooth and frosty.
Spoon into footed glasses and serve immediately.

3 servings (yield: 1½ cups)   *1 serving: ½ cup*

			Nutritive values per serving:			
CHO (g)	PRO (g)	FAT (g)	CAL —	Fiber (g)	Sodium (mg)	Chol (mg)
26	1	0	100	3.3	3	0

Food Exchanges per serving: 2 Fruit Exchanges.

Low-sodium diets: This recipe is excellent.

PUDDINGS, CUSTARDS, AND MOLDS

Cranberry Tapioca Pudding

2 tablespoons quick-cooking tapioca
1½ cups water
2 cups fresh cranberries
½ teaspoon pure orange extract
Sugar substitute equivalent to ½ cup sugar

Combine tapioca and water in a saucepan; let stand 5 minutes.
Bring to a boil and simmer 3 minutes, stirring frequently. Add
cranberries and cook until all berries have popped, then remove from heat. Add orange extract and sweetener and mix
well. Allow to cool before putting in refrigerator. Chill
thoroughly.

4 servings (yield: 2 cups)   *1 serving: ½ cup*

			Nutritive values per serving:			
CHO (g)	PRO (g)	FAT (g)	CAL —	Fiber (g)	Sodium (mg)	Chol (mg)
13	0	0	50	0.6	1	0

Food Exchange per serving: 1 Fruit Exchange.

Low-sodium diets: This recipe is excellent.

Cream Puff Shells

These shells are lovely with pudding and fruit fillings but are also delightful stuffed with tuna or chicken salad.

¼ cup margarine
½ cup boiling water
¹⁄₁₆ teaspoon salt
½ cup sifted all-purpose flour
2 large eggs

Preheat oven to 450°F. Prepare baking sheet with vegetable pan-coating. Cut margarine into pieces; boil water and salt in a saucepan; add margarine and bring to a vigorous boil. Add flour all at once. Keeping heat low, stir rapidly to blend; then beat strenuously with a wooden spoon until the mixture forms a ball and pulls away from the sides of the pan. Remove from heat; allow to cool a few minutes. Add eggs, one at a time, beating vigorously after each addition. Drop 2 level table-spoons onto prepared sheet for each shell; place batter at least 2 inches apart. Bake for 10 minutes; reduce heat to 400°F and continue baking until puffs are firm and browned, about 25 minutes. Transfer to wire rack; slit each puff with the tip of a sharp knife to allow steam to escape. Let cool before filling.

9 servings   *1 serving: 1 puff shell*

Nutritive values per serving:

CHO (g)	PRO (g)	FAT (g)	CAL —	Fiber (g)	Sodium (mg)	Chol (mg)
5	2	6	86	0.2	88	61

Food Exchanges per serving (unfilled shell): 1 Fat Exchange plus ½ Starch Exchange.

Low-sodium diets: Omit salt. Substitute unsalted margarine.

Rice Pudding

This is a favorite way of using extra rice after Chinese meals.

2 cups skim milk
2 medium eggs, beaten
2 tablespoons sugar
¼ teaspoon salt
¼ teaspoon ground cinnamon
1 teaspoon pure vanilla extract
1 cup cold cooked rice
2 tablespoons seedless raisins

Preheat oven to 350°F. Prepare a 1-quart casserole with vegetable pan-coating. Scald (heat) milk in the top of a double boiler over simmering water. Combine eggs, sugar, salt, cinnamon, and vanilla. Pour hot milk on top slowly, stirring to mix well. Spread rice in the bottom of the casserole; scatter raisins evenly over rice; pour milk mixture carefully on top. Place casserole in pan of hot water with hot water coming almost up to the top of the casserole. Bake about 45 minutes or until knife tip inserted in center comes out clean. Remove casserole from water and chill in refrigerator. This pudding may be served warm or chilled, as you prefer.

4 servings (yield: 3 cups)   *1 serving: ¾ cup*

Nutritive values per serving:

CHO (g)	PRO (g)	FAT (g)	CAL —	Fiber (g)	Sodium (mg)	Chol (mg)
25	8	3	159	0.8	221	139

Food Exchanges per serving: 1½ Starch Exchanges plus 1 Lean Meat Exchange.

Low-sodium diets: Omit salt when cooking rice; omit salt from recipe.

Bread Pudding

Use white or whole-wheat bread for this old favorite. Try serving it with our Fluffy Lemon Sauce (see Index) or with a tablespoon of one of the sweet spreads (see Index).

    2 slices bread
    2 teaspoons margarine, softened
    2 tablespoons seedless raisins
    2 cups skim milk
    2 large eggs
    ¼ teaspoon salt
    2 tablespoons sugar
    ¼ teaspoon ground cinnamon
    1 teaspoon pure vanilla extract

Preheat oven to 350°F. Prepare a 1½-quart casserole with vegetable pan-coating. Spread bread with margarine and cut each slice into 16 cubes. Place bread cubes in bottom of prepared casserole. Scatter raisins evenly on top. Scald (heat) milk in the top of a double boiler over simmering water; remove from heat. Beat eggs until light; beat in remaining ingredients. Pour hot milk on top, stirring to blend well; pour carefully on top of bread cubes. Place casserole in a pan of hot water (enough to come up to half the depth of the casserole). Bake 50 minutes or until knife inserted halfway between center and outside edge comes out clean. Remove dish from water. Chill pudding in refrigerator 3 hours or longer or serve warm.

4 servings (yield: 3 cups)   *1 serving: ¾ cup*

Nutritive values per serving:

CHO (g)	PRO (g)	FAT (g)	CAL —	Fiber (g)	Sodium (mg)	Chol (mg)
22	8	5	169	0.7	307	139

Food Exchanges per serving: 1 Starch Exchange plus ½ Whole Milk Exchange.

Low-sodium diets: Omit salt. Use unsalted margarine.

Baked Custard

If you want to unmold this Baked Custard, leave cups in the refrigerator 2 to 3 extra hours.

    1½ cups skim milk
    2 large eggs, beaten slightly
    2 tablespoons sugar
    ⅛ teaspoon salt
    1 teaspoon pure vanilla extract
    ⅛ teaspoon ground nutmeg (optional)

Preheat oven to 325°F. Heat milk in the top of a double boiler over simmering water until surface begins to wrinkle. Blend together the eggs, sugar, salt, and vanilla. Add hot milk gradually, stirring to mix well. Pour into four 6-ounce individual custard cups. Sprinkle surface lightly with nutmeg. Set cups in a deep pan; pour hot water around cups to come to within ½ inch of tops of custard cups. Bake 50–60 minutes or until knife tip inserted in center of custard comes out clean. Remove from heat and water pan. Chill for several hours before serving.

4 servings (yield: 2 cups)   *1 serving: ½ cup*

Nutritive values per serving:						
CHO (g)	PRO (g)	FAT (g)	CAL —	Fiber (g)	Sodium (mg)	Chol (mg)
11	6	3	95	0	143	139

Food Exchange per serving: 1 Low-Fat Milk Exchange.

Low-sodium diets: Omit salt.

NEW Pudding in Cookie Flowers

These cookie shells can also be filled with fresh fruits or other fillings.

COOKIES
- ½ cup margarine
- ½ cup sugar
- 3 packets Sweet'n Low or other heat-stable sugar substitute
- 1 teaspoon pure vanilla extract
- 1 cup all-purpose flour
- 4 egg whites

FILLING
- 1 1.7-ounce package sugar-free vanilla or chocolate pudding
- 3 cups skim milk
- ¼ cup fresh blueberries or raspberries

Preheat oven to 350°F. Prepare cookies: Cream together margarine, sugar, Sweet'n Low, and vanilla. Add flour alternately with egg whites, mixing well after each addition. Measure 1 heaping tablespoonful dough for each cookie. Place 3 inches apart on a nonstick cookie sheet, pressing cookie batter with back of spoon in circular motion to extend circle to 4 inches. Six cookies will fit on each pan. Have muffin pan available for shaping after baking. Bake cookies for 8–10 minutes or until golden around edges. Remove cookies immediately with a spatula and gently form into the muffin tin with hands, giving the cookie a cup shape. Return to oven and cook 5 minutes more. Allow cookie shells to cool, remove from pan, and store in a tightly covered tin.

Prepare filling: Prepare pudding with skim milk according to package directions. Refrigerate until it is set.

When ready to serve, fill each cookie cup with about 3 tablespoons pudding. Garnish each filled cup with a few fresh berries. Serve immediately.

16 servings   *1 serving: 1 filled cookie cup*

Nutritive values per serving:

CHO (g)	PRO (g)	FAT (g)	CAL —	Fiber (g)	Sodium (mg)	Chol (mg)
17	3	6	135	0.3	239	1

Food Exchanges per serving: 1 Starch Exchange plus 1 Fat Exchange.

Low-sodium diets: Suitable for occasional use if sodium restriction is not severe. Substitute unsalted margarine.

NEW Lemon Yogurt Cups

Try this as a dessert or in the center of a fresh fruit salad plate.

    2 tablespoons granulated gelatin
    ½ cup water
    2 6-ounce cartons lemon yogurt
    2 teaspoons grated lemon rind
    4 fresh mint sprigs (optional)

Dissolve gelatin in water in small saucepan. Cook over medium heat, stirring often, until gelatin is dissolved. Stir in yogurt and lemon rind. Pour yogurt mixture into four 4-ounce molds. Refrigerate until firm. When ready to serve, run a knife around edge and unmold onto serving plate. Garnish with fresh mint leaves.

4 servings (yield: 2 cups)   *1 serving: ½ cup*

Nutritive values per serving:

CHO (g)	PRO (g)	FAT (g)	CAL —	Fiber (g)	Sodium (mg)	Chol (mg)
15	5	1	85	0	67	4

Food Exchange per serving: 1 Skim Milk Exchange.

Low-sodium diets: This recipe is excellent.

Chocolate Chiffon Mold

The kids aren't the only ones who like this yummy dessert!

1 tablespoon granulated gelatin
½ cup cold water
3 medium eggs, separated
¼ cup cocoa powder
⅛ teaspoon salt
1 cup skim milk
1½ teaspoons pure vanilla extract
½ teaspoon pure chocolate extract
Sugar substitute equivalent to ⅔ cup sugar
6 small ladyfingers
⅛ teaspoon cream of tartar

Soak gelatin in cold water. Beat egg yolks until light; add cocoa, salt, and milk; beat until smooth. Turn into the top of a double boiler. Cook over simmering water, stirring constantly until thick and smooth. Remove from heat. Add vanilla, chocolate extract, and sweetener; mix well. Add chocolate mixture to gelatin and stir until gelatin is completely dissolved. Chill in refrigerator, stirring occasionally, until mixture sets to the consistency of unbeaten egg whites. Meanwhile, split ladyfingers. Place halves upright (flat side in) around outer sides of a 4-cup mold. When chocolate mixture is partially thickened, beat egg whites with cream of tartar until stiff. Fold into chocolate mixture; blend thoroughly. Carefully spoon into mold. Cover with clear plastic wrap. Chill for 3–4 hours or until set. Unmold onto a serving plate. To serve, cut into six slices.

*6 servings (yield: 1 mold)   1 serving: ⅔ cup chocolate mold
plus 2 ladyfinger halves*

Nutritive values per serving:

CHO (g)	PRO (g)	FAT (g)	CAL —	Fiber (g)	Sodium (mg)	Chol (mg)
14	7	4	109	0	106	141

Food Exchanges per serving: 1 Starch Exchange plus
½ Medium-Fat Meat Exchange.

Low-sodium diets: Omit salt.

Tapioca Nectar Fluff

¼ cup quick-cooking tapioca
6 ounces apricot nectar
6 ounces unsweetened pineapple juice
1 tablespoon fresh lemon juice
¾ cup water
1 egg, separated
Sugar substitute equivalent to ½ cup sugar
½ teaspoon pure vanilla extract
¼ teaspoon pure orange extract
1 egg white
3 maraschino cherries, sliced thin

Mix tapioca, apricot nectar, pineapple juice, lemon juice, water, and beaten egg yolk in a heavy pan; let stand 5 minutes. Bring to a full boil over medium heat; cook and stir constantly 6–8 minutes. Remove from heat; add sweetener and flavorings; mix well. Beat egg white to soft peaks. Gradually add tapioca, stirring quickly only until blended. Serve warm or chilled. Garnish with sliced maraschino cherries.

5 servings (yield: 2½ cups)   *1 serving: ½ cup*

Nutritive values per serving:

CHO (g)	PRO (g)	FAT (g)	CAL —	Fiber (g)	Sodium (mg)	Chol (mg)
21	2	1	99	0.2	137	54

Food Exchanges per serving: 1 Fruit Exchange plus ½ Starch Exchange.

Low-sodium diets: This recipe is suitable.

Rich Strawberry Trifle

1¼ cups Phony Whipped Cream (*see* Index)
1 pint fresh strawberries
Sugar substitute equivalent to 1 tablespoon sugar
2 tablespoons Grand Marnier
1½ cups whole milk
4 medium eggs
⅛ teaspoon salt
1¼ teaspoons pure vanilla extract
¼ teaspoon pure orange extract
Sugar substitute equivalent to ¼ cup sugar
24 vanilla wafers

Chill Phony Whipped Cream. Meanwhile, wash strawberries, reserving six whole berries with hulls for garnish. Slice and quarter remaining berries and mix with sweetener to substitute for 1 tablespoon sugar; add Grand Marnier; mix well, cover, and set aside. Scald milk in the top of a double boiler. Beat eggs and salt slightly. Pour hot milk on top of egg mixture very slowly, stirring constantly. Return mixture to the top of the double boiler. Place over simmering water (water should not touch bottom of top part). Cook, stirring constantly, until mixture coats a metal spoon. Immediately remove from over simmering water; add vanilla, orange extract, and sweetener to substitute for ¼ cup sugar. Cool custard well; fold in 1 cup of Phony Whipped Cream; blend carefully. Arrange 16 vanilla wafers on bottom and around sides of a large glass dessert bowl (or three in each of six individual dessert servers). Spread half of the strawberries on top, then half of the custard mixture. Repeat with remaining vanilla wafers, then strawberries, and finally custard. Cover with clear plastic. Chill for several hours. When ready to serve, garnish with spoonfuls of remaining Phony Whipped Cream and reserved whole strawberries.

6 servings   *1 serving: ½ cup plus 4 vanilla wafers*
(yield: 3 cups)

			Nutritive values per serving:			
CHO (g)	PRO (g)	FAT (g)	CAL —	Fiber (g)	Sodium (mg)	Chol (mg)
25	8	10	231	3.9	171	201

Food Exchanges per serving: 1 Whole Milk Exchange plus 1 Fruit Exchange.

Low-sodium diets: Omit salt.

Port Parfait

1 tablespoon granulated gelatin
¼ cup cold water
½ cup boiling water
1 tablespoon fresh lemon juice
¾ cup unsweetened orange juice
½ cup port wine
¼ teaspoon pure orange extract
¼ teaspoon pure almond extract
Sugar substitute equivalent to 2 tablespoons sugar
1 small orange, peeled and sectioned

Soak gelatin in cold water; dissolve in boiling water. Add all remaining ingredients except orange segments; mix well. Chill until it is the consistency of unbeaten egg whites; stir gently and spoon into four parfait or wine glasses. Chill until set. Just before serving, garnish each with three orange sections.

4 servings (yield: 2 cups)   *1 serving: ½ cup*

			Nutritive values per serving:			
CHO (g)	PRO (g)	FAT (g)	CAL —	Fiber (g)	Sodium (mg)	Chol (mg)
13	2	0	88	0.5	4	0

Food Exchanges per serving: 1 Fruit Exchange plus ½ Fat Exchange (to account for calories from the alcohol in the wine).

Low-sodium diets: This recipe is excellent.

Heavenly Mold

1 tablespoon granulated gelatin
½ cup cold water
1½ cups buttermilk, made from skim milk
1 teaspoon grated lemon rind
1 teaspoon grated orange rind
2 teaspoons fresh lemon juice
$\frac{1}{16}$ teaspoon ground mace
Sugar substitute equivalent to ¼ cup sugar
2 maraschino cherries, sliced *or* 4 small
    strawberries for garnish

Combine gelatin and cold water in a small bowl; place bowl in a small amount of hot water to dissolve gelatin completely. Add to buttermilk with all remaining ingredients except garnish; mix well. Pour into four ½-cup molds. Chill for a few hours. Unmold into small dessert dishes; garnish each with slices of a maraschino cherry or a whole strawberry.

4 servings (yield: 2 cups)   *1 serving: ½ cup*

Nutritive values per serving:						
CHO (g)	PRO (g)	FAT (g)	CAL —	Fiber (g)	Sodium (mg)	Chol (mg)
7	5	1	53	0.1	99	3

Food Exchange per serving: ½ Skim Milk Exchange.

Low-sodium diets: Substitute 1½ cups skim milk mixed with 1½ tablespoons additional lemon juice for the buttermilk if sodium restriction is severe.

Snow Pudding

1 tablespoon granulated gelatin
½ cup cold water
1 tablespoon grated lemon rind
¼ cup fresh lemon juice
1¼ cups boiling water
Sugar substitute equivalent to ½ cup sugar
2 medium egg whites
¼ teaspoon pure vanilla extract
¼ teaspoon pure lemon extract

Soak gelatin in cold water. Meanwhile, combine lemon rind, juice, and boiling water in a saucepan; bring to a boil, then remove from heat. Add softened gelatin and sweetener; mix well to dissolve both. Chill until it is the consistency of unbeaten egg whites. Then add unbeaten egg whites, vanilla extract, and lemon extract. Beat with a rotary beater until it is very fluffy and holds its shape. Pile into six serving dishes. Chill until firm.

6 servings (yield: 3 cups)   *1 serving: ½ cup*

Nutritive values per serving:

CHO (g)	PRO (g)	FAT (g)	CAL —	Fiber (g)	Sodium (mg)	Chol (mg)
3	2	0	19	0	16	0

Food Exchange per serving: Up to ½ cup may be considered "free"; 1 cup should be counted as ½ Skim Milk Exchange.

Low-sodium diets: This recipe is excellent.

FRUIT-FLAVORED GELS

Because sugar-free gelatin desserts are so tasty and popular on menus for diabetics, the following recipes are included. Most people will use the sugar-free gelatins now on the market. Our gelatins are particularly tasty; try them.

Here are a few simple rules to guide you in making fruit-flavored gelatin desserts. Our recipes are tested and are successful as well as delicious, but if you want to try other combinations, these rules will help you:

- All recipes calling for gelatin are made with unflavored, granulated gelatin sold in 1-pound tins or in individual envelopes in boxes.
- Use either 1 tablespoon (7 grams) of the bulk gelatin or 1 envelope of the unflavored gelatin; either amount will gel 2–2½ cups of liquid.
- The basic fruit-flavored gel desserts that follow are to be molded in one 2- to 2½-cup bowl for serving by spoonfuls or in four to five individual dessert dishes. Serve them plain, with toppings such as frozen whipped topping or Phony Whipped Cream (see Index) or use a bit of fresh fruit as a garnish.
- Do not use the full 2 cups of the liquid if you want to make gel molds. Decrease the amount of water by ¼ cup; but always use the same amount of fruit juice and never less than ¼ cup cold water to soak the gelatin at the beginning of the recipe.
- When you want to add some cut or chopped fresh fruit, decrease liquid by ¼ cup, chill the mixture until it is the consistency of unbeaten egg whites, then fold in up to, but no more than, 1½ cups cut or chopped fruit. Turn into a 3-cup fancy mold or six individual dessert dishes. Be sure to add ½ Fruit Exchange (CHO 7.5 g and 30 Calories) to the individual fruit-flavored gel's food values.
- You can prepare whipped gels, and the result will be double the amount of the basic recipes. To do this, prepare the basic fruit-flavored gelatin, turn it into a deep bowl, chill it

until it is almost set but still lumpy; stir it occasionally during the chilling period. Beat it at high speed with an electric mixer until it is very frothy and three times its original volume. Turn it into a 6-cup dessert serving bowl or into eight individual dessert dishes. Chill until firm and garnish just before serving.

Pretty Apple Gel

This one is so delicious it needs nothing added to it. But if you are a yogurt or Phony Whipped Cream (see Index) fan, then you might want to add a dollop.

2 teaspoons granulated gelatin
¼ cup cold water
½ cup boiling water
Sugar substitute equivalent to 1 tablespoon sugar
1¼ cups unsweetened apple juice
1 teaspoon fresh lemon juice
4 drops red food color (optional)
Fresh mint leaves if available

Soak gelatin in cold water. Add boiling water and sweetener and stir until dissolved. Combine hot liquid with apple juice and lemon juice; mix well and stir in red food color. Chill in a covered bowl or jar until it is the consistency of unbeaten egg whites. Pour carefully into four individual dessert dishes. Chill until set. Garnish each with two leaves of fresh mint if available.

4 servings (yield: 2 cups)   *1 serving: ½ cup*

Nutritive values per serving:

CHO (g)	PRO (g)	FAT (g)	CAL —	Fiber (g)	Sodium (mg)	Chol (mg)
10	1	0	42	0.2	3	0

Food Exchange per serving: 1 Fruit Exchange.
Low-sodium diets: This recipe is excellent.

Pineapple Gelatin

2 teaspoons granulated gelatin
¼ cup cold water
½ cup boiling water
1 teaspoon fresh lemon juice
1¼ cups unsweetened pineapple juice
Sugar substitute equivalent to 1 tablespoon sugar
4 fresh strawberries (optional)

Soak gelatin in cold water. Add boiling water and lemon juice
and stir to dissolve. Add pineapple juice and sweetener; stir to
dissolve. Chill until partially set, stirring occasionally. Spoon
into a 2-cup dessert bowl or four individual dessert dishes.
Chill until set. A pretty garnish of a whole or sliced strawberry
on each may be added.

4 servings (yield: 2 cups)   *1 serving: ½ cup*

Nutritive values per serving:						
CHO (g)	PRO (g)	FAT (g)	CAL —	Fiber (g)	Sodium (mg)	Chol (mg)
11	1	0	46	0	2	0

Food Exchange per serving: 1 Fruit Exchange.
Low-sodium diets: This recipe is excellent.

26
Little Extras

SAUCES AND GRAVIES

Barbecue Sauce

This sauce is excellent for basting chicken or meats prior to grilling or for barbecued beef or pork sandwiches.

> ½ cup finely chopped onion
> ¼ cup finely chopped green pepper
> ½ cup water
> ⅓ cup catsup
> 3 tablespoons vinegar
> 2 teaspoons Worcestershire sauce
> 2–3 drops hot pepper sauce

Cook onion and green pepper in water over low heat about 8 minutes, stirring frequently. Add remaining ingredients and mix well; cook 2 more minutes.

4 servings (yield: 1 cup)   *1 serving: ¼ cup*

Nutritive values per serving:

CHO (g)	PRO (g)	FAT (g)	CAL —	Fiber (g)	Sodium (mg)	Chol (mg)
8	0	0	33	0.5	232	0

Food Exchange per serving: 1 Vegetable Exchange if using ¼ cup, "free" if using 2 tablespoons or less.

Low-sodium diets: Use dietetic unsalted catsup and low-sodium Worcestershire sauce if available.

Creole Gumbo Sauce

This sauce might be served with braised veal cutlets or broiled or baked fish or used in making Shrimp Creole (see Index). Because veal, fish, and shrimp are particularly low in fat, count ½ cup Creole Gumbo Sauce only as 1 Vegetable Exchange and do not count the fat value.

    2 tablespoons margarine
    ½ cup chopped onion
    ½ cup chopped green pepper
    ½ cup thinly sliced okra (optional)
    1 16-ounce can tomatoes with liquid
    2 tablespoons tomato paste
    1 cup tomato juice
    2 tablespoons chopped green olives
    1/16 teaspoon cayenne pepper
    ½ teaspoon salt
    2 beef bouillon cubes
    1½ teaspoons sugar

Melt margarine in a heavy saucepan; add onion, green pepper, and okra; cook gently, stirring frequently until onions are tender. Cut up tomatoes and add with tomato liquid; add all other ingredients to onion mixture; mix well. Bring to a boil; simmer gently for 8–10 minutes.

6 servings (yield: 3 cups)   *1 serving: ½ cup*

Nutritive values per serving:

CHO (g)	PRO (g)	FAT (g)	CAL —	Fiber (g)	Sodium (mg)	Chol (mg)
9	2	4	79	1.6	865	0

Food Exchanges per serving: 1 Vegetable Exchange plus 1 Fat Exchange.

Low-sodium diets: Omit salt. Substitute low-sodium bouillon cubes.

Curry Sauce

This sauce can be used over cooked chicken, fish, or lamb.

2 tablespoons margarine
1 cup thinly sliced mushrooms
¼ cup chopped onion
2 tablespoons all-purpose flour
1 chicken bouillon cube
1 teaspoon salt
1½ teaspoons curry powder
1 cup skim milk
1 cup water
1 cup finely diced red apple with skin
1½ tablespoons dried parsley *or* ¼ cup minced fresh
    parsley

Melt margarine and add mushrooms and onion; sauté until onion is tender, stirring frequently. Stir in the flour, bouillon cube, salt, and curry powder; mix well. Add milk and water gradually, stirring until smooth. Add apple and parsley; boil gently until mixture is thick and apples are tender but not mushy.

8 servings (yield: 2 cups)   *1 serving: ¼ cup*

			Nutritive values per serving:			
CHO (g)	PRO (g)	FAT (g)	CAL —	Fiber (g)	Sodium (mg)	Chol (mg)
7	2	3	59	0.8	403	1

Food Exchanges per serving: 1 Vegetable Exchange plus ½ Fat Exchange.

Low-sodium diets: Omit salt. Use unsalted margarine and low-sodium chicken bouillon cube.

Cooked Cranberry Sauce

This is a soft sauce or spread. If you want it firm enough to mold, increase the amount of granulated gelatin.

    1 pound fresh or frozen cranberries
    2½ cups cold water
    1 teaspoon grated fresh orange rind
    2 teaspoons granulated gelatin
    ½ teaspoon pure orange extract
    Sugar substitute equivalent to ¾ cup sugar

Pick over and wash cranberries. Place in a deep saucepan with 2 cups water and orange rind. Bring to a boil and cook briskly until all berries have "popped." Meanwhile, soak gelatin in ½ cup cold water and remove cranberries from heat. Add gelatin, orange extract, and sweetener; stir until gelatin is dissolved and blended. Turn into jars, cover, chill, and store in refrigerator.

8 servings (yield: 4 cups)   *1 serving: ½ cup*

Nutritive values per serving:

CHO (g)	PRO (g)	FAT (g)	CAL —	Fiber (g)	Sodium (mg)	Chol (mg)
10	1	0	38	0.7	1	0

Food Exchange per serving: ½ Fruit Exchange. Up to ¼ cup may be considered "free."

Low-sodium diets: This recipe is excellent.

Caper Sauce

Serve this as dip for chilled cooked scallops or shrimp or as a topping on seafood cocktails.

    ⅔ cup plain low-fat yogurt
    1 tablespoon drained capers
    1 tablespoon prepared mustard

1 tablespoon fresh lemon juice
½ teaspoon Worcestershire sauce
3 drops hot pepper sauce
¼ teaspoon salt

Combine all ingredients; turn into a half-pint jar; cover. Chill a few hours before serving.

6 servings (yield: ¾ cup)   *1 serving: 2 tablespoons*

Nutritive values per serving:

CHO (g)	PRO (g)	FAT (g)	CAL —	Fiber (g)	Sodium (mg)	Chol (mg)
2	1	0	19	0	167	2

Food Exchange per serving: Up to 2 tablespoons may be considered "free."

Low-sodium diets: Use only 1 tablespoon. Omit salt.

Cucumber Sauce

This is wonderful over poached fish or over chilled canned salmon.

Puree the Cucumber Salad (*see* Index) at low speed in blender until thoroughly chopped. Chill mixture 1 hour before serving.

7 servings (yield: 1¾ cups)   *1 serving: ¼ cup*

Nutritive values per serving:

CHO (g)	PRO (g)	FAT (g)	CAL —	Fiber (g)	Sodium (mg)	Chol (mg)
4	2	1	28	0.6	164	2

Food Exchange per serving: 1 Vegetable Exchange. Half a serving, or 1 ounce (2 tablespoons), may be considered "free."

Low-sodium diets: Omit salt in Cucumber Salad recipe.

Dill Sauce

This sauce is especially good when served on cooked cauliflower, peas, broccoli, small boiled onions, or carrots.

- 1½ tablespoons margarine
- 2 tablespoons all-purpose flour
- 1 teaspoon seasoned salt
- ⅛ teaspoon ground white pepper
- 1 teaspoon instant chicken bouillon *or* 1 chicken bouillon cube
- ½ cup hot water
- 1 cup plain low-fat yogurt
- 1 tablespoon minced fresh dill weed *or* 1 teaspoon dried dill weed

Melt margarine; stir in flour, salt, and pepper and blend until smooth. Add bouillon, then hot water, gradually stirring to blend. Cook over low heat, stirring constantly until thick and smooth. Remove from heat. Stir in yogurt and dill weed; blend well. Stir over low heat but do not allow to boil.

8 servings (yield: 1½ cups)   *1 serving: 3 tablespoons*

			Nutritive values per serving:			
CHO (g)	PRO (g)	FAT (g)	CAL —	Fiber (g)	Sodium (mg)	Chol (mg)
4	2	3	45	0.1	275	2

Food Exchange per serving: ½ Low-Fat Milk Exchange.

Low-sodium diets: Omit salt. Use unsalted margarine and a low-sodium chicken bouillon cube

Lean Chicken Gravy

Canned or fresh chicken broth can be substituted for the bouillon cubes and water.

2 chicken bouillon cubes
1 cup water
1 tablespoon finely minced onion
1 tablespoon cornstarch
¼ cup cold water
⅛ teaspoon salt
2 dashes freshly ground pepper

In a small saucepan combine bouillon cubes, water, and onion. Simmer gently 2–3 minutes, stirring occasionally to dissolve bouillon cubes. Meanwhile, combine cornstarch and cold water, stirring with a fork until smooth and well blended. Add gradually to boiling bouillon, stirring constantly. Cook and stir over medium heat until thick, smooth, and transparent. Stir in salt and pepper. May be seasoned with additional desired herbs.

4 servings (yield: 1 cup)   *1 serving: ¼ cup*

			Nutritive values per serving:			
CHO (g)	PRO (g)	FAT (g)	CAL —	Fiber (g)	Sodium (mg)	Chol (mg)
2	0	0	11	0	491	0

Food Exchange per serving: Up to ¼ cup is "free."

Low-sodium diets: Omit salt. Use low-sodium bouillon cubes. Add additional herbs or spices (compatible with meat served) to flavor gravy.

Lean Beef Gravy

2 beef bouillon cubes
1 cup water
1 tablespoon finely minced onion
1 tablespoon cornstarch
¼ cup cold water
⅛ teaspoon salt
2 dashes freshly ground pepper

In a small saucepan combine bouillon cubes, water, and onion. Simmer gently 2–3 minutes, stirring occasionally to dissolve bouillon cubes. Meanwhile, combine cornstarch and cold water, stirring with a fork until smooth and well blended. Add gradually to boiling bouillon, stirring constantly. Cook and stir over medium heat until thick, smooth, and transparent. Stir in salt and pepper. May be seasoned with additional desired herbs.

4 servings (yield: 1 cup)   *1 serving: ¼ cup*

Nutritive values per serving:

CHO (g)	PRO (g)	FAT (g)	CAL —	Fiber (g)	Sodium (mg)	Chol (mg)
2	0	0	11	0	491	0

Food Exchange per serving: Up to ¼ cup is "free."

Low-sodium diets: Omit salt. Use low-sodium bouillon cubes. add additional herbs or spices (compatible with meat served) to flavor gravy.

Real Italian Sauce

1 12-ounce can tomato paste
2 cups water
1 12-ounce can V-8 Juice
1 tablespoon minced onion
1 tablespoon wine vinegar
1 teaspoon minced garlic
½ teaspoon dried oregano
½ teaspoon dried basil
Pinch crushed red pepper

Combine all ingredients in a medium pot. Simmer gently for 25 minutes, stirring occasionally. This sauce keeps well in refrigerator or may be frozen in 1-cup containers and used as needed.

7 servings (yield: 3½ cups)   *1 serving: ½ cup*

Nutritive values per serving:

CHO (g)	PRO (g)	FAT (g)	CAL —	Fiber (g)	Sodium (mg)	Chol (mg)
12	2	0	53	0.6	548	0

Food Exchanges per serving: 2 Vegetable Exchanges.

Low-sodium diets: Substitute unsalted V-8 Juice.

Mock Hollandaise Sauce

This is very similar to a light hollandaise sauce. It is excellent on a variety of cooked vegetables and especially fine for making deviled eggs.

1 egg yolk
¾ cup plain low-fat yogurt
2 tablespoons fresh lemon juice
¼ teaspoon salt
⅛ teaspoon dry mustard

Beat egg yolk slightly in a heavy saucepan with ¼ cup yogurt, lemon juice, salt, and mustard. Cook over low heat, stirring constantly until thick and smooth. Remove from heat. Slowly stir in remaining ½ cup yogurt; blend well. Serve warm over vegetables or store in a covered jar in refrigerator. Reheat gently over low flame.

8 servings (yield: ¾ cup)   *1 serving: 1½ tablespoons*

Nutritive values per serving:						
CHO (g)	PRO (g)	FAT (g)	CAL —	Fiber (g)	Sodium (mg)	Chol (mg)
2	1	1	22	0	77	35

Food Exchange per serving: A "free" food unless large amounts are used.

Low-sodium diets: Omit salt.

Mustard Sauce

This is delicious served with ham, pork, or Canadian bacon.

2 egg yolks
½ teaspoon dry mustard
3 tablespoons white vinegar
3 tablespoons skim milk
1 tablespoon prepared mustard
1 tablespoon fresh lemon juice,
Sugar substitute equivalent to 1 teaspoon sugar

Beat egg yolks with dry mustard in the top of a double boiler until blended. Add vinegar gradually, beating after each addition. Cook over simmering water, stirring constantly until thick and smooth. Add milk gradually, beating it in with a fork or wire whip. Cook 5 more minutes over simmering water. Remove from heat. Let cool 10 minutes. Add remaining ingredients and blend well.

8 servings (yield: ½ cup)   *1 serving: 1 tablespoon*

Nutritive values per serving:						
CHO (g)	PRO (g)	FAT (g)	CAL —	Fiber (g)	Sodium (mg)	Chol (mg)
1	1	1	20	0	29	68

Food Exchange per serving: Up to 1 tablespoon may be considered "free." If you use 3 tablespoons, count it as 1 Fat Exchange.

Low-sodium diets: This recipe is suitable but should be used with fresh pork, hot ham, or Canadian-style bacon.

Sunshine Sauce

An easy and excellent sauce for fish.

½ cup unsweetened orange juice
1 tablespoon margarine
½ teaspoon grated fresh orange rind
½ teaspoon salt
Dash ground nutmeg
1 tablespoon minced fresh parsley

Combine all ingredients in small pan. Heat until warmed through. Serve over poached or broiled fillets.

4 servings (yield: ½ cup)   *1 serving: 2 tablespoons*

			Nutritive values per serving:			
CHO (g)	PRO (g)	FAT (g)	CAL —	Fiber (g)	Sodium (mg)	Chol (mg)
3	0	3	40	0.1	278	0

Food Exchange per serving: 1 Fat Exchange. Fish that is poached or baked or broiled without added fat is generally so low in fat that this sauce may be served and counted as a free food to enhance the fish.

Low-sodium diets: Omit salt.

Sweet and Sour Sauce

This may be served with cooked shrimp, chicken, ham, or pork.

1½ tablespoons cornstarch
½ teaspoon ground ginger *or* 1 teaspoon grated
    fresh gingerroot
¼ teaspoon salt
1 8½-ounce can pineapple tidbits canned in
    pineapple juice
¼ cup cider vinegar
1 tablespoon soy sauce
1¼ cups chicken broth
Sugar substitute equivalent to ¼ cup sugar

Mix cornstarch, ginger, and salt in a small heavy saucepan.
Drain pineapple tidbits, saving liquid; set pineapple aside.
Combine drained pineapple liquid, vinegar, soy sauce, and
chicken broth; add gradually to cornstarch mixture, stirring
until smooth. Bring to a boil and cook over medium heat,
stirring constantly until thick and smooth. Add pineapple;
simmer gently 4–5 minutes. Add sweetener shortly before
serving.

8 servings (yield: 2 cups)   *1 serving: ¼ cup*

Nutritive values per serving:

CHO (g)	PRO (g)	FAT (g)	CAL —	Fiber (g)	Sodium (mg)	Chol (mg)
7	1	0	32	0.2	311	0

Food Exchange per serving: ½ Fruit Exchange.

Low-sodium diets: Omit salt. Substitute reduced-sodium (light)
    soy sauce.

Strawberry Sauce

Serve on Baking Powder Biscuits, or ladyfingers. This sauce is also very nice with Tapioca Nectar Fluff or Rice Pudding (see Index).

 1½ cups whole fresh strawberries
 Sugar substitute equivalent to 2 teaspoons sugar
   (optional)
 1 tablespoon water

Wash berries; remove hulls and bad spots. Cut berries into bite-sized pieces. Place in a bowl, crushing bottom layer slightly with a fork. If desired, add sweetener, mixing thoroughly with water and then adding to berries, and mix well. Cover lightly. Chill until required.

2 servings (yield: 1⅓ cups)   *1 serving: ⅔ cup*

Nutritive values per serving:

CHO (g)	PRO (g)	FAT (g)	CAL —	Fiber (g)	Sodium (mg)	Chol (mg)
8	1	0	36	2.4	1	0

Food Exchange per serving: ½ Fruit Exchange. Up to ⅓ cup may be considered "free."

Low-sodium diets: This recipe is excellent.

RELISHES

Raw Apple Relish

1 medium red-skinned apple, cored and chopped
  fine
1 tablespoon fresh lemon juice
3 tablespoons finely diced onion
2 tablespoons chopped sweet gherkins
2 tablespoons chopped ripe olives
¼ cup low-calorie French dressing

Combine all ingredients well. Pack into a pint container. Cover
and chill for a few hours before serving.

7 servings (yield: 1¼ cups)   *1 serving: 3 tablespoons*

Nutritive values per serving:						
CHO (g)	PRO (g)	FAT (g)	CAL —	Fiber (g)	Sodium (mg)	Chol (mg)
5	0	1	28	0.7	116	0

Food Exchange per serving: 1 Vegetable Exchange or ½ Fruit
                              Exchange. Up to 1½ tablespoons
                              may be considered "free."

Low-sodium diets: This recipe is excellent.

NEW Pickled Ginger

This ginger relish is used in the Chicken Breast with Pickled Ginger recipe. It can also be used as a spicy relish with roast pork or lamb chops.

½ cup sliced peeled fresh gingerroot (paper thin)
1 cup boiling water
½ cup rice vinegar
Sugar substitute equivalent to 2 tablespoons sugar
1 tablespoon water
¼ teaspoon salt

Place ginger slices in a bowl and cover with boiling water; allow ginger to stand for 1 minute and drain. Add remaining ingredients and stir well until sugar substitute dissolves. Refrigerate until ready to serve. Drain pickled ginger before serving.

8 servings   1 serving: 1 rounded teaspoon
(yield: ¼ cup pickled ginger)

Nutritive values per serving:						
CHO (g)	PRO (g)	FAT (g)	CAL —	Fiber (g)	Sodium (mg)	Chol (mg)
2	0	0	8	1.4	100	0

Food Exchange per serving: A "free" food.

Low-sodium diets: Omit salt.

Sweet Pickled Cherries

*A delightful treat for everyone and so easy to make! Serve with
a salad, as a tasty, unusual garnish, or as finger food on relish
trays.*

> 3 cups (1 pound) sweet Bing cherries with stems
> 1 cup cold water
> 1 cup white vinegar
> 1 teaspoon brown sugar
> 1 tablespoon salt

Pick over cherries to select firm, ripe ones. Leave on as many
stems as possible. Carefully wash and drain cherries. Pack
easily into a 1-quart jar, shaking but not pressing down. Combine remaining ingredients until salt dissolves, then pour on
top of cherries. Seal jar tightly and turn upside down. Leave for
2 hours in a cool place. Turn upright. Store in refrigerator. Do
not use for at least 24 hours. Use within 1 month.

8 or more servings   *1 serving: 6–8 cherries*
(yield: 1 quart, 50–60 cherries)

Nutritive values per serving:

CHO (g)	PRO (g)	FAT (g)	CAL —	Fiber (g)	Sodium (mg)	Chol (mg)
12	1	1	47	0.8	367	0

Food Exchange per serving: 6–8 cherries—1 Fruit Exchange; 1–2
cherries may be considered "free."

Low-sodium diets: This recipe is not suitable.

Tomato Relish

Serve this as a relish with hot or cold meats or as a sauce on seafood cocktails.

1 16-ounce can tomatoes with liquid
¼ cup finely chopped onion
1 teaspoon salt
¼ cup finely chopped celery
¼ cup finely chopped green pepper
1 teaspoon celery seed
1 tablespoon white vinegar
Dash cayenne pepper
Sugar substitute equivalent to 1 teaspoon sugar

Turn tomatoes and liquid into a small bowl; cut tomatoes into very small pieces. Add all remaining ingredients and mix well. Turn into a pint jar; cover tightly. Store in refrigerator several hours before using. Use within 10 days.

12 servings (yield: 1½ cups)   1 serving: 2 tablespoons

Nutritive values per serving:						
CHO (g)	PRO (g)	FAT (g)	CAL —	Fiber (g)	Sodium (mg)	Chol (mg)
2	0	0	11	0.4	227	0

Food Exchange per serving: Up to 2 tablespoons may be considered "free."

Low-sodium diets: Omit salt. Use unsalted canned tomatoes.

Pickled Cucumber Strips

These pickles are suitable for refrigerator storage only up to one week.

    3 small (about ½ pound) pickling cucumbers,
        3-4 inches long
    1 cup cider vinegar
    ½ cup water
    1 teaspoon mixed pickling spices
    ½ teaspoon salt
    ½ teaspoon celery seed
    1 stick cinnamon, 3-4 inches long
    Sugar substitute equivalent to 4 tablespoons sugar

Scrub cucumbers; remove and discard ends; cut cucumbers lengthwise into eight strips each; set aside. Combine vinegar, water, spices, salt, celery seed, and cinnamon. Bring to a boil, reduce heat to low, and let simmer for 5 minutes. Add cucumber strips; return to a boil and simmer for 3 minutes. Add sweetener and mix well. Pack strips upright in a hot pint jar. Strain vinegar and pour on top of cucumber strips. Cover jar, cool, and store in refrigerator. Do not use for 24 hours. Use within week.

8 servings (yield: 1 pint jar)   *1 serving: 3 strips*

Nutritive values per serving:						
CHO (g)	PRO (g)	FAT (g)	CAL —	Fiber (g)	Sodium (mg)	Chol (mg)
4	0	0	7	0.4	64	0

Food Exchange per serving: Up to five strips may be considered "free."

Low-sodium diets: Acceptable for occasional use unless sodium restriction is severe. They are far lower in salt than most pickles.

Dilly Vegetable Pickles

¾ cup white vinegar
¾ cup cold water
1 teaspoon salt
1½ teaspoons dill seed
1 cup small cauliflowerets
1 small (3-ounce) pickling cucumber
4–5 small white pickling onions, peeled
Sugar substitute equivalent to 2 tablespoons sugar

Combine vinegar, cold water, salt, and dill seeds and bring to a boil; simmer for 5 minutes. Prepare vegetables; slice cucumber crosswise and measure ¾ cup; slice onions crosswise into thin slices and separate into rings. Add cauliflowerets, cucumbers, and onions to hot vinegar; bring to a boil and cook gently for 1 minute. Remove from heat. Add sweetener and stir until dissolved. Spoon vegetables carefully into a hot, clean pint jar. Pour vinegar mixture on top. Cover and cool. Seal jar and store in refrigerator. Do not use for 24 hours. Use within a week—no longer.

8 servings (yield: 1 pint)   *1 serving: ¼ cup*

			Nutritive values per serving:			
CHO (g)	PRO (g)	FAT (g)	CAL —	Fiber (g)	Sodium (mg)	Chol (mg)
2	0	0	12	0.6	124	0

Food Exchange per serving: Up to ¼ cup may be considered "free."

Low-sodium diets: May be used occasionally if sodium restriction is not severe. These contain far less sodium than traditional pickles.

Raisins Indienne

Keep this raisin chutney in the refrigerator to serve with roast duckling, chicken, lamb, or pork or on top of hot cooked rice (plain or curried). One tablespoon over cottage cheese adds a wonderful flavor and color contrast. Mary likes to serve it with chicken salad, too.

1 cup seedless raisins
½ cup finely chopped green pepper
½ cup finely chopped celery
½ cup finely chopped green onion
1½ tablespoons margarine
¼ cup boiling water
2 tablespoons chopped Major Grey's chutney
¼ cup slivered blanched almonds
3 tablespoons diced pimiento
1½ tablespoons vinegar
1½ tablespoons brown sugar

Combine first six ingredients in a heavy frying pan. Bring to a boil, reduce heat to low, cover, and simmer gently until crisp-tender. Add all remaining ingredients. Stir over moderate heat to blend and heat together. Store in the refrigerator up to 1 month.

24 servings (yield: 1½ cups)   *1 serving: 1 tablespoon*

Nutritive values per serving:						
CHO (g)	PRO (g)	FAT (g)	CAL —	Fiber (g)	Sodium (mg)	Chol (mg)
7	1	1	41	0.8	15	0

Food Exchange per serving: ½ Fruit Exchange *or* ½ Starch Exchange.

Low-sodium diets: This recipe is excellent.

Cranberry and Orange Relish

Serve with hot or cold sliced baked poultry or ham. To freeze this relish, omit sweetener and add it at time of serving.

    2 cups (½ pound) fresh or frozen cranberries
    1 medium orange
    Sugar substitute equivalent to 4 tablespoons sugar

Wash and pick over cranberries; discard overripe berries. Wash orange, cut into small chunks, and discard seeds and center core. Put both fruits through a food grinder using coarse blade or chop in a food processor. Add sweetener; mix well. Chill in a covered container.

8 servings (yield: 1½ cups)   *1 serving: 3 tablespoons*

Nutritive values per serving:						
CHO (g)	PRO (g)	FAT (g)	CAL —	Fiber (g)	Sodium (mg)	Chol (mg)
7	0	0	26	0.7	0	0

Food Exchange per serving: ½ Fruit Exchange.

Low-sodium diets: This recipe is excellent.

TOPPINGS

Vanilla Crème Fraîche

Use this as a topping for berries, other fruits, and desserts.

¼ cup whipping cream
¼ cup plain low-fat yogurt
1 teaspoon pure vanilla extract

In a small chilled bowl whip cream until almost stiff. Gently fold in the yogurt and vanilla. Chill in a covered container at least two hours to allow flavors to blend. Store in refrigerator no longer than two days.

6 servings (yield: ¾ cup)   *1 serving: 2 tablespoons*

Nutritive values per serving:						
CHO (g)	PRO (g)	FAT (g)	CAL —	Fiber (g)	Sodium (mg)	Chol (mg)
1	1	4	40	0	10	14

Food Exchange per serving: 1 Fat Exchange.
Low-sodium diets: This recipe is excellent.

Phony Whipped Cream

This recipe can be used instead of real whipped cream or frozen whipped topping. It contains about half the calories, cholesterol, protein, and fat as Cool-Whip. In other words, you can use 2 tablespoons of this for the same calories as 1 tablespoon of Cool-Whip. Either can be used in moderation by individuals with diabetes.

    1 teaspoon granulated gelatin
    1 tablespoon cold water
    ½ cup iced water
    ½ cup instant nonfat dry milk
    Sugar substitute equivalent to 3 tablespoons sugar
    ½ teaspoon pure vanilla extract
    2 tablespoons vegetable oil

Chill a small mixing bowl and beaters. Meanwhile, soften gelatin in cold water, then dissolve it over boiling water. Allow it to cool until tepid. Place iced water and nonfat dry milk in chilled bowl and beat at high speed until stiff peaks form. Continue beating, adding remaining ingredients and gelatin, until blended. Place bowl in freezer for 15 minutes, then transfer to refrigerator. Occasionally stir gently to keep mixture smooth and well blended. Store in refrigerator for no longer than two days.

24 servings (yield: 3 cups)   *1 serving: 2 tablespoons*

Nutritive values per serving:

CHO (g)	PRO (g)	FAT (g)	CAL —	Fiber (g)	Sodium (mg)	Chol (mg)
1	1	1	16	0	8	0

Food Exchange per serving: Up to 2 tablespoons may be considered "free."

Low-sodium diets: This recipe is excellent.

SWEET SPREADS

All of the sweet spreads are really fruit concentrates. Since they do not have sugar, which acts as a preservative, they are more perishable than commercial jams and jellies. Keep them in the refrigerator.

Apricot Spread

2 cups chopped pitted fresh apricots (small bite-sized pieces)
¾ cup cold water
1 teaspoon fresh lemon juice
1½ teaspoons granulated gelatin
½ teaspoon pure almond extract
Sugar substitute equivalent to 3 tablespoons sugar

Put apricots in a heavy saucepan with ½ cup water and the lemon juice. Bring to a boil; lower heat and simmer gently for 8–10 minutes, stirring frequently with a wooden (not metal) spoon. Meanwhile, soak gelatin in remaining ¼ cup cold water. When apricots are cooked, remove from heat. Add gelatin, almond extract, and sweetener; mix thoroughly. Pack into two or three small, hot jars; cover lightly and allow to cool. Cover tightly and store in refrigerator. Use within two weeks.

10 servings (yield: 1¼ cups)   *1 serving: 2 tablespoons*

Nutritive values per serving:						
CHO (g)	PRO (g)	FAT (g)	CAL —	Fiber (g)	Sodium (mg)	Chol (mg)
3	1	0	15	0.5	1	0

Food Exchange per serving: Up to 2 tablespoons may be considered "free."

Low-sodium diets: This recipe is excellent.

Apple Jelly Spread

When Kay developed this recipe, she said it reminded her of her grandmother's Dolga crab apple jelly!

2 cups unsweetened apple juice
1 teaspoon fresh lemon juice
6 large *or* 8 small whole cloves
2 teaspoons granulated gelatin
½ cup cold water
Sugar substitute equivalent to ¾ cup sugar
Few drops red food color (optional)

Combine apple and lemon juices and whole cloves in a heavy saucepan. Bring to a boil; simmer gently 10 minutes. Meanwhile, soak gelatin in cold water. Remove apple juice from heat; discard cloves; add gelatin and sweetener and mix well to dissolve. Add about three drops red food color; mix well. Pour carefully into two small, hot jars. Cover lightly until cooled. Then cover tightly and store in refrigerator no longer than two weeks.

32 servings (yield: 2 cups)   *1 serving: 1 tablespoon*

Nutritive values per serving:

CHO (g)	PRO (g)	FAT (g)	CAL —	Fiber (g)	Sodium (mg)	Chol (mg)
2	0	0	10	0	1	0

Food Exchange per serving: Up to 2 tablespoons may be
                            considered "free."

Low-sodium diets: This recipe is excellent.

Fresh Peach Spread

This was one of Kay's favorite toast spreads. It can also be used on bread, muffins, or crackers.

   2 cups chopped peeled pitted fresh peaches (small
       bite-sized pieces) (about 1 pound)
   1 teaspoon fresh lemon juice
   ¾ cup cold water
   1½ teaspoons granulated gelatin
   Sugar substitute equivalent to 3 tablespoons of
       sugar
   ⅛ teaspoon pure orange extract

Place peaches in a heavy saucepan with lemon juice and add ½ cup cold water. Bring to a boil; simmer gently for about 8 minutes, stirring frequently. Meanwhile, soak gelatin in remaining ¼ cup cold water. Remove cooked peaches from heat. Add gelatin, sweetener, and orange extract; mix well to blend flavors and dissolve gelatin. Turn into two or three small, hot jars; cover lightly and allow to cool. Cover tightly and store in refrigerator no longer than two weeks.

24 servings (yield: 1½ cups)   *1 serving: 1 tablespoon*

			Nutritive values per serving:			
CHO (g)	PRO (g)	FAT (g)	CAL —	Fiber (g)	Sodium (mg)	Chol (mg)
2	0	0	8	0.4	0	0

Food Exchange per serving: Up to 2 tablespoons may be
                           considered "free."

Low-sodium diets: This recipe is excellent.

NEW Pear Butter

If you like it sweeter, add sweetener to taste after cooking. Pears vary considerably in sweetness. Use Pear Butter as a topping or on toast, as you would use butter. For a special taste treat, use pear butter spread over chicken breasts or a pork chop before grilling or after cooking.

2½ pounds firm, ripe pears
⅔ cup water
2 tablespoons fresh lemon juice
1 teaspoon ground cinnamon
¼ teaspoon ground nutmeg
1 teaspoon julienned lemon rind

Wash, core, and cut pears into quarters. Place pieces in a 4-quart saucepan. Add water and lemon juice and bring mixture to boil over medium heat. Cover pot and simmer for 35 minutes or until pears are tender. Puree pears using a food processor fitted with steel blade or a food mill. Return the puree to pot, including cooking liquid, and add the cinnamon, nutmeg, and lemon rind. Simmer pear mixture, uncovered, for 40–50 minutes, stirring occasionally until mixture thickens. Pour cooled pear butter into small, hot jars, cover, and refrigerate. Store in refrigerator no longer than three weeks.

72 servings (yield: 3 cups)   *1 serving: 2 teaspoons*

			Nutritive values per serving:			
CHO (g)	PRO (g)	FAT (g)	CAL —	Fiber (g)	Sodium (mg)	Chol (mg)
2	0	0	10	0.4	0	0

Food Exchange per serving: Up to 4 teaspoons may be considered "free."

Low-sodium diets: This recipe is excellent.

Fresh Strawberry Spread

When Rachel's friend, Peter Geyer, discovered that he had diabetes he received several copies of this book as a gift. This recipe is one of his favorites.

2 pints fresh strawberries
2 tablespoons cold water
1½ tablespoons fresh lemon juice
2 teaspoons granulated gelatin
¼ cup cold water
Sugar substitute equivalent to 4 tablespoons sugar

Wash and clean berries; discard hulls and measure 3 cups. Cut berries into small, bite-sized pieces and place in a heavy pan with 2 tablespoons cold water and the lemon juice. Partially crush berries. Bring to a boil. Stir and cook rapidly about 5 minutes until berries are just cooked. Meanwhile, soak gelatin in ¼ cup cold water. Remove berries from heat. Add gelatin and sweetener and stir to dissolve and blend. Remove scum from surface and discard. Turn into small, hot jars; cover lightly and cool. Then cover tightly and store in refrigerator no longer than two weeks.

18 servings (yield: 2¼ cups)   *1 serving: 2 tablespoons*

Nutritive values per serving:						
CHO (g)	PRO (g)	FAT (g)	CAL —	Fiber (g)	Sodium (mg)	Chol (mg)
2	0	0	10	0.5	1	0

Food Exchange per serving: Up to 2 tablespoons may be considered "free."

Low-sodium diets: This recipe is excellent.

Blueberry Spread

2 cups blueberries
¾ cup cold water, divided
2 teaspoons fresh lemon juice
1½ teaspoons granulated gelatin
Sugar substitute equivalent to 3 tablespoons sugar

Combine blueberries, ½ cup water, and lemon juice in a heavy saucepan. Bring to a boil; simmer gently for about 8 minutes, stirring frequently. Meanwhile, soak gelatin in remaining ¼ cup cold water. Remove blueberries from heat; add gelatin and sweetener and mix well to dissolve. Turn into small, hot jars; cover lightly and allow to cool. Cover tightly and store in refrigerator no longer than two weeks.

24 servings (yield: 1½ cups)   *1 serving: 1 tablespoon*

Nutritive values per serving:

CHO (g)	PRO (g)	FAT (g)	CAL —	Fiber (g)	Sodium (mg)	Chol (mg)
2	0	0	8	0.3	1	0

Food Exchange per serving: Up to 2 tablespoons may be considered "free."

Low-sodium diets: This recipe is excellent.

Red Plum Spread

1¼ cups chopped pitted fresh red plums (small bite-
     sized pieces) (about 1 pound)
¾ cup cold water, divided
1 teaspoon fresh lemon juice
1¼ teaspoons granulated gelatin
Sugar substitute equivalent to 4 tablespoons sugar

Combine plums with ½ cup water and the lemon juice in a
heavy saucepan. Bring to a boil, then simmer gently about 8
minutes, stirring frequently. Meanwhile, soak gelatin in remaining ¼ cup cold water. Remove cooked plums from heat;
stir in gelatin and sweetener and mix well. Turn into clean,
small, hot jars; cover lightly until cool. Then cover tightly and
store in the refrigerator no longer than two weeks.

20 servings (yield: 1¼ cups)   *1 serving: 1 tablespoon*

			Nutritive values per serving:			
CHO (g)	PRO (g)	FAT (g)	CAL —	Fiber (g)	Sodium (mg)	Chol (mg)
2	0	0	8	0.2	0	0

Food Exchange per serving: Up to 2 tablespoons may be
                              considered "free."

Low-sodium diets: This recipe is excellent.

Concord Grape Jelly Spread

This spread for bread, toast, muffins, or crackers has a real grapey flavor. You may use red or white grape juice in place of purple if you like.

1½ cups pure Concord grape juice
1 teaspoon fresh lemon juice
2 teaspoons granulated gelatin
½ cup cold water
Sugar substitute equivalent to ¼ cup sugar

Combine grape juice and lemon juice in a heavy saucepan. Bring to a boil; simmer 3–4 minutes. Meanwhile, soak gelatin in cold water. Remove grape juice from heat. Add gelatin and sweetener; mix well to dissolve. Pour into two small, hot jars, cover lightly, and cool. Cover tightly and store in refrigerator no longer than two weeks.

24 servings (yield: 1½ cups)   *1 serving: 1 tablespoon*

			Nutritive values per serving:			
CHO (g)	PRO (g)	FAT (g)	CAL —	Fiber (g)	Sodium (mg)	Chol (mg)
3	0	0	11	0	1	0

Food Exchange per serving: Up to 2 tablespoons may be considered "free."

Low-sodium diets: This recipe is excellent.

27
Beverages

Orange Fizz

6 ice cubes
½ cup orange juice
1 teaspoon fresh lemon juice
½ teaspoon pure orange extract
Sugar substitute equivalent to 2 teaspoons sugar
   (optional)
1 10-ounce bottle club soda
1 thin slice orange

Crush ice cubes and divide between two 10-ounce glasses. Mix together orange juice, lemon juice, and orange extract; dissolve sweetener in fruit juices. Pour ¼ cup of mixed juices into each glass. Pour half bottle club soda into each glass. Stir briskly. Cut orange slice in half crosswise, then fit onto edge of glass. Serve immediately.

2 servings   *1 serving: 1 large glass*

Nutritive values per serving:

CHO (g)	PRO (g)	FAT (g)	CAL —	Fiber (g)	Sodium (mg)	Chol (mg)
8	0	0	34	0.6	31	0

Food Exchange per serving: ½ Fruit Exchange.

Low-sodium diets: This recipe is excellent.

Foamy Orange Cup

½ cup skim milk or buttermilk made from skim
    milk
½ cup unsweetened orange juice
Sugar substitute equivalent to 1 teaspoon sugar
¼ teaspoon pure vanilla extract
⅛ teaspoon pure almond extract
Dash salt
3 ice cubes, cracked into small pieces

Place all ingredients in blender; cover. Blend on low speed until
ice cubes are crushed and the drink is foamy.

2 servings (yield: 1½ cups)   *1 serving: ¾ cup*

Nutritive values per serving:

CHO (g)	PRO (g)	FAT (g)	CAL —	Fiber (g)	Sodium (mg)	Chol (mg)
10	3	0	50	0.2	32	1

Food Exchange per serving: 1 Fruit Exchange *or* ½ Skim Milk
                    Exchange.

Low-sodium diets: This recipe is excellent.

Pink Lady

1 cup skim milk
3 ice cubes, cracked into small pieces
½ teaspoon imitation rum extract
1–2 drops red food color
Sugar substitute equivalent to 1 teaspoon sugar
⅛ teaspoon pure vanilla extract

Chill two serving glasses. Measure all ingredients into blender
container; cover. Blend at low speed, then switch to high until
ice cubes are crushed and mixture is foamy and well blended.
Pour into glasses.

2 servings (yield: 1½ cups)   *1 serving: ¾ cup*

		Nutritive values per serving:				
CHO (g)	PRO (g)	FAT (g)	CAL —	Fiber (g)	Sodium (mg)	Chol (mg)
6	4	0	44	0	63	2

Food Exchange per serving: ½ Skim Milk Exchange.

Low-Sodium diets: This recipe is suitable.

Champagne Fooler

Bubble, bubble, no toil, no trouble!

⅓ cup chilled unsweetened apple juice
¼ teaspoon fresh lemon juice
About ½ cup chilled club soda

Chill a champagne glass or wineglass. Measure apple and lemon juices into a measuring cup. Add enough club soda to make a total of ¾ cup; stir gently to blend. Pour into chilled champagne glass or wineglass. Serve immediately.

1 serving   *1 serving: ¾ cup*

		Nutritive values per serving:				
CHO (g)	PRO (g)	FAT (g)	CAL —	Fiber (g)	Sodium (mg)	Chol (mg)
10	0	0	38	0.1	18	0

Food Exchange per serving: ½ Fruit Exchange.

Low-sodium diets: This recipe is excellent.

Lime Fizz

6 ice cubes
Sugar substitute equivalent to 2 tablespoons sugar
¼ cup fresh or bottled unsweetened lime juice
1 10-ounce bottle club soda

Crush ice cubes and divide between two 10-ounce glasses. Dissolve sweetener in lime juice, then pour 2 tablespoons of mixture on top of crushed ice. Pour half bottle club soda on top of each; stir briskly with spoon. Serve immediately.

2 servings   *1 serving: 1 large glass*

Nutritive values per serving:

CHO (g)	PRO (g)	FAT (g)	CAL —	Fiber (g)	Sodium (mg)	Chol (mg)
4	0	0	14	0	30	0

Food Exchange per serving: One large glass may be considered "free."

Low-sodium diets: This recipe is excellent.

Lemon Fizz

6 ice cubes
Sugar substitute equivalent to 2 tablespoons sugar
⅓ cup fresh lemon juice
1 10-ounce bottle club soda
2 slices lemon

Crush ice cubes and divide between two 10-ounce glasses. Dissolve sweetener in lemon juice, then pour 2½ tablespoons of mixture on top of crushed ice. Pour half bottle club soda into each glass; stir briskly. Cut lemon slices halfway through to core and garnish side of each glass with a lemon slice.

2 servings   *1 serving: 1 large glass*

Nutritive values per serving:						
CHO (g)	PRO (g)	FAT (g)	CAL —	Fiber (g)	Sodium (mg)	Chol (mg)
6	0	0	18	0.2	31	0

Food Exchange per serving: One large glass may be considered "free."

Low-sodium diets: This recipe is excellent.

Chocolate-Flavored Drinks

These chocolate-flavored drinks are all made using the Chocolate-Flavored Syrup recipe that follows. You may use 1–2 tablespoons of the Chocolate-Flavored Syrup, depending upon your own taste for chocolate. There are several good sugar-free cocoa mixes at your supermarket, but our Chocolate-flavored Syrup is equally tasty and economical.

Chocolate-Flavored Syrup

½ cup firmly packed cocoa powder
1¼ cups cold water
¼ teaspoon salt
Sugar substitute equivalent to ½ cup sugar
2½ teaspoons pure vanilla extract

Mix cocoa, water, and salt in a heavy saucepan until smooth. Bring to a boil and simmer gently, stirring constantly for 3 minutes. Remove from heat; let cool 10 minutes. Add sweetener and vanilla and mix well. Pour into a jar, cover, and store in refrigerator. Stir in jar before measuring to use.

20 servings (yield: 1¼ cups)   *1 serving: 1 tablespoon*

Nutritive values per serving:						
CHO (g)	PRO (g)	FAT (g)	CAL —	Fiber (g)	Sodium (mg)	Chol (mg)
2	1	0	11	0.1	25	0

Food Exchange per serving: Up to 2 tablespoons may be considered "free." If ¼ cup is used, count as 1 Vegetable Exchange *or* ½ Fruit Exchange.

Low-sodium diets: Omit salt.

Chocolate Milk

1 cup chilled skim milk
1–2 tablespoons Chocolate-Flavored Syrup (*see* Index)

Combine ingredients in a tall, cold glass and stir vigorously to mix well.

1 serving   *1 serving: 8 ounces*

Nutritive values per serving:

CHO (g)	PRO (g)	FAT (g)	CAL —	Fiber (g)	Sodium (mg)	Chol (mg)
13	9	1	97	0.1	151	4

Food Exchange per serving (1 tablespoon syrup): 1 Skim Milk Exchange.

Low-sodium diets: Omit salt from Chocolate-Flavored Syrup.

Hot Milk Chocolate

1 cup (8 ounces) skim milk
1–2 tablespoons Chocolate-Flavored Syrup (*see* preceding recipe)

Heat milk and syrup together in the top of a double boiler over simmering water, stirring frequently until very hot. Serve immediately in a warmed mug or cup.

1 serving   *1 serving: 8 ounces*

Nutritive values per serving:

CHO (g)	PRO (g)	FAT (g)	CAL —	Fiber (g)	Sodium (mg)	Chol (mg)
13	9	1	97	0.1	151	4

Food Exchange per serving (1 tablespoon syrup): 1 Skim Milk Exchange.

Low-sodium diets: Omit salt from Chocolate-Flavored Syrup.

Mocha Milk Drink

1 tablespoon Chocolate-Flavored Syrup (*see* Index)
1 teaspoon instant coffee powder
1 cup (8 ounces) skim milk

Measure Chocolate-Flavored Syrup into a tall glass, add instant coffee, and pour milk on top slowly, stirring vigorously to blend well. If you have a blender, measure ingredients into blender, cover, and mix at low speed for about 30 seconds.

1 serving   —   *1 serving: 8 ounces*

			Nutritive values per serving:			
CHO (g)	PRO (g)	FAT (g)	CAL —	Fiber (g)	Sodium (mg)	Chol (mg)
14	9	1	100	1.1	152	4

Food Exchange per serving: 1 Skim Milk Exchange.

Low-sodium diets: Omit salt from Chocolate-Flavored Syrup.

Double Chocolate Soda

Some call this drink a chocolate phosphate. It's perfect for the chocolate lovers among us—and it's "legal."

2–3 ice cubes, cracked into small pieces
2 tablespoons Chocolate-Flavored Syrup (*see* Index)
6–8 ounces chilled club soda

Place ice cubes in a tall beverage glass. Measure Chocolate-Flavored Syrup on top of ice. Add club soda slowly; stir vigorously with a long-handled beverage spoon to blend well. Serve at once.

1 serving *1 serving: 8–10 ounces*

Nutritive values per serving:

CHO (g)	PRO (g)	FAT (g)	CAL —	Fiber (g)	Sodium (mg)	Chol (mg)
3	1	1	22	0.2	109	0

Food Exchange per serving: One serving may be considered "free."

Low-sodium diets: Omit salt from Chocolate-Flavored Syrup recipe.

Appendix
Sources of Information

Everyone with diabetes can benefit from understanding the disease and how it affects him or her personally. You are not alone. There are many individuals and organizations that can help you. The more you know, the more in control you will feel. The more in control you feel, the easier it will be to make wise day-to-day decisions about food choices, exercise, or medication adjustments. For most people, primary sources of information are their doctor and dietitian. This book augments their advice.

Your relationship with your doctor and diet counselor becomes quite personal; being absolutely frank and honest about your concerns and problems is essential if you are to get the individualized care you need. If you are dissatisfied with the quality of your care, find another professional who can help you. It's your life—take charge!

The local chapter of the American Diabetes Association, Inc., is one source of referral to physicians and dietitians who specialize in diabetes care. Some major medical centers have diabetes centers that are wonderful sources for information and counseling. Ask the American Diabetes Association where the nearest Diabetes Education and Training Center is and call for an appointment if you have recently diagnosed diabetes or problems in managing your condition.

Your library is another good source of information. You can

also let the library come to your mailbox by phoning the American Diabetes Association, Inc., and receiving its publications and information about local programs. When you join the national group, you will automatically become a member of the local affiliated organization. For many people, discussions with and support of others with diabetes at meetings and while working together are enormously helpful.

Organizations

All of these organizations will send you information about materials and/or programs they offer for individuals with diabetes.

American Association of Diabetes Educators
Ste. 1400
500 N. Michigan Ave.
Chicago, IL 60611

The American Diabetes Association, Inc.
National Service Center
1660 Duke St.
Alexandria, VA 22314

The American Dietetic Association
Ste. 1100
208 S. LaSalle St.
Chicago, IL 60604

American Heart Association
National Center
7320 Greenville Ave.
Dallas, TX 75231

Canadian Diabetic Association
Ste. 601
123 Edward St.
Toronto, ON
Canada M5G 1E2

Diabetes Center
Northwestern Memorial Hospital
Superior and Fairbanks Ct.
Chicago, IL 60611

International Diabetes Center
5000 W. 39th St.
Minneapolis, MN 55436
Order its books from:
Diabetes Center, Inc.
Ste. 251
13911 Ridgedale Dr.
Minnetonka, MN 55343

Joslin Diabetes Center
1 Joslin Pl.
Boston, MA 02215

Juvenile Diabetes Foundation International
432 Park Ave.
New York, NY 10016-8013
  Ask for local affiliate's name and address.

National Diabetes Information Clearinghouse
Box NDIC
Bethesda, MD 20202
  The clearinghouse has listings of material on specific diabetes-related topics.

Magazines for Those with Diabetes

Diabetes Forecast
  A monthly magazine that is a membership benefit upon joining the American Diabetes Association, Inc.

Diabetes in the News
Box 3105
Elkhart, IN 46515
  A bimonthly magazine that provides articles and news about diabetes management.

The SugarFree Center Health-O-Gram
Box 114
Van Nuys, CA 91408
   A newsletter and mail-order catalog for diabetics.

Books for Those with Diabetes

The American Diabetes Association/The American Dietetic Association, Family Cookbooks I, II, and III.
   These books are available from either organization; see organizations list for addresses.

Biermann, June, and Toohey, Barbara. *The Diabetics Book*. New York: St. Martins Press, 1981.

Biermann, June, and Toohey, Barbara. *The Peripatetic Diabetic*. Boston: Houghton Mifflin, 1984.

Coustan, Donald R., and Garvey, Shiela. *The Baby Team: A Positive Approach to Pregnancy with Diabetes*. St. Louis: Monoject, Division of Sherwood Medical Department, T.I., 1979. 1831 Olive Street, St. Louis, MO, 63103.

Diabetes in the Family. American Diabetes Association, Inc. (Robert J. Brady Co., Prentice-Hall Publishing and Communications Company, Bowie, MD 20715), 1982.

Ducat, Lee, and Cohen, Sherry Suib. *Diabetes: A New and Complete Guide to Parents, Children, and Young Adults Who Have Insulin-Dependent Diabetes*. New York: Harper and Row, 1983.

Etzwiler, Donnel D., et al. *Learning to Live Well with Diabetes*. Minnetonka, MN: Diabetes Center, Inc., 1985. Ste. 250, 13911 Ridgedale Dr. 55343

Franz, Marion J. *Exchanges for All Occasions: Meeting the Challenge of Diabetes*. Minnetonka, MN: Diabetes Center, Inc., 1987. Ste. 250, 13911 Ridgedale Dr. 55343

Franz Marion J. *Fast Food Facts*. Minnetonka, MN: Diabetes Center, Inc., 1987. Ste. 250, 13911 Ridgedale Dr. 55343

Pennington, J. A. T., and Church, H. N. *Bowes and Church's Food Values of Portions Commonly Used.* Philadelphia: J. B. Lippincott Company, 1985.
   This book tells food values in grams and milligrams if you want to compute your own recipes. The massive USDA series is used by professionals and is more than most consumers need.

Powers, Margaret A. *Handbook of Diabetes Nutritional Management.* Rockville, MD: Aspen Publishers, Inc., 1987.
   This book is the most important and current source for professionals and those needing technical information.

Sims, Dorothea F., ed. *Diabetes: Reach for Health and Freedom.* St. Louis: American Diabetes Association, C. V. Mosby Company, 1984.

Traisman, Howard. *Management of Juvenile Diabetes Mellitus,* 3rd edition, St. Louis: C. V. Mosby Company, 1980.
   A text for professionals by a great pediatrician/diabetologist.

Travis, Luther B. *An Instructional Aid on Juvenile Diabetes Mellitus,* 7th ed. Fort Worth, TX: Stafford-Lowden (American Diabetes Association, Texas Affiliate), 1985.

Word Power

Alcohol: A substance produced when carbohydrates are fermented. Alcohol is an ingredient of beer, wine, and liquors. Each gram of pure alcohol yields seven calories. See Chapter 10, "Alcohol for Diabetics?"

Amino acids: The building units of proteins. There are 22 amino acids, 9 of which must be supplied by the diet; others can be made in the body.

Aspartame: The chemical name of a sugar substitute derived from amino acids. Marketed as NutraSweet, it is an ingredient in Equal, many sugar-free sodas, and other products. See the section titled "Sugar Substitutes" in Chapter 3.

Atherosclerosis: Deposits of fat and other substances in the walls of arteries that cause loss of elasticity and decreased blood flow.

Blood glucose: Sugar (glucose) in the blood. The amount can be determined by a simple test, using only a drop of blood from a finger.

Calorie: A unit to measure heat or energy provided by food. Carbohydrates, proteins, fats, alcohol, and sugar alcohols provide calories; vitamins, minerals, and pure cellulose fiber do not provide calories.

Carbohydrates: Compounds containing carbon, hydrogen, and oxygen found in sugars and starches. They yield four calories per gram and are a major source of energy for the body. The abbreviation for carbohydrate in our recipes is *CHO*. See Chapter 3, "The Great Sugar Masquerade."

Cardiovascular: Referring to the heart and blood vessels.

Cholesterol: A fatlike substance (sterol) found in animals; a part of the brain, hormones, cells, bile, nerve tissue, and blood. When too much cholesterol is present, it deposits in artery walls causing atherosclerosis. Cholesterol is made in the human body but is also found in foods of animal origin, particularly egg yolks and organ meats. Every recipe here has a cholesterol value listed as *Chol.*

Diabetes Mellitus: The failure of the body cells to use carbohydrates due to lack of insulin in a usable form; often referred to simply as *diabetes.*

Diabetologist: A doctor who specializes in the treatment of individuals with diabetes mellitus.

Dietetic Foods: Foods for special diets, including low-sodium, fat-modified, water-packed, or reduced-sugar foods. These foods are not necessarily intended for diabetic diets. See the section titled "Looking at Labels" in Chapter 12.

Dietitian: (Diet counselor) A registered dietitian (R.D.) is recognized by the medical profession as the primary provider of nutritional care, education, and counseling. The initials *R.D.* after a dietitian's name ensure that she or he has met the standards of the American Dietetic Association and has passed a national registration exam. Look for this credential when you seek advice on nutrition. Some states also have licensed dietitians (L.D.). This is an additional credential and does not replace the R.D.

Enrichment: The addition of nutrients to a food to increase the consumption of those nutrients. Enriched bread, for example, has added thiamine, riboflavin, niacin, and iron.

Fat: Oily substance found in meat, fish, poultry, eggs, cheese, milk, and some vegetables; a concentrated source of calories yielding nine calories per gram. See Chapter 4, "A New Look at Fats."

  Polyunsaturated fats are fats found in vegetable oils that contain several double bonds in the main carbon chain. See Chapter 4, "A New Look at Fats."

Saturated fats tend to raise blood cholesterol levels. Saturated fat comes primarily from animals and is often hard at room temperature. Examples of saturated fats are butter, lard, meat fat, solid shortening, palm oil, and coconut oil.

Unsaturated fats tend to lower blood cholesterol levels. Unsaturated fats may be monounsaturated or polyunsaturated. They come from plants and are usually liquid at room temperature. Examples of unsaturated fats are vegetable oils such as corn, cottonseed, sunflower, safflower, soybean, olive, and peanut oil.

Fiber: Indigestible carbohydrates that are found in whole grains, nuts, fruits, and vegetables. After digestion, fiber yields bulk but no calories. Different types of fiber have different benefits to the body as discussed in Chapter 5, "Fantastic Fiber." The amount of dietary fiber is included in each recipe calculation in Part III.

Soluble fiber has high water-holding capability and turns to gel during digestion, thus slowing digestion and the rate of nutrient absorption from the stomach and intestine. This type of fiber is found in oat bran, pectins (from fruits and vegetables) and various gums that are found in nuts, seeds, and legumes. Soluble fiber may play a role in smoothing out the elevation of blood sugar after eating and in reducing the likelihood of atherosclerosis by reducing blood cholesterol levels.

Insoluble fiber (cellulose) is found in foods such as wheat bran and other whole grains and has poor water-holding capability. Insoluble fiber appears to speed the passage of foods through the stomach and intestines and to increase fecal bulk. This type of fiber probably does not affect elevation of blood sugar after eating or atherosclerosis.

Food Exchanges: Lists of foods with similar nutrient values. Refer to Chapter 2, "The Exchange System."

Food habits: Your pattern of choosing and cooking the foods you have learned to eat; a result of cultural, economic, family, and religious influences.

Fortification: The addition of nutrients to foods that do not naturally have those nutrients. Milk is often fortified with vitamins A and D; many cereals, breakfast drinks, and processed foods are fortified.

"Free" Foods: Contain few calories and carbohydrates. "Free" foods may be used in the diabetic diet without controlling quantity or may be used in limited quantities without counting as an exchange. Usually, "free" foods have fewer than 20 calories per serving. Those that contain calories should be limited to three servings per day because even small numbers of calories do add up. Herbs, spices, and other ingredients that contain no calories may be used safely in any amount. See list 7: Free Foods, in Chapter 2.

Fructose: A type of simple sugar naturally found in fruits. See Chapter 3, "The Great Sugar Masquerade."

Gastrointestinal: Referring to the entire digestive tract.

Glucagon: A hormone produced by the pancreas that raises blood sugar by breaking down glycogen by the liver; its activity is opposite that of insulin.

Gluconeogenesis: The conversion of amino acids to glucose by the liver.

Glucose: A simple sugar that results from the digestion of carbohydrate-containing foods. Glucose is the form of sugar used by the body for energy. See Chapter 3, "The Great Sugar Masquerade."

Glycogen: Stored form of carbohydrates in the liver as a reserve source of fuel. During fasting or in an insulin reaction, glycogen breaks down to glucose and is released into the bloodstream.

Glycosylated Hemoglobin: A test that gives information about blood glucose levels during the preceding one to two months. When blood glucose is above normal, more glucose attaches to the hemoglobin in red blood cells; these altered cells last for about 100 days, and the amount of glucose in the hemoglobin can be measured.

Gram: A unit of mass and weight in the metric system. An ounce is about 28 grams. In recipe calculations, *g* is the abbreviation for gram.

Hormones: Chemical messengers that work in the blood-stream to regulate processes throughout the body. Insulin and glycogen are examples of hormones.

Hydrogenation: The process of adding hydrogen to a liquid fat (oil) that makes the fat more solid and saturated. This process is used to make margarine or shortening from oil.

Hyperglycemia: An abnormally high blood sugar level. Hyperglycemia can lead to diabetic emergencies and/or long-term complications of diabetes mellitus.

Hypoglycemia: An abnormally low blood sugar level that can lead to insulin reaction or insulin shock.

IDDM: Insulin-dependent diabetes mellitus (Type I diabetes). Individuals with IDDM are ketosis-prone and will develop ketoacidosis if they do not take insulin regularly. This type of diabetes was formerly called *juvenile-onset diabetes* because it usually begins in childhood or adolescence.

Ideal weight: The best weight of an individual based on sex, height, and bone structure. People of ideal weight statistically live longer and are healthier. Also called *desirable weight.*

Insulin: A hormone produced by the beta cells of the pancreas. Insulin regulates glucose going from the blood into body cells. If not enough insulin is made, or if it cannot be used properly, injections of insulin must be given.

Ketoacidosis: An excess of blood sugar and deficiency of available insulin that results in an increase in ketones in the blood, causing the body's acid balance to shift to abnormal levels. Ketoacidosis is an emergency situation that may result in coma and death if untreated.

Ketone: An acid (such as acetone) formed in the body when fats are burned for energy because the cells do not have enough carbohydrate to use as fuel.

Lipids: Another term for fats. Aside from stored body fats, there are several types of lipids (cholesterol and triglycerides) that circulate in the bloodstream. See Chapter 4, "A New Look at Fats."

Lipoproteins: Complexes of fat and protein. Lipoproteins are the transport form of fat in the bloodstream. See Chapter 4, "A New Look at Fats."

Very low-density lipoproteins (VLDLs) are the transport form of certain types of lipoproteins. High VLDL levels increase risk of coronary heart disease.

Low-density lipoproteins (LDLs) are the lipoprotein complex that transports cholesterol and are somewhat different in structure from VLDL.

High-density lipoproteins (HDLs) are the "good" type of cholesterol that protects against coronary heart disease. HDL can be raised by increasing exercise.

Low-sodium diet: A modified diet that may be prescribed by a physician. A dietitian can help with your meal plans and may mark this book so you can select foods and recipes with limited amounts of sodium. Follow the directions at the end of each recipe if you are on a low-sodium diet. This diet may also be called a salt-free, low-salt, or sodium-restricted diet.

Low-sodium foods: Foods that are processed or prepared without the addition of salt or other sodium products. Foods that are normally high-sodium may be labeled *unsalted, salt-free, or dietetic low-sodium* when they are modified to be low in sodium. When foods are high in sodium (soy sauce, canned vegetables, cereals, catsup, baking powder, cheese, etc.), a reduced-sodium (unsalted) product may be available at your grocery store.

Meal plan: A specific plan prepared by a dietitian that considers the dietary prescription and the food habits of an individual. Typically, exchanges are used, but some types of meal plans count calories, carbohydrates, or other units. See Chapter 1, "The Diabetic Meal Plan."

Metabolism: The chemical and physical processes of all cells of the body.

Milligram: A metric weight equal to 1/1,000 of a gram. In the recipe calculations, sodium and cholesterol are measured in milligrams, the abbreviation for which is *mg.*

Mineral: Chemically inorganic substances found in nature that are needed in small amounts to build and repair body tissue or control metabolism. Calcium, iron, magnesium, phosphorus, potassium, sodium, and zinc are minerals.

NIDDM: Non-insulin-dependent diabetes mellitus (Type II diabetes). Individuals with NIDDM may or may not take insulin for better control of their blood glucose levels; however, they are not ketosis-prone. NIDDM is the current terminology that has generally replaced *adult-onset (maturity-onset) diabetes*. NIDDM is generally less severe than IDDM and usually begins after the age of 40.

Monounsaturated fat: An unsaturated fat with only one double bond in its carbon chain. Olive, rapeseed, and peanut oils are primarily monounsaturated. See Chapter 4, "A New Look at Fats."

Nutrients: Substances necessary to life that are found in food; carbohydrates, proteins, fats, vitamins, minerals, and water are nutrients.

Nutrition: The taking in and utilization of food to nourish the body.

Omega-3 fatty acids: A particular structure of healthful fatty acids found in the oil of fish. These fatty acids have been shown to reduce levels of blood cholesterol. See Chapter 4, "A New Look at Fats."

Oral hypoglycemic agents: Several drugs, taken by mouth, that lower blood sugar by promoting insulin formation; sometimes called *antidiabetic pills*.

Pancreas: A gland in the upper abdomen that secretes digestive enzymes into the intestine. The pancreas contains cells that produce two hormones, insulin and glucagon, that are released directly into the bloodstream.

Postprandial: After eating.

Preprandial: Before eating.

Protein: A major nutrient made up of amino acids that are necessary to maintain life. Protein provides four calories per gram. The abbreviation for protein in our recipes is PRO.

    Animal protein is protein from animal sources—milk, meat, poultry, fish, egg, cheese. All animal proteins contain all nine essential amino acids that cannot be manufactured by the body.

Vegetable protein (plant protein) is protein from soybeans, nuts, dried peas and beans, seeds, oatmeal, wheat germ, and grains. These proteins usually contain some, but not all, of the essential amino acids. Combinations of vegetable proteins can provide all essential amino acids.

P/S ratio: A ratio obtained by dividing polyunsaturated fat by the number of grams of saturated fat in a food. Most fats contain both types of fatty acids. See Chapter 4, "A New Look at Fats."

Reasonable weight: An attainable and maintainable weight for an individual based upon body frame and other factors. Ideal weight is often too low to be realistic; thus, counseling is often geared to maintaining a reasonable weight.

Saccharin: An artificial sweetener that provides no carbohydrate or calories. See the section titled "Sugar Substitutes" in Chapter 3.

Salt: Sodium chloride, a compound containing about 40 percent sodium, that is used as a food flavoring and preservative.

Saturated fat: Fats, mostly from animal foods, that tend to raise the level of blood cholesterol and triglycerides. See Chapter 4, "A New Look at Fats."

Sodium: A mineral, needed by the body to maintain life, found mainly as a component of salt. Many individuals need to cut down the amount of sodium (and salt) they eat to help control high blood pressure. Each recipe calculation in Part III includes a sodium value and instructions on how to reduce the sodium level if a low-sodium diet is prescribed.

Starch: One of the two major types of carbohydrate. Foods consisting mainly of starch come from the Starch/Bread Exchanges list.

Sugar: One of the two major types of carbohydrate. Foods consisting mainly of simple sugars are those from the Milk, Vegetable, and Fruit Exchanges lists. Other simple sugars include table sugar and the sugar alcohols. See Chapter 3, "The Great Sugar Masquerade."

Sugar alcohols: Sorbitol, mannitol, and xylitol are chemical substances that taste sweet but are more slowly absorbed by the body than sugars. In excess, they can act as a laxative. See Chapter 3, "The Great Sugar Masquerade."

Triglycerides: The form of fat found in food and manufactured by the body. Excess weight, consuming too much fat, alcohol, and sugar may increase the blood triglycerides to an unacceptably high level. See Chapter 4, "A New Look at Fats."

Urinalysis: Chemical analysis of the urine. Urine can be tested for sugar, an indication of diabetes.

Vitamins: Chemically organic substances found in food that are needed in very small amounts for normal body functions; includes vitamins A, B Complex, C, D, E, and K. Vitamins do not provide calories.

Index

1-800-363-6539